Congenital Heart Disease in Adolescents and Adults

Endorsed by
The ESC Working Group on Grown-up Congenital Heart Disease
AEPC Adult with Congenital Heart Disease Working Group

Series Editors

Massimo Chessa
San Donato Milanese, Italy

Helmut Baumgartner
Münster, Germany

Andreas Eicken
Munich, Germany

Alessandro Giamberti
San Donato Milanese, Italy

The aim of this series is to cast light on the most significant aspects – whether still debated or already established – of congenital heart disease in adolescents and adults and its management. Advances in the medical and surgical management of congenital heart disease have revolutionized the prognosis of infants and children with cardiac defects, so that an increasing number of patients, including those with complex problems, can reach adolescence and adult life. The profile of the adult population with congenital heart disease (ACHD) is consequently changing, and in future many adult patients will present different hemodynamic and cardiac problems from those currently seen. A cure is rarely achieved, and provision of optimal care is therefore dependent on ongoing surveillance and management in conjunction with experts in this highly specialized field. Specialists in ACHD management need to have a deep knowledge not only of congenital cardiac malformations and their treatment in infancy and childhood, but of general medicine, too. A training in adult cardiology, including coronary artery disease, is also essential. Similarly, surgeons need to acquire expertise and good training in both adult and pediatric cardiosurgery. Readers will find this series to be a rich source of information highly relevant to daily clinical practice.

More information about this series at http://www.springer.com/series/13454

Pastora Gallego · Israel Valverde
Editors

Multimodality Imaging Innovations In Adult Congenital Heart Disease

Emerging Technologies and Novel Applications

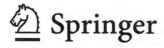 Springer

Editors
Pastora Gallego
Institute of Biomedicine of Seville
Virgen del Rocío University Hospital
Seville
Spain

Israel Valverde
Pediatric Cardiology Unit
Virgen del Rocío University Hospital
Institute of BioMedicine of Seville
Seville
Spain

ISSN 2364-6659   ISSN 2364-6667   (electronic)
Congenital Heart Disease in Adolescents and Adults
ISBN 978-3-030-61929-9   ISBN 978-3-030-61927-5   (eBook)
https://doi.org/10.1007/978-3-030-61927-5

This Springer imprint is published by the registered company Springer Nature Switzerland AG
The registered company address is: Gewerbestrasse 11, 6330 Cham, Switzerland

Preface to the Series

In Europe, we are currently faced with an estimated ACHD population of 4.2 million; adults with congenital heart disease now outnumber children (approximately 2.3 million). The vast majority cannot be considered cured but rather having a chronic heart condition that requires further surveillance and timely re-intervention for residual or consequent anatomical and/or functional abnormalities. ACHD patients have very special needs, and the physicians taking care of them need expert training. Special health care organization and training programs for those involved in ACHD care are therefore required to meet the needs of this special population.

ACHD problems remain a small part of general cardiology training curricula around the world, and pediatric cardiologists are trained to manage children with CHD and may, out of necessity, continue to look after these patients when they outgrow pediatric age.

There are clearly other health issues concerning the adult with CHD, beyond the scope of pediatric medicine, that our patients now routinely face. Adult physicians with a non-CHD background are therefore increasingly involved in the day-to-day management of patients with CHD.

Experts in congenital heart disease should work to improve the health care system, so that teens and young adults have an easier time making the transition from receiving health care in pediatric cardiology centers to receiving care from specialists in adult cardiology.

The aim of this series is to cast light on the most significant aspects of congenital heart disease in adolescents and adults and its management, such as transition from pediatric to adulthood, pregnancy and contraception, sport and physical activities, pulmonary hypertension, burning issues related to surgery, interventional catheterization, electrophysiology, intensive care management, and heart failure.

This series wishes to attract the interest of cardiologists, anesthesiologists, cardiac surgeons, electrophysiologists, psychologists, GPs, undergraduate and postgraduate students, and residents, and would like to become relevant for courses of cardiology, pediatric cardiology, cardiothoracic surgery, and anesthesiology.

We thank both the wonderful groups of leading cardiovascular experts from around the world for donating their precious time, producing excellent textbooks, and making this book series a reality, and the members of the two Working Groups (ESC and AEPC ACHD/GUCH Working Group) for the invaluable suggestions and support without which this work would not be possible.

San Donato Milanese, Italy   Massimo Chessa
Münster, Germany   Helmut Baumgartner
Munich, Germany   Andreas Eicken
San Donato Milanese, Italy   Alessandro Giamberti

Preface

Innovations and emerging technologies for diagnosis, evaluation and treatment in congenital heart defects are continually evolving. Thanks to these advancements in non-invasive diagnosis there has been an improvement in the survival of patients born with a congenital heart disease and most of them are now reaching adulthood.

Novel approaches to transcatheter interventions and advances in echocardiography, MRI and CT imaging are being developed. This is now possible because novel imaging techniques have overcome traditional trade-offs such as low spatial and temporal resolution and because multimodality imaging fusion is now a reality. Even more, non-medical technologies used in the field of engineering and aeronautical industry such as computational fluid dynamics and 3D printing are now being incorporated into clinical practice. All these emerging technologies are profoundly transforming our clinical practice guidelines, research, trainee education and interactions among multidisciplinary teams. Now we hoard a tremendous amount of physiological data unimaginable long time ago which will help us to better understand complex congenital cardiac defect pathophysiology and will provide new treatment options for this unique population. Patient management will continue evolving towards patient-specific strategies such as individualized virtual design and testing technologies. All these advancements warrant a dedicated textbook to cover congenital heart disease and emerging imaging technologies.

This book will cover all clinically relevant aspects of the fascinating new cardiac imaging technologies: including an overview of the fundamental principles and technical concepts of recent advances in cardiovascular imaging modalities, an evaluation of novel techniques for a better understanding of the anatomy and pathophysiology and a detailed description of their specific uses in the broad spectrum of clinically important congenital heart disease in adults with congenital heart disease. Our purpose is to provide trainees, clinical imaging practitioners and surgeons with a comprehensive and integrated summary of all the contemporary and novel imaging technologies and how they can guide future management of adults with congenital heart disease.

The text is the result of the excellent contribution from the best experts in each field, involving a multidisciplinary team of engineers, adult and paediatric cardiologists and radiologists, who addressed complex topics in a simplified format. It is organized into two major parts. The first involves familiarizing the reader with the new imaging technologies. The second part deals with the use of these novel and conventional imaging technologies in the broad categories of congenital heart disease.

We hope this book will not only be used for reference, but will inspire about new research on imaging applications which will help us better predict outcome and manage our clinical decision.

Seville, Spain   Pastora Gallego
Seville, Spain   Israel Valverde

Contents

Part I

Emerging Imaging Techniques and Modalities

3D Echocardiography

Inger Olson, Jerrid Brabender, Kelly Thorson, and Leo Lopez

1.1 Introduction

Three-dimensional (3D) echocardiography (3DE) complements the routine two-dimensional (2D) echocardiography (2DE) in clinical practice by providing additional volumetric information that 2DE cannot [1], and guidelines for its use in adult and pediatric cardiology have been established over the past decade [2, 3]. Ever since the establishment of echocardiography as a diagnostic tool, clinicians have used 2DE to gain knowledge about cardiac anatomy and physiology in patients with suspected and known heart disease. Most clinicians have utilized the multiple planes of 2DE to mentally create a virtual 3D reconstruction of a particular heart. This then allows clinicians to understand the pathology for that heart and formulate a therapeutic approach. The ability to render a 3D reconstruction from 2DE data in one's mind is established only after significant training and experience, and many care providers never develop this ability. 3DE has provided the tools to overcome this limitation by providing actual 3D reconstructions of a heart from 2DE data that can then be visualized and manipulated in order to improve understanding of the anatomy and physiology [4, 5] (Fig. 1.1).

I. Olson (✉) · L. Lopez
Division of Pediatric Cardiology, Lucile Packard Children's Hospital Stanford, Palo Alto, CA, USA
e-mail: iolson@stanford.edu; leolopez@stanford.edu

J. Brabender · K. Thorson
Echocardiography Department, Lucile Packard Children's Hospital Stanford, Palo Alto, CA, USA
e-mail: jbrabender@stanfordchildrens.org; kthorson@stanfordchildrens.org

© Springer Nature Switzerland AG 2021
P. Gallego, I. Valverde (eds.), *Multimodality Imaging Innovations In Adult Congenital Heart Disease*, Congenital Heart Disease in Adolescents and Adults, https://doi.org/10.1007/978-3-030-61927-5_1

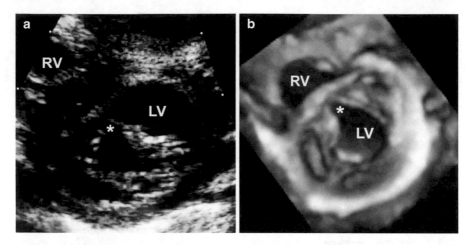

Fig. 1.1 (**a**) 2DE image of a mitral valve with a cleft (*) in the anterior leaflet. (**b**) 3DE image of the same mitral valve in which the cleft (*) is more easily visualized due to the added depth of the three-dimensional image (*LV* left ventricle, *RV* right ventricle)

Fig. 1.2 Live 3D image of a mitral valve in which the narrow angle only includes a small portion of the left atrium and ventricle on either side of the valve

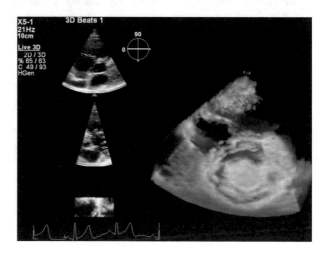

1.2   3DE Acquisition Modes

2DE image optimization is the most important aspect in the acquisition of a good 3DE dataset. Appropriate use of data presentation settings will avoid artifacts and misdiagnoses as discussed below. Most ultrasound systems have three acquisition modes: **real time or live 3D** (narrow angle), **3D zoom** (magnified), and **full volume** (wide angle).

The **live 3D** mode acquires data within a narrow angle, producing a 3DE volume sector that does not span the entire heart [6] (Fig. 1.2). It is most useful for real-time imaging, such as during interventional procedures when the region of interest is only one particular segment of the heart. Live 3D is simple and fast because complex cropping maneuvers are not necessary with this mode.

3D zoom involves magnification of a segment of the narrow-angle acquisition used in live 3D, so it evaluates an even smaller 3DE volume sector (Fig. 1.3). Images obtained with this mode have high spatial and temporal resolution. Because of the limited amount of data acquired, it is mainly useful for looking at specific structures, such as valve pathology, atrial septal defects (ASDs), ventricular septal defects (VSDs), and small, fast-moving structures.

The **full-volume 3DE** mode has the largest acquisition sector of all the modes, usually encompassing the entire heart (Fig. 1.4). This wide-angle mode is ideal for imaging complex anatomy with display of the spatial relationships of multiple structures. The full-volume mode is also useful for analysis of left ventricular (LV) function. Although this mode has the highest spatial resolution, it has lower temporal resolution compared to narrow-angle 3DE modes. Higher temporal resolution can be achieved by stitching together several narrow pyramidal scans obtained over multiple consecutive heartbeats. This acquisition requires ECG gating and is best during suspended respiration to avoid a stitch artifact in the image (Fig. 1.5). The three-view multiplanar reconstruction (MPR) image display can help avoid stitch artifacts since it allows for display of the imaging plane perpendicular to the plane of acquisition and visualization of stitch artifacts in real time, thereby providing a rapid assessment of the quality of the dataset (Fig. 1.6). The default setting for full-volume acquisitions is 1 beat. This can be optimized to increase the volume rate and size for specific clinical needs, involving 2, 4, or 6 beats or the high-volume-rate (HVR) setting. HVR is live imaging in a full volume.

Fig. 1.3 3D zoom image of a common atrioventricular valve showing well-defined leaflets; high resolution is obtained by focusing on the specific region of interest, excluding other structures

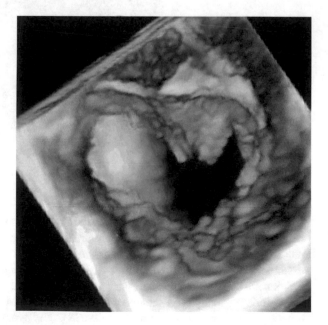

Fig. 1.4 Full-volume 3DE image from the right heart perspective of a subarterial VSD (*); because this is a larger dataset than live 3D and 3D zoom datasets, it has lower resolution (*PA* pulmonary artery, *RA* right atrium, *RV* right ventricle)

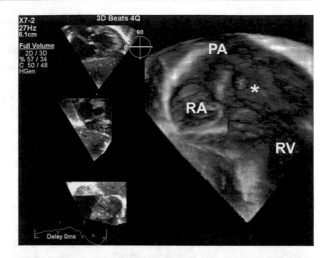

Fig. 1.5 Multiple stitch artifacts in a 4-beat 3DE image

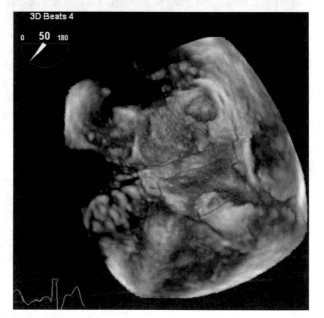

1.3   3DE Image Optimization

Once the 3DE volume dataset is acquired, manipulation can begin with a goal of presenting a 3D image that showcases the anatomy of interest as well as surrounding anatomic structures. Refined 3DE images should be presented in a consistent anatomic manner so that the regions of interest are easily recognizable by other clinicians. The tools include software that exists on the ultrasound system, can be loaded independently on a separate computer, or as part of the cardiology picture archival and communications system (PACS). The workflow for the tools varies

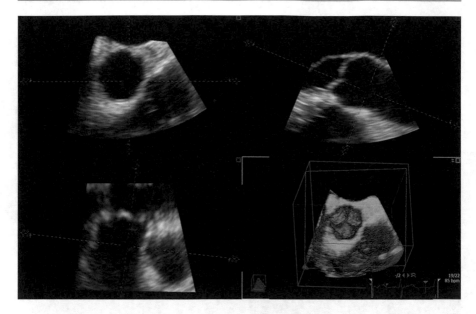

Fig. 1.6 Multiplanar reconstruction (MPR) of a full-volume 3DE dataset showing a trileaflet aortic valve; the MPR display helps ensure a high-quality dataset without stitch artifact

among systems, with tasks performed as the study is conducted or as off-line manipulation of acquired datasets after the procedure.

1.3.1 Volume Manipulation Tools

A 3D volume dataset can be evaluated from virtually any plane, allowing for presentation using an anatomically correct view or a surgical view [3, 7]. It may be rotated to display any side of the dataset, including the top and bottom, with the anchor point typically at the dataset center. The **axial rotation** tool allows the user to rotate the 3DE image like the hands on a clock. The **frontal plane rotation** tool allows the user to rotate the image from the frontal plane with the center axis as the anchor point, much like rotating a globe.

Tools that allow for enhancement of the 3DE image include **gain, brightness, dynamic range/compression, 3D tissue maps,** and **light sources.** These tools function somewhat independently but together can enhance the image. The **gain** function allows for better understanding of the anatomy. If the gain is too high, the surface details will be obscured, and the lumen of the chambers may appear small. An over-gained 3DE image will lose depth perspective by filling in those areas that allow for a perception of depth. A gain setting that is too low will introduce artificial holes in the anatomy and reduce surface detail. An under-gained 3DE image will allow for visualization through the image from the frontal plane to the back of the image (Fig. 1.7). Fine-tuning of the 3DE gain should result in a balance between the

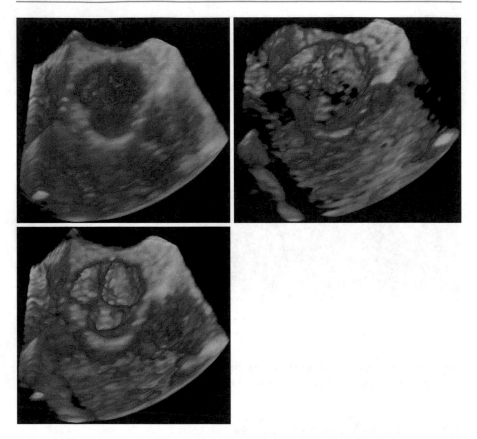

Fig. 1.7 3DE showing an en face view of a trileaflet aortic valve in various gain settings: (**a**) inappropriately high-gain settings result in a poorly defined valve with loss of depth; (**b**) inappropriately low-gain setting results in a significant loss of information; (**c**) ideal-gain settings result in a well-defined image of the aortic valve leaflets with appropriate depth

two extremes, leaving enough detail of the anatomic surfaces without introducing artificial image dropout [2, 3]. The general recommendation is to slightly over gain the image using the time-gain controls rather than the power-output gain, as the gain can then be reduced during postprocessing.

The image **brightness** setting changes the surface brightness of the image and affects the perceived depth of the image. After the optimal gain setting is achieved, the brightness can be fine-tuned to allow for perception of contours across the region of interest and throughout the complete volume dataset.

The **dynamic range/compression** settings expand or contract the number of light-to-dark colors in an image and are similar to image contrast. An image with high compression or dynamic range will result in a softer appearance at the edges, while an image with low dynamic range will result in a sharper edge and better differentiation between the lumen and wall of an anatomic structure. A dynamic range or compression that is too low may eliminate fine structures, while a dynamic

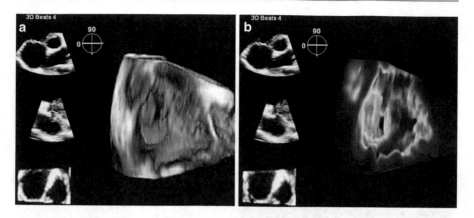

Fig. 1.8 3DE image of a secundum ASD as well as the ostium of the coronary sinus: (**a**) tissue mapping displays structures in the foreground with a lighter color, while the posteriorly located left atrial wall is blue; (**b**) using simulated light source and natural color tissue mapping highlights the ASD

range or compression setting that is too high will not allow for subtle contours and may not allow for visualization of discrete edges. Some anatomy favors lower versus higher dynamic range, and modulation of these settings should be based on the region of interest. Anatomy that favors a lower dynamic range or compression setting includes structures such as the atrial cavity or the aorta, where the lower dynamic range may help differentiate the lumen from the wall. Valves and fine anatomic structures with irregular borders typically will be improved by a higher dynamic range or compression setting.

3DE tissue or color maps are similar to 2DE B-mode maps with the addition of different colors or shades to represent depth. Available maps have been optimized to enhance the perception of depth, typically using a lighter color to represent structures that are closest to the viewer and a different, usually darker, color for those that are farther away. Newer maps utilize colors that more closely represent the natural tissue. A new feature of 3D imaging utilizes a **simulated light source** (Fig. 1.8) that adds light and shadow to present a real sense of depth and topography and can be oriented to best visualize the region of interest. For instance, a mitral valve can have the light source directed from the ventricle toward the valve, illuminating the underside and enhancing subtle details of the valvular apparatus.

1.3.2   Volume Slice and Edit Tools

The presentation of a 3DE volume image frequently requires the user to remove material or data from the volume dataset in order to highlight the region of interest. The volume editing tools available on most systems include **box plane edit**, **freestyle plane edit**, **draw plane inclusion removal**, and **draw plane exclusion removal**.

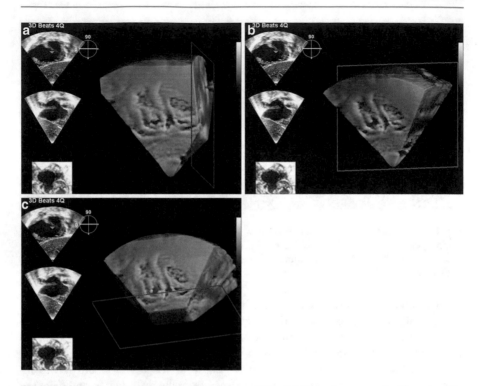

Fig. 1.9 Full-volume 3DE dataset with box plane editing: (**a**) the *x*-plane crops data from the right or left aspect of the image; (**b**) the *y*-plane crops data from the front or back; and (**c**) the *z*-plane crops data from the bottom or top surface

A 3DE volume exists as a pyramidal shape, and this pyramid exists within a virtual cube. The cube can be modified to show the region of interest by removing unnecessary information in three standard planes using **box plane edit**. The *x*-plane (lateral or sagittal plane) can remove material from the left or right aspect of the cube; the **y-plane** (axial or frontal plane) can be used to remove material from the front or back; and the **z-plane** (azimuthal plane) can be used to remove material from the top or bottom (Fig. 1.9). The box plane edit function is somewhat limited because these standard planes are often not in line with the anatomy and region of interest.

The **freestyle plane edit tool** is based on the same concept, but the editing plane is not limited to the *x*-, *y*-, or *z*-plane. It can be rotated at any angle and is a powerful tool for precision editing [8, 9]. Other cut tools include the **draw plane inclusion** and **draw plane exclusion** tools. Both use a virtual pen to draw around the region of interest and are valuable for small revisions of a dataset. The exclusion tool cuts the drawn planes away from within the drawn lines, and the inclusion tool removes data outside of the drawn lines (Fig. 1.10). For example, the exclusion tool can remove an artifact within the left atrium proximal to the mitral valve by drawing a circle around the artifact and cutting it from the dataset. Similarly, the inclusion tool can be used to draw a circle around the mitral valve and exclude all data outside the circle.

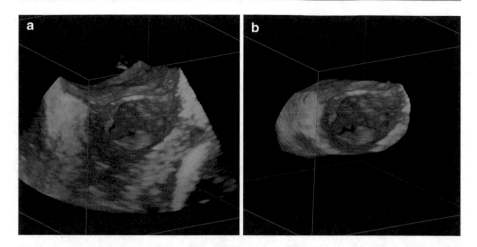

Fig. 1.10 3DE image of an aortic valve (**a**) before and (**b**) after using the draw plane inclusion tool to remove excess data and focus attention on the valve

1.3.3   Volume Viewing Functions

The 3DE volume dataset can be viewed using different methods in conjunction with the cut plane tools, and these include the **MPR focus view, perspective view, dual view**, and **spin and rotate view**. The **MPR focus** view shows a view of each orthogonal plane, allowing the user to center the region of interest within the MPR crosshairs and rotate each view to enable 3D alignment of the region of interest [3, 10, 11] (Fig. 1.6). This view also allows an autorotation into each of the MPR planes. For users who are less familiar with the advanced tools, the **perspective view** enables the user to define the perspective and depth from which to view the region of interest, typically as a ball and arrow function, where the ball is the viewer and the arrow points toward and extends beyond the region of interest to a specified depth (volume thickness).

Dual view exists in two forms. One displays half of the volume pyramid on one side of the screen and the opposite half on the other side of the screen, displaying the differences (or similarities) between each side of the 3DE volume dataset. The second transects the anatomy using a perspective plane, allowing visualization of the anatomy from two complementary perspectives. For example, this method can allow a user to view an atrioventricular valve from the ventricle and the atrium simultaneously. This view is also useful for septal defects and semilunar valves.

The majority of the 3DE volumes exist as a cine loop containing one or more cardiac cycles. The **spin** or **rotation mode** can use a cine loop or still image of a volume dataset and rotate it back and forth with a user-defined degree and speed of rotation. The rotation angle is typically around 20°, and the speed should be slow enough for easy evaluation of the region of interest and its surrounding anatomy.

1.3.4   3DE Perspective and Viewing Planes

Standardization of views is essential for effective understanding and communication of anatomic information. Standard views include **anatomic** and **surgical views**, which can be further stratified into the **right heart view**, **left heart view**, **atrial view**, **ventricular view**, and **arterial view** [2, 3, 7]. Specific **en face** views can also be frequently helpful.

The **anatomic view** is essentially a frontal plane, similar to the anteroposterior chest X-ray view. The **surgical view** is distinctly different from the anatomic view and displays the anatomy from the perspective of a cardiothoracic surgeon standing on the right side of the patient with the superior structures on the left side of the screen [2, 3]. The surgical view generally requires identification of several landmarks, such as the left atrial appendage, aorta, or superior vena cava.

The **right heart view** shows structures as viewed from the right heart and is optimal for displaying the inlet, outlet, membranous, and apical trabecular ventricular septum as well as the right atrial perspective of the atrial septum. It is also helpful for viewing the tricuspid valve apparatus [8, 9]. The **left heart view** shows structures as viewed from the left heart and can be helpful in delineating the location, size, and geometry of VSDs (especially given the smooth wall of the LV septum) and the distance of these defects from important structures such as the aortic valve or papillary muscles. It can also show the location of an ASD relative to the mitral valve and pulmonary veins.

The **LV-to-free wall view** shows the LV free wall as imaged from the ventricular septum. This is useful for demonstrating mitral valve papillary muscle position and structure as well as LV noncompaction and aneurysms. The **left atrial-to-posterior wall view** is a similar view showing the posterior atrial wall as imaged from the atrial septum and is useful for characterizing the pulmonary vein ostia.

The **atrial view** originates from either atrium and looks toward the respective ventricle, thereby an ideal view for demonstrating the atrial aspect of the mitral and tricuspid valves, particularly as it relates to the mechanism of regurgitation (Figs. 1.11a and 1.12a). Care should be taken to start the perspective fairly close to the valve to avoid artifacts and optimize spatial resolution. In contrast, the **ventricular view** originates from the ventricles and looks toward the atria (Figs. 1.11b and 1.12b). It is helpful in evaluating atrioventricular valvular pathology as well as the ventricular outflow tracts [2, 3, 7].

The **arterial view** utilizes an imaging perspective either from the great arteries or from the ventricles looking toward the semilunar valves (Fig. 1.13). It is an excellent way to characterize the semilunar valves cusps, including their excursion and distal commissural attachments. The arterial view from the aorta can also demonstrate the location and shape of the coronary ostia [2].

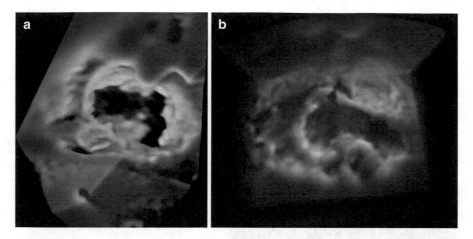

Fig. 1.11 3DE image of a common atrioventricular valve using natural color tissue mapping (**a**) as viewed from the atria showing a well-defined annulus and (**b**) as viewed from the ventricle showing well-defined leaflet edges

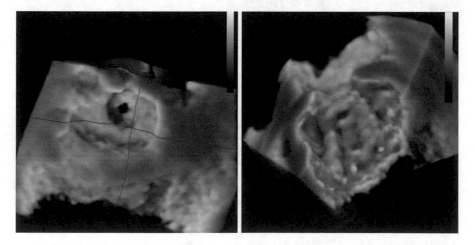

Fig. 1.12 3DE image of a mitral valve arcade using natural color tissue mapping (**a**) as viewed from the left atrium showing a very small valvular orifice and (**b**) as viewed from the left ventricle showing the arcade chordal structure

1.4   3D Echocardiography and Interventions

3DE is especially helpful when imaging structures with asymmetric shapes, septal defects in unusual locations, or multiple defects, which can be difficult to accurately delineate by 2DE alone [12–16]. With 3DE, a defect or valve can be imaged en face, allowing better assessment of the shape of the defect, location of valve regurgitation, or potential impact of any proposed intervention on adjacent structures [8, 9, 12, 14–21] (Fig. 1.14).

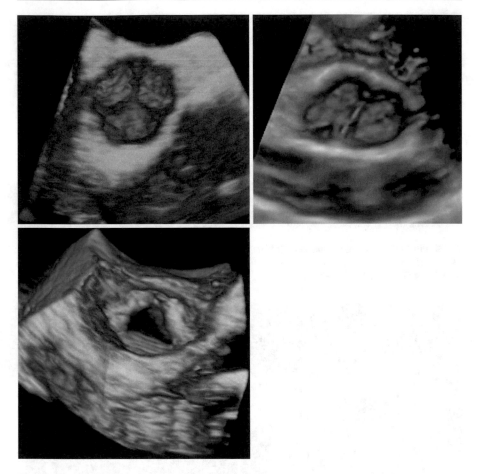

Fig. 1.13 Arterial views of the aortic valve: (**a**) a trileaflet aortic valve, looking from the aorta; (**b**) a bicuspid aortic valve, looking from the aorta; and (**c**) a trileaflet aortic valve, looking from the left ventricle

The presentation of 3DE images must account for the lesion being evaluated and the potential intervention. Ideally, a 3DE image should include all pertinent structures in one view. For example, images of an ASD before device closure should demonstrate all of the rims as well as nearby structures that might be impacted by the device, such as the right pulmonary veins and the mitral valve [12].

Live 3D acquires data during one beat, eliminating the need for a breath hold, but more data can be obtained by acquiring a full-volume dataset if time permits. However, during the interventional procedure, it is much more efficient to use live 3D, 3D zoom, or MPR to image the specific area of interest without the need for postprocessing.

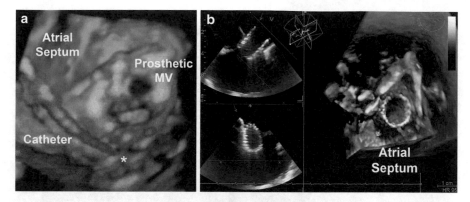

Fig. 1.14 3DE images during interventional procedures: (**a**) a mechanical mitral valve with a catheter crossing a paravalvular leak (*), and (**b**) a stent placed in the atrial septum as viewed from the left atrium in a different patient (*MV* mitral valve)

Fig. 1.15 3DE anatomic view of Ebstein anomaly of the tricuspid valve showing tethered leaflets that are displaced beyond the atrioventricular groove (*) (*LV* left ventricle, *TVPL* tricuspid valve posterior leaflet, *TVSL* tricuspid valve septal leaflet)

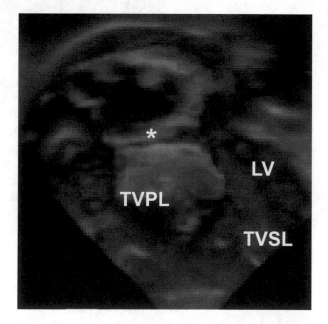

1.4.1   Surgical Guidance

For surgical intervention in adult patients with congenital heart disease, 3DE is most useful in evaluating the mitral, tricuspid, and aortic valves [3, 7–9, 19]. The valves can be displayed en face from above or below, allowing better visualization of valvular morphology and localization of coaptation defects. For example, the tricuspid valve in Ebstein anomaly typically has complex attachments and multiple coaptation defects; evaluation is difficult by 2DE alone and enhanced by 3DE (Fig. 1.15). 3DE can display valvular regurgitation en face with better visualization

Fig. 1.16 En face view of a prosthetic mitral valve as seen from the left atrium with good visualization of the sewing ring (*) (*LA* left atrium, *RV* right ventricle)

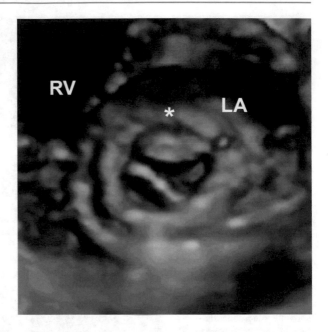

and more accurate planimetry of the vena contracta, which is helpful in comparing pre and postoperative regurgitation. 3DE is also useful for prosthetic valves and can provide more accurate information of the location and extent of paravalvular leaks than 2DE alone (Fig. 1.16). Lastly, it can help localize baffle leaks in patients with complex repairs such as the atrial switch or the Rastelli procedure (Fig. 1.17).

In patients with multiple or unusual VSDs or ASDs, 3DE allows for imaging of the defects from the right or left side of the heart and better characterization prior to surgical intervention [12, 14–16]. 3DE can also be particularly helpful in complex subaortic stenosis, where it can identify the mechanism and severity of the obstruction [10], and double outlet right ventricle (Fig. 1.18), where it can determine suitability for biventricular repair [22].

1.4.2   Interventional Cath Guidance

3DE is also useful in guiding catheter interventions [11], particularly for complex ASDs or VSDs with irregular or asymmetric shape [3, 13] (Fig. 1.19). En face views of an ASD can help evaluate the size, shape, number, and location of ASDs as well as the adequacy of the rims [12, 13]. Imaging from the right atrium can demonstrate the relationship of the ASD with the vena cava, and imaging from the left atrium can demonstrate its relationship with the pulmonary veins. The MPR 4-panel view, live 3D, and 3D zoom are all useful for performing measurements. A full-volume dataset can be used for planning, but real-time 3D transesophageal echocardiography (TEE) is generally used for guidance during device placement [13]. Here, 3DE can evaluate

Fig. 1.17 3DE image of a patient status post-Mustard procedure with two baffle leaks (*) as seen from the perspective of the pulmonary venous pathway (*Pulm Vein Pathway* pulmonary venous pathway, *SVC* superior vena cava). (Courtesy of Brian Soriano, MD, Seattle Children's Hospital, USA)

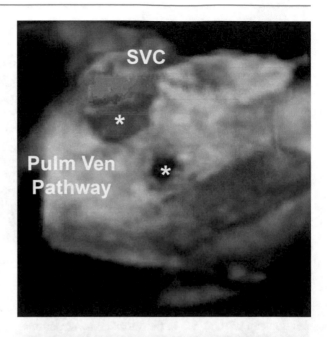

Fig. 1.18 3DE image of a patient with double outlet right ventricle and subaortic VSD (*) (*AO* aorta, *PA* pulmonary artery, *RA* right atrium, *RV* right ventricle). (Courtesy of Kuberan Pushparajah, MD, Evelina Children's Hospital, London, UK)

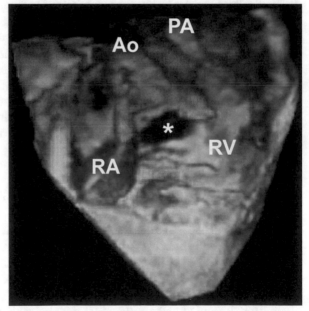

device position relative to the aortic, mitral, tricuspid valves, vena cava, and pulmonary veins. And color Doppler can evaluate for residual defects (Fig. 1.20).

During VSD device closures, 3DE from a 4-chamber TEE view can demonstrate the VSD en face from either the RV or the LV side (Fig. 1.21), allowing for evaluation of the size, shape, number, and location of the VSD, the anatomy of the tricuspid

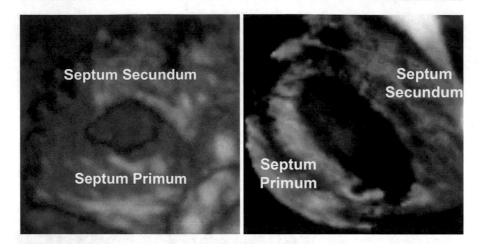

Fig. 1.19 3DE images of different secundum ASDs as viewed from the left atrium with (**a**) a round shape and (**b**) an elliptical shape

aneurysmal pouch frequently associated with a perimembranous VSD, and the relationship of the VSD to the surrounding structures. This view can also assist in device deployment. After device placement, color Doppler imaging with live 3D, MPR, or biplane views can exclude residual defects or new aortic regurgitation.

3D TEE can be useful in transcatheter mitral valve repair with a mitral clip by characterizing the severity and mechanism of mitral regurgitation before the procedure [17, 18] (Fig. 1.22). It can then provide an expanded view of the valve, left atrium, and atrial septum, localize with the transseptal puncture to avoid damaging the mitral valve, and help guide positioning of the clip with an en face view of the valve [23]. 3DE has also been used to assist in aortic valve implantation, particularly in terms of improved characterization of the aortic annular size and geometry [24–26].

1.4.3 Echocardiographic-Fluoroscopic Fusion

Interventional procedures are frequently performed under both TEE and fluoroscopic guidance, using two different systems and two different screens. Echocardiographic-fluoroscopic fusion imaging combines images from both modalities by overlaying them on a single screen in real time [27]. This allows for improved localization and characterization of devices and catheters within the heart (Fig. 1.23). After the TEE probe tip is identified and registered by the application, it detects all changes in probe position and updates the combined images on the screen while maintaining anatomic orientation. Changes in C-arm orientation also modify the TEE images live. If the probe leaves the field of view, it will be automatically resynchronized when it returns.

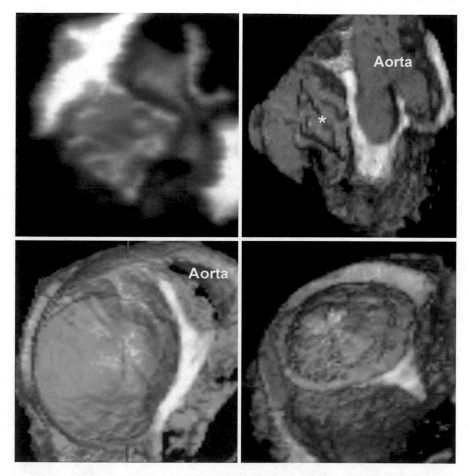

Fig. 1.20 3DE images of different atrial septal defect devices: (**a**) Angel Wings septal occluder, (**b**) CardioSEAL septal occluder (*), (**c**) HELEX septal occlude, and (**d**) Amplatzer septal occluder

For example, a 3D TEE image of an ASD can be displayed on the fluoroscopy screen with additional markers to identify the center of the defect or surrounding structures like the aortic and mitral valves. This modality can also help ensure guidewire advancement through a larger defect in cases of multiple ASDs and VSDs [28]. In aortic stenosis, markers can be placed at the valvular opening and anterior mitral valve leaflet to help guide the catheter across the stenotic valve and assist with proper placement for balloon dilation. In procedures requiring a transseptal puncture, a marker can identify the optimal location to cross the atrial septum, especially when there is an aneurysmal atrial septum or when a mitral intervention requires precise location of the puncture relative to the mitral valve.

Fig. 1.21 3DE image of a small outlet muscular VSD (*) as seen from the LV view (*LA* left atrium, *LV* left ventricle, *AO* aorta)

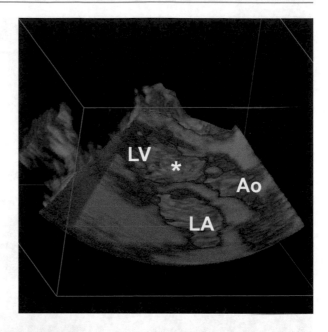

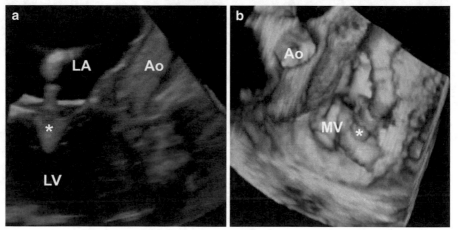

Fig. 1.22 3DE images of the MitraClip delivery system (*) used for mitral regurgitation: (**a**) left heart view showing open device arms and (**b**) atrial view showing the system (*) at the mitral orifice (*LA* left atrium, *LV* left ventricle, *MV* mitral valve, *AO* aorta). (Courtesy of Rebecca Hahn, MD, Columbia University Medical Center, New York, USA)

1.5   Future Directions

Continued advances in transducer technology, data processing, and electronic storage capacity with better spatial and temporal resolution have increased the capabilities and potential applications of 3DE, particularly in terms of chamber quantification, evaluation of heart disease, and guidance during interventional procedures [29, 30].

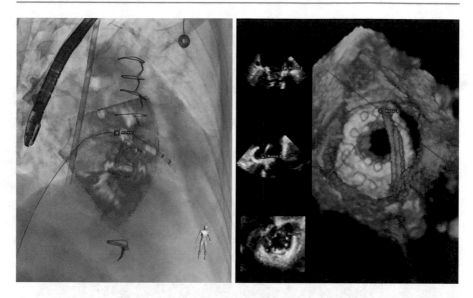

Fig. 1.23 Echocardiographic-fluoroscopic fusion imaging during device closure of a paravalvular leak, where a target is placed at the site of the leak on the 3D TEE image (Marker 2) and displayed in the same anatomic location on the fluoroscopy screen. (Courtesy of Pei-Ni Jone, MD, Children's Hospital Colorado, USA)

In addition, 3DE is continuing to provide better tools to describe normal and abnormal anatomy to clinicians who are not experienced with 2DE or 3DE. The future of 3DE is likely to include more advances in the use of **artificial intelligence**, **3DE deformation analysis**, **3D printing**, **virtual reality**, and **holography**.

Semiautomated chamber quantification algorithms using 3DE datasets of heart chambers have been available for a few years. **Artificial intelligence** and deep learning have been used to enable fully automated quantification of LV and left atrial size, using either a knowledge-based contouring algorithm [31] or an adaptive analytics algorithm [32]. The results of the latter have been validated against the semiautomated approach using manual tracing [32] though there are still limitations in terms of feasibility and vendor-related differences [33]. Artificial intelligence has also been used for automated evaluation of mitral valve contours with some success [34].

2D speckle tracking echocardiography to evaluate segmental and global myocardial deformation has evolved as a valuable modality to evaluate cardiac function over the past two decades, but it is limited by the inability to evaluate speckle motion outside of the 2D plane of interest. With improving 3DE technology, **3DE deformation analysis** using 3D speckle tracking may soon emerge as a solution to the out-of-plane speckle motion problem, please see Chap. 6. Although some studies have suggested clinical value [35], work is still needed to evaluate the feasibility, reproducibility, and impact of this emerging technology.

3D printing has been used increasingly over the past decade to better understand structural heart diseases and simulate potential interventions. However, most reports have involved high-resolution data from computed tomography or magnetic resonance imaging. Improved spatial resolution has allowed for the use of 3DE to create 3D printed models for simulated surgical interventions [36], potentially paving the way for other scenarios, where 3DE data will suffice for 3D printing. For more information, see Chap. 10.

Virtual reality was first used in the 1970s for educational purposes such as flight simulations. The gaming industry subsequently produced headsets to simulate artificial realities, eventually developing stereoscopic headsets that allow a user to explore, interact with, and manipulate a simulated environment. Just as 3DE data have been used to print models for various purposes, the same data are available for computer-generated 3D environments that can be used for education and surgical planning [37] (Fig. 1.24). **Holography** is another technology that can also use a

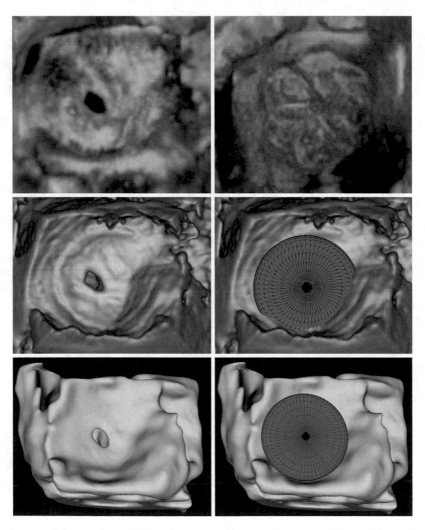

Fig. 1.24 Volume rendering of an ASD from a 3DE dataset with simulated device closure using a virtual reality modeling tool. (Courtesy of Matthew Jolley, MD, and Hannah Nam, BS, Children's Hospital of Philadelphia, USA)

Fig. 1.25 3DE dataset projected above the monitor by holography, which can then be manipulated to better understand the anatomy (*AO* aortic valve, *MV* mitral valve). (Courtesy of Sergio Aguirre, MSc, EchoPixel, Santa Clara, USA)

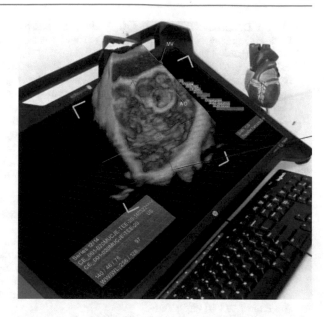

3DE dataset and project an external model of a heart either on a monitor or "floating" in space (in contrast to the internal heart model that one sees within the virtual reality headsets) that can be manipulated to improve understanding of the anatomy and plan for therapeutic intervention [38, 39] (Fig. 1.25).

References

1. Hung J, Lang R, Flachskampf F, Shernan SK, McCulloch ML, Adams DB, et al. 3D echocardiography: a review of the current status and future directions. J Am Soc Echocardiogr. 2007;20(3):213–33.
2. Lang RM, Badano LP, Tsang W, Adams DH, Agricola E, Buck T, et al. EAE/ASE recommendations for image acquisition and display using three-dimensional echocardiography. J Am Soc Echocardiogr. 2012;25(1):3–46.
3. Simpson J, Lopez L, Acar P, Friedberg MK, Khoo NS, Ko HH, et al. Three-dimensional echocardiography in congenital heart disease: an expert consensus document from the European Association of Cardiovascular Imaging and the American Society of Echocardiography. J Am Soc Echocardiogr. 2017;30(1):1–27.
4. Dekker DL, Piziali RL, Dong E Jr. A system for ultrasonically imaging the human heart in three dimensions. Comput Biomed Res. 1974;7(6):544–53.
5. Sheikh K, Smith SW, von Ramm O, Kisslo J. Real-time, three-dimensional echocardiography: feasibility and initial use. Echocardiography. 1991;8(1):119–25.
6. Xie MX, Wang XF, Cheng TO, Lu Q, Yuan L, Liu X. Real-time 3-dimensional echocardiography: a review of the development of the technology and its clinical application. Prog Cardiovasc Dis. 2005;48(3):209–25.
7. Del Pasqua A, Sanders SP, de Zorzi A, Toscano A, Iacobelli R, Pierli C, et al. Impact of three-dimensional echocardiography in complex congenital heart defect cases: the surgical view. Pediatr Cardiol. 2009;30(3):293–300.

8. Muraru D, Hahn RT, Soliman OI, Faletra FF, Basso C, Badano LP. 3-Dimensional Echocardiography in Imaging the Tricuspid Valve. JACC Cardiovasc Imaging. 2019;12(3):500–15.

9. Faletra FF, Leo LA, Paiocchi VL, Schlossbauer SA, Borruso MG, Pedrazzini G, et al. Imaging-based tricuspid valve anatomy by computed tomography, magnetic resonance imaging, two and three-dimensional echocardiography: correlation with anatomic specimen. Eur Heart J Cardiovasc Imaging. 2019;20(1):1–13.

10. Bharucha T, Ho SY, Vettukattil JJ. Multiplanar review analysis of three-dimensional echocardiographic datasets gives new insights into the morphology of subaortic stenosis. Eur J Echocardiogr. 2008;9(5):614–20.

11. Perk G, Lang RM, Garcia-Fernandez MA, Lodato J, Sugeng L, Lopez J, et al. Use of real time three-dimensional transesophageal echocardiography in intracardiac catheter based interventions. J Am Soc Echocardiogr. 2009;22(8):865–82.

12. Roberson DA, Cui W, Patel D, Tsang W, Sugeng L, Weinert L, et al. Three-dimensional transesophageal echocardiography of atrial septal defect: a qualitative and quantitative anatomic study. J Am Soc Echocardiogr. 2011;24(6):600–10.

13. Johri AM, Witzke C, Solis J, Palacios IF, Inglessis I, Picard MH, et al. Real-time three-dimensional transesophageal echocardiography in patients with secundum atrial septal defects: outcomes following transcatheter closure. J Am Soc Echocardiogr. 2011;24(4):431–7.

14. Cheng TO, Xie MX, Wang XF, Wang Y, Lu Q. Real-time 3-dimensional echocardiography in assessing atrial and ventricular septal defects: an echocardiographic-surgical correlative study. Am Heart J. 2004;148(6):1091–5.

15. van den Bosch AE, Ten Harkel DJ, McGhie JS, Roos-Hesselink JW, Simoons ML, Bogers AJ, et al. Feasibility and accuracy of real-time 3-dimensional echocardiographic assessment of ventricular septal defects. J Am Soc Echocardiogr. 2006;19(1):7–13.

16. Mercer-Rosa L, Seliem MA, Fedec A, Rome J, Rychik J, Gaynor JW. Illustration of the additional value of real-time 3-dimensional echocardiography to conventional transthoracic and transesophageal 2-dimensional echocardiography in imaging muscular ventricular septal defects: does this have any impact on individual patient treatment? J Am Soc Echocardiogr. 2006;19(12):1511–9.

17. Biner S, Perk G, Kar S, Rafique AM, Slater J, Shiota T, et al. Utility of combined two-dimensional and three-dimensional transesophageal imaging for catheter-based mitral valve clip repair of mitral regurgitation. J Am Soc Echocardiogr. 2011;24(6):611–7.

18. Faletra FF, Pedrazzini G, Pasotti E, Petrova I, Drasutiene A, Dequarti MC, et al. Role of real-time three dimensional transoesophageal echocardiography as guidance imaging modality during catheter based edge-to-edge mitral valve repair. Heart. 2013;99(16):1204–15.

19. Sadagopan SN, Veldtman GR, Sivaprakasam MC, Keeton BR, Gnanapragasam JP, Salmon AP, et al. Correlations with operative anatomy of real time three-dimensional echocardiographic imaging of congenital aortic valvar stenosis. Cardiol Young. 2006;16(5):490–4.

20. van den Bosch AE, Ten Harkel DJ, McGhie JS, Roos-Hesselink JW, Simoons ML, Bogers AJ, et al. Surgical validation of real-time transthoracic 3D echocardiographic assessment of atrioventricular septal defects. Int J Cardiol. 2006;112(2):213–8.

21. Hlavacek AM, Crawford FA Jr, Chessa KS, Shirali GS. Real-time three-dimensional echocardiography is useful in the evaluation of patients with atrioventricular septal defects. Echocardiography. 2006;23(3):225–31.

22. Pushparajah K, Barlow A, Tran VH, Miller OI, Zidere V, Vaidyanathan B, et al. A systematic three-dimensional echocardiographic approach to assist surgical planning in double outlet right ventricle. Echocardiography. 2013;30(2):234–8.

23. Poon J, Leung JT, Leung DY. 3D echo in routine clinical practice - state of the art in 2019. Heart Lung Circ. 2019;28(9):1400–10.

24. Khalique OK, Kodali SK, Paradis JM, Nazif TM, Williams MR, Einstein AJ, et al. Aortic annular sizing using a novel 3-dimensional echocardiographic method: use and comparison with cardiac computed tomography. Circ Cardiovasc Imaging. 2014;7(1):155–63.

25. Otto CM, Kumbhani DJ, Alexander KP, Calhoon JH, Desai MY, Kaul S, et al. 2017 ACC expert consensus decision pathway for transcatheter aortic valve replacement in the management of adults with aortic stenosis: a report of the American College of Cardiology Task Force on Clinical Expert Consensus Documents. J Am Coll Cardiol. 2017;69(10):1313–46.
26. Bleakley C, Monaghan MJ. The pivotal role of imaging in TAVR procedures. Curr Cardiol Rep. 2018;20(2):9.
27. Jone PN, Ross MM, Bracken JA, Mulvahill MJ, Di Maria MV, Fagan TE. Feasibility and safety of using a fused echocardiography/fluoroscopy imaging system in patients with congenital heart disease. J Am Soc Echocardiogr. 2016;29(6):513–21.
28. Hadeed K, Hascoet S, Karsenty C, Ratsimandresy M, Dulac Y, Chausseray G, et al. Usefulness of echocardiographic-fluoroscopic fusion imaging in children with congenital heart disease. Arch Cardiovasc Dis. 2018;111(6–7):399–410.
29. Lafitte S. Revolution in echocardiography: from M-mode to printing. Arch Cardiovasc Dis. 2018;111(6–7):389–91.
30. Lang RM, Addetia K, Narang A. Mor-Avi V. 3-Dimensional echocardiography: latest developments and future directions. JACC Cardiovasc Imaging. 2018;11(12):1854–78.
31. Yang L, Georgescu B, Zheng Y, Foran DJ, Comaniciu D. A fast and accurate tracking algorithm of left ventricles in 3d echocardiography. Proc IEEE Int Symp Biomed Imaging. 2008;5:221–4.
32. Medvedofsky D, Mor-Avi V, Amzulescu M, Fernandez-Golfin C, Hinojar R, Monaghan MJ, et al. Three-dimensional echocardiographic quantification of the left-heart chambers using an automated adaptive analytics algorithm: multicentre validation study. Eur Heart J Cardiovasc Imaging. 2018;19(1):47–58.
33. Spitzer E, Ren B, Zijlstra F, Mieghem NMV, Geleijnse ML. The role of automated 3D echocardiography for left ventricular ejection fraction assessment. Card Fail Rev. 2017;3(2):97–101.
34. Jeganathan J, Knio Z, Amador Y, Hai T, Khamooshian A, Matyal R, et al. Artificial intelligence in mitral valve analysis. Ann Card Anaesth. 2017;20(2):129–34.
35. Guedes H, Moreno N, Dos Santos RP, Marques L, Seabra D, Pereira A, et al. Importance of three-dimensional speckle tracking in the assessment of left atrial and ventricular dysfunction in patients with myotonic dystrophy type 1. Rev Port Cardiol. 2018;37(4):333–8.
36. Scanlan AB, Nguyen AV, Ilina A, Lasso A, Cripe L, Jegatheeswaran A, et al. Comparison of 3D echocardiogram-derived 3D printed valve models to molded models for simulated repair of pediatric atrioventricular valves. Pediatr Cardiol. 2018;39(3):538–47.
37. Currie ME, McLeod AJ, Moore JT, Chu MW, Patel R, Kiaii B, et al. Augmented reality system for ultrasound guidance of transcatheter aortic valve implantation. Innovations. 2016;11(1):31–9; Discussion 9.
38. Ballocca F, Meier LM, Ladha K, Qua Hiansen J, Horlick EM, Meineri M. Validation of quantitative 3-dimensional transesophageal echocardiography mitral valve analysis using stereoscopic display. J Cardiothorac Vasc Anesth. 2019;33(3):732–41.
39. Bruckheimer E, Rotschild C, Dagan T, Amir G, Kaufman A, Gelman S, et al. Computer-generated real-time digital holography: first time use in clinical medical imaging. Eur Heart J Cardiovasc Imaging. 2016;17(8):845–9.

Ultrafast Ultrasound Imaging

2

Matthew Henry, Olivier Villemain, and Luc Mertens

2.1 Introduction to Ultrasound

The development of ultrasound technology has significantly impacted the field of medical diagnosis, especially in cardiology. This started with the discovery of the piezoelectric effect by Pierre and Jacques Currie in the 1880s. It was found that crystal deformation results in conversion of kinetic or mechanical energy into electrical energy. This is at the basis how ultrasound waves received by the crystals in the transducers generate electric signals that can be processed into images. The application of an electric field to a crystal results in crystal lengthening or contraction, converting electrical energy into kinetic or mechanical energy. This is how transducers produce ultrasound waves.

The introduction of ultrasound in cardiology started in Lund with Edler and Hertz in the 1950s. Echocardiography quickly developed as one of the key diagnostic techniques to assess cardiac structure and function structure and function evolving from M-mode imaging [1] to 2D and then 3D/4D imaging [2–4]. Doppler imaging allowed visualization of blood or tissue motion [5–7], and more recently, speckle-tracking echocardiography allowed imaging of myocardial deformation as a novel method to quantify myocardial function [8–10]. These technical evolutions were made possible by advances in electronics, computer science, and through improved ultrasound transducer technology.

M. Henry · O. Villemain · L. Mertens (✉)
Labatt Family Heart Centre, The Hospital for Sick Children, University of Toronto, Toronto, ON, Canada

Division of Cardiology, Hospital for Sick Children, Toronto, ON, Canada
e-mail: Matthew.henry@sickkids.ca; Olivier.Villemain@sickkids.ca; Luc.Mertens@sickkids.ca

© Springer Nature Switzerland AG 2021
P. Gallego, I. Valverde (eds.), *Multimodality Imaging Innovations In Adult Congenital Heart Disease*, Congenital Heart Disease in Adolescents and Adults, https://doi.org/10.1007/978-3-030-61927-5_2

2.2   Ultrafast Ultrasound Imaging

Conventional ultrasound uses single-line acquisition, whereby a single focused beam is emitted and then received prior to the next pulse being emitted (Fig. 2.1). An image is constructed by combining each of the beams into a coherent image (beamforming). As the speed of an acoustic beam through soft tissue is around 1530 m/s [11], the rate of image formation is largely dependent on the number of focused beams transmitted to create the image. Larger beams result in higher frame rates at the expense of spatial resolution. Smaller beams improve spatial resolution, but the maximal frame rate typically achieved by conventional beamforming ranges between 25 and 150 frames per second (FPS). This is sufficient to capture valve, blood, and tissue motion but is too low to record fast- and short-lived events such as those occurring during isovolumetric periods. When applying focused emission, it is possible to modify the transmission/reception mode to increase temporal resolution and while different approaches, such as multiline transmit beamforming or multiline acquisition beamforming, have been developed (improving frame rates), all still have significant limitations in temporal resolution [12].

Ultrafast (UF) imaging further builds on the concept that reducing the number of transmissions increases frame rate. UF imaging is based on the use of broad, unfocused beams called plane or divergent waves instead of the focused beams described above [13]. Plane and divergent waves are generated by applying a plane or circular delay algorithm to the transducer elements (Fig. 2.2). This makes it possible to reconstruct an image with a single emission, which is not possible with conventional ultrasound imaging. The result is a frame rate increase up to 10,000 f/s (depending on the acquisition depth), yet this occurs at the expense of lower spatial resolution and lower image contrast. To overcome this limitation, a coherent recombination of compounded plane-wave transmissions (also called coherent plane-wave compounding) is used to construct high-quality echocardiographic images without losing the frame rate [14]. When compared to conventional B-mode imaging, this provides

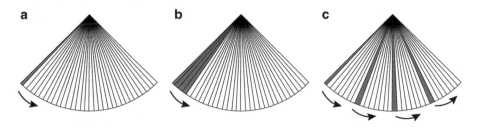

Fig. 2.1 Conventional beamforming. Image beam forming methods. (**a**) Single-line acquisition used in conventional beamforming. (**b**) Beamforming using multiline acquisitions with four lines. (**c**) Beamforming using multiline transmits beamforming. Green areas represent areas covered by transmit beam and arrows the direction of scanning. (Courtesy of Cikes et al.: Cikes M, Tong L, Sutherland GR, D'Hooge J (2014) Ultrafast cardiac ultrasound imaging: Technical principles, applications, and clinical benefits. JACC Cardiovasc Imaging 7:812–823)

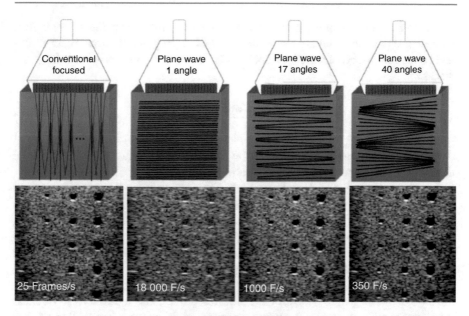

Fig. 2.2 Plane-wave imaging. Conventional ultrasound uses focused beams resulting in an image with good spatial resolution yet a frame rate of only 25 FPS. Plane-wave imaging with a single plane wave allows for exceptional temporal resolution (18,000 FPS) yet poor spatial resolution. Compounding plane waves result in spatial resolution comparable to conventional imaging yet much higher frame rates. (Courtesy of Tanter and Fink: Tanter M, Fink M (2014) Ultrafast imaging in biomedical ultrasound. IEEE Trans Ultrason Ferroelectr Freq Control 61:102–119)

similar image quality in terms of contrast, signal-to-noise ratio, and spatial resolution [15]. UF imaging is thus possible with good image quality (Fig. 2.2).

UF is a revolutionary ultrasound technique used clinically for different noncardiac applications including breast [16] and prostate [17] cancer, imaging of cerebral vessels in neonates [18], and liver stiffness assessment [19].

2.3 Limitations of Conventional Ultrasound Imaging in Congenital and Pediatric Cardiology

Conventional ultrasound techniques suffer from technical limitations that have significant clinical implications. One of the well-known limitations is the angle dependence of all Doppler techniques used to assess blood flow and tissue velocities. Velocities measured by this method are derived using the Doppler equation (Eq. 2.1), which represents the relationship between the measured Doppler shift (f_D) and the velocity (v). However, as the angle of insonification increases from 0° (where $\cos(0) = 1$) to 90° ($\cos(90) = 0$), velocities measured are underestimated, and are unmeasurable at 90°. Pressure gradients based on this velocity are estimated using the simplified Bernoulli equation which takes into account velocity measured only at a single point, assuming that the velocity before the narrowing is negligible. However, this is not accurate for small vessels, long segment narrowing, or multi-level obstructions, all of which are commonly seen in patients with congenital heart disease.

$$\mathcal{F}_D = -\frac{2v\cos\ominus\,\mathcal{F}_T}{c} \tag{2.1}$$

v = velocity, $\mathcal{F}_T$ = transmit frequency, $\ominus$ = angle between tissue/blood direction and ultrasound beam, and c = velocity of sound through tissue (1530 m/s).

Measurement of blood flow is also limited to a single plane (i.e. towards or away from the ultrasound probe). This is particularly important in patients with a narrowing such as valvular stenosis, where jet direction may be eccentric, and, therefore, the peak velocity may be out of plane and underestimated. More complex flow patterns such as vortices, which have been shown to be important for hemodynamic efficiency, can also not be visualized [20].

Finally, imaging of short-lived cardiac events such as myocardial changes during the isovolumetric periods, electromechanical coupling, and measurement of shear wave propagation is not feasible using conventional frame rates. Tissue Doppler has been used to study isovolumetric contraction (isovolumetric acceleration), but the technique is angle-dependent, and time resolution is a limiting factor.

Conventional frame rate ultrasound also has limitations in studying myocardial function. Ventricular contractility and especially ventricular compliance/stiffness measurements are based on surrogate measures. Conventional assessment of systolic function largely relies upon methods that study dimensional changes which are often based on geometric assumptions (fractional shortening and 2D-based ejection fraction) and are influenced by loading conditions. Direct measurements of myocardial motion (tissue Doppler velocities) and deformation (speckle-tracking echocardiography) avoid geometrical assumptions by directly assessing the myocardium, but these methods are also affected by loading conditions. 3D echocardiography [21, 22] avoids geometric assumptions, but its temporal resolution remains limited with frame rates between 10 and 50 volumes/s for real-time imaging and even lower for color-Doppler assessment. Limited temporal resolution is an important limitation in pediatric heart disease, where typically heart rates are high. Diastolic functional assessment is even more challenging, especially in children and patients with congenital heart disease. Current LV diastolic assessment is dependent on interpretation of combined transmitral and pulmonary venous Doppler, LA volume, and TDIs [23–25]. In patients with variable anatomy and highly variable loading conditions, these parameters are generally very difficult to interpret. This limits assessment of diastolic function, which is an essential component of functional assessment.

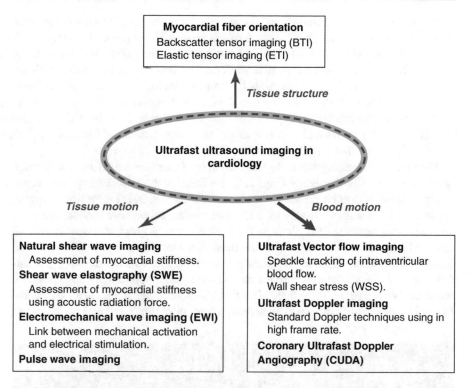

Fig. 2.3 Clinical applications of ultrafast imaging. Applications possible using ultrafast ultrasound. (Courtesy of Villemain et al.: Villemain O, Baranger J, Friedberg MK, Papadacci C, Dizeux A, Messas E, Tanter M, Pernot M and Mertens L. Ultrafast Ultrasound Imaging in Pediatric and Adult Cardiology: Techniques, Applications and Perspectives. JACC Cardiovasc Imaging. 2019)

2.4   Technological Tools Now Available Using Ultrafast Imaging

UF ultrasound is a novel method of image acquisition, which overcomes some of the frame rate limitations of conventional ultrasound, allowing very high temporal resolution. It enables novel imaging approaches to blood motion, tissue motion, and tissue characteristics (Fig. 2.3).

2.4.1   Visualization of Blood Flow

2.4.1.1 Vector Flow Imaging

Color flow imaging visualizes blood flow based on measuring Doppler shifts. These are color-coded and superimposed on B-mode images representing direction of flow and mean flow velocities. Measurement of flow is limited to one dimension (i.e., toward or away from the transducer). Flow patterns in the circulation are, however, typically more complex with formation of vortices as blood passes through an orifice like the mitral valve [26]. The vortex ring associated with flow through the mitral valve can be visualized as two vortices. The first one is associated with the anterior mitral valve leaflet and rotates counter clockwise. The second smaller vortex is associated with the posterior mitral valve leaflet and rotates clockwise. As vortices conserve kinetic energy, in contrast to turbulent flow in which kinetic energy is rapidly dissipated, the formation and maintenance of vortices play an important role in efficient flow mechanics [27].

Different echocardiographic approaches have been developed to image these more complex flow dynamics (Fig. 2.4). Particle image velocimetry uses echocontrast infusion to enhance blood flow visualization [28, 29]. Vector flow mapping combines Doppler flow imaging with LV wall motion assessment to visualize more complex flow patterns [30]. Both methods have intrinsic limitations as they both acquire flow data at relatively low frame rates. A novel method has been introduced based on UF ultrasound in which Doppler combined with speckle-tracking technology allows the user to image complex blood flow without contrast injection or mathematical assumptions [31–33]. In this method, speckles are correlated frame-by-frame, and the speckle displacement over time is used to calculate

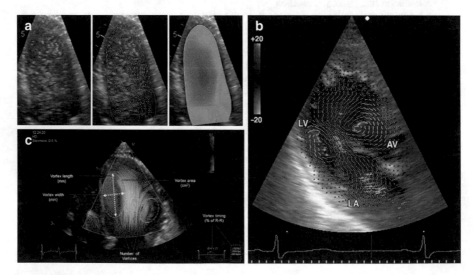

Fig. 2.4 Imaging techniques for blood flow. Imaging techniques for assessing blood flow. (**a**) Particle image velocimetry using contrast courtesy of Prinz et al. (**b**) Blood velocity mapping courtesy of Sengupta et al. (**c**) Blood speckle imaging. (Courtesy of de Waal et al.: Prinz C, Faludi R, Walker A, Amzulescu M, Gao H, Uejima T, Fraser AG, Voigt JU (2012) Can echocardiographic particle image velocimetry correctly detect motion patterns as they occur in blood inside heart chambers? A validation study using moving phantoms. Cardiovasc. Ultrasound 10. Sengupta PP, Pedrizzetti G, Kilner PJ, Kheradvar A, Ebbers T, Tonti G, Fraser AG, Narula J (2012) Emerging trends in CV flow visualization. JACC Cardiovasc Imaging 5:305–316. de Waal K, Crendal E, Boyle A (2019) Left ventricular vortex formation in preterm infants assessed by blood speckle imaging. Echocardiography. doi: https://doi.org/10.1111/echo.14391)

velocities in 2D. As decorrelation occurs quickly, high frame rates are needed to accurately image speckle movements. This method is less angle-dependent, allows imaging flows in two dimensions without using assumptions of wall motion, and has been validated for pediatric use on higher frequency curvilinear pediatric probes [34]. The obtained flow velocity information can be used to calculate energy losses, vorticity parameters, and intraventricular pressure gradients. Energy loss can be calculated based on vector velocities throughout the cardiac cycle and is a marker of flow turbulence representing kinetic energy loss into heat due to friction between blood viscosity and wall shear [35]. Vortex analysis includes describing vortex location, morphology, formation time, and vorticity [36], which is a measure of local rotation representing areas with increased shear stress. Finally, intraventricular pressure gradients may be estimated throughout the cardiac cycle, and in diastole, provides an estimate of the diastolic suction force [37]. One of the challenges of blood speckle-tracking technologies is the very large datasets that makes the technique computationally challenging and also challenges the storage capacity of current ultrasound scanners. Penetration of the UF ultrasound plane waves is a second challenge that currently limits application for mainly pediatric use. In vivo and in vitro validation has demonstrated that with the current techniques, velocity estimation using UF ultrasound is only reliably to a depth of 10 cm [38]. We expect that blood speckle-tracking technologies will be further developed and will likely replace current color Doppler techniques as technology evolves.

2.4.1.2 Coronary Ultrafast Doppler Angiography (CUDA)

Conductive coronary vessels are imaged using the methods of cardiac catheterization or CT angiography. To date, however, neither of these modalities allow for imaging of blood flow in the more distal prearteriolar coronary vessels. Coronary ultrafast Doppler angiography (CUDA) is a novel, noninvasive method based on UF ultrasound technology that allows for visualization and quantification of these more distal coronary vessels. This was introduced by Maresca [7] using spatiotemporal filters to separate myocardial movement from blood flow which provides the ability to reconstruct the vessel morphology and flows separate from the tissue as illustrated in Fig. 2.5. Both venous and arterial coronary flow can be imaged within the myocardium and this technique has been validated in pig models and in humans using linear array probes. By adding power Doppler technology, coronary flow reserve may be quantified, which could be used as a powerful noninvasive tool to diagnose ischemic heart disease.

2.4.2 Visualization of Tissue Motion

UF ultrasound technology allows acquiring tissue motion at very high frame rates, which offer opportunities for studying tissue motion in more detail. Different applications have been developed for studying cardiac function and tissue characteristics. Shear wave imaging is one of the better developed applications.

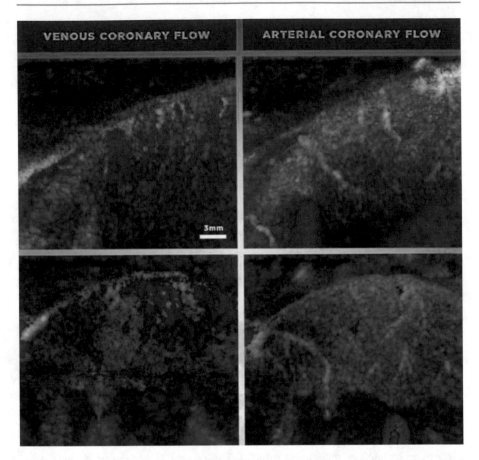

Fig. 2.5 CUDA imaging in open-chest swine. Subepicardial arterioles are successfully detected using ultrafast Doppler imaging. Upper panels show a long-axis view of venous coronaries in mid-systole (left) and arterial coronaries in mid-diastole (right). Lower panels show a mid-level short-axis view of venous coronaries in mid-systole (left) and arterial coronaries in mid-diastole (right). (Courtesy of Maresca et al.: Maresca D, Correia M, Villemain O, Bizé A, Sambin L, Tanter M, Ghaleh B, Pernot M (2018) Noninvasive Imaging of the Coronary Vasculature Using Ultrafast Ultrasound. JACC Cardiovasc Imaging 11:798–808)

2.4.2.1 Shear Wave Imaging

A shear wave is a transverse wave occurring as a result of an applied force (e.g., an acoustic radiation force). In the heart, this wave travels with a velocity of approximately 1–10 m/s, which is able to be imaged and quantified using UF ultrasound (>1000 FPS). Shear wave speed is directly linked to tissue stiffness through the shear modulus (Eq. 2.2), and thus measuring the velocity of shear waves can be used to assess myocardial stiffness in different parts of the cardiac cycle. Shear waves can be externally generated by applying an external force (acoustic radiation force) to the myocardium [39], but shear waves also occur naturally in the myocardium and are caused by an internal force such as induced in the myocardium at the time of valve closure [40].

$$V_c = \sqrt{\frac{\mu}{\rho}} \qquad (2.2)$$

V_c = shear wave velocity, μ = stiffness, ρ = local density (which is almost constant in soft tissue at around 1000 kg/m³).

Shear wave imaging using acoustic radiation force uses a short burst (several hundred microseconds) of focused ultrasound to induce tissue displacement in a region of interest (Fig. 2.6). The shear wave generated by this force is propagated perpendicular with a speed that is proportional to tissue stiffness [39]. The shear wave speed Vc may be computed at each depth of the image, allowing for

External stimulus and UF imaging

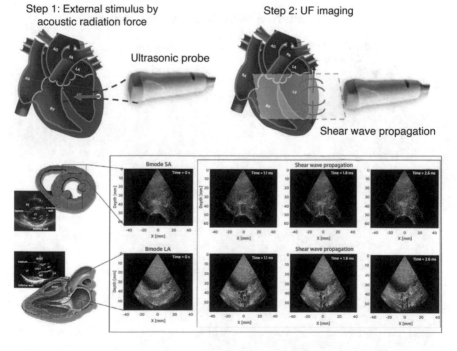

Fig. 2.6 Shear wave imaging using external stimulus. An external stimulus is used to generate a shear wave, which is then visualized with ultrafast ultrasound. Propagation of the shear wave can be seen on B-mode, allowing for calculation of shear wave speed. (Courtesy of Villemain et al.: Villemain O, Baranger J, Friedberg MK, Papadacci C, Dizeux A, Messas E, Tanter M, Pernot M and Mertens L. Ultrafast Ultrasound Imaging in Pediatric and Adult Cardiology: Techniques, Applications and Perspectives. JACC Cardiovasc Imaging. 2019)

calculation of stiffness μ using the shear modulus. Shear wave imaging using an externally induced radiation force allows to estimate myocardial stiffness at every moment of the cardiac cycle [41], both during systole and diastole, which is useful for studying end systolic elastance as a contractility parameter and end-diastolic stiffness as a diastolic parameter. The main disadvantage is that it is only possible to analyze a specific myocardial region, as defined by the push area (limited spatial resolution). Full-chamber stiffness assessment in one cardiac cycle is thus not possible using this approach. Further limitations relate to the anisotropy of the myocardial tissue as the myocardium is a complex three-dimensional-layered structure where fiber orientation varies with layer. Myocardial shear waves propagate preferentially in the direction of the fibers, which implicate that 2D assessment of shear waves needs to be very well standardized.

Shear waves are also generated throughout the cardiac cycle as a result of *intrinsic* mechanical events [42] such as valve closure (Fig. 2.7). The closure of the aortic valve, for instance, induces a measurable shear wave [43], which can be used to estimate myocardial stiffness at this specific time in the cardiac cycle (end-systole

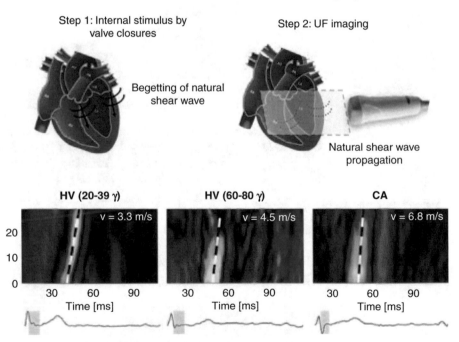

Fig. 2.7 Shear wave imaging using internal stimulus. This shear wave is generated by an internal stimulus (valve closure). Ultrafast ultrasound allows for imaging of its propagation and estimation of the shear wave speed. (Courtesy of Villemain et al.: Villemain O, Baranger J, Friedberg MK, Papadacci C, Dizeux A, Messas E, Tanter M, Pernot M and Mertens L. Ultrafast Ultrasound Imaging in Pediatric and Adult Cardiology: Techniques, Applications and Perspectives. JACC Cardiovasc Imaging. 2019)

or early relaxation). Similarly, the atrial contraction causes myocardial stretch from which stiffness may be derived [44]. Shear wave imaging relying on natural shear waves enables a more global MS assessment as the natural shear waves propagate in the heart over larger distances. However, natural shear waves in the myocardium are complex phenomena. By nature, its source is uncontrolled in terms of location, wavelength, and amplitude, as it mainly depends on valve morphology. Furthermore, propagation occurs in three dimensions along unknown directions. Natural shear waves are generated at fixed time points in the cardiac cycle, restricting stiffness estimates to a limited number of cardiac events. Shear waves generated from aortic and mitral valve closure represent only isovolumetric relaxation and contraction periods, respectively. Finally, stiffness estimates during end-diastole (which would be a useful surrogate of end-diastolic pressure) must be derived using myocardial stretch and are not true shear waves.

2.4.2.2 Electromechanical Wave Imaging (EWI)

Electromechanical coupling is the direct link between electrical and mechanical activation occurring approximately between 20 and 50 ms, depending on the myocardial segment evaluated [45]. Electrical depolarization leads to electromechanical activation as the muscles change to a contractile state. The myocardium produces a transient deformation at the time of activation, which can be imaged at very high frame rates. Based on this, electromechanical activation times can be derived. The feasibility of this approach has been demonstrated in human patients in both 2D as well as in [46] 3D [47] and 4D [48].

2.4.3   Tissue Structure and Fiber Orientation

Previous work on myocardial fiber orientation has largely been done on ex vivo specimens using diffraction-tensor MRI techniques. Recent work based on UF ultrasound demonstrated that imaging fiber orientation by ultrasound is feasible. Two different techniques have been described. Backscatter tensor imaging (BTI) uses the spatial coherence (i.e., the degree of resemblance) of speckle echoes to deduce myocardial fiber direction. Fibers parallel with the ultrasound wave show the highest spatial coherence, whereas those at 90° show the lowest. Based on this principle, myocardial fiber vectors can be created according to the degree of spatial coherence. This was first performed using fiber-reinforced composites showing that fiber direction relates to spatial coherence [49] with feasibility subsequently demonstrated in 2D and 3D models of cardiac tissue [50, 51] (Fig. 2.8).

Elastic tensor imaging (ETI) uses shear wave velocities to deduce myocardial fiber direction. Shear wave velocities are maximal when propagation occurs along the length of a fiber and minimal when traversing it. ETI exploits this phenomenon and constructs fiber maps using the shear wave velocities obtained from multiple angulations. This method has shown good correlation with MR DTI in ex vivo and in vivo animal models [52] but remains somewhat laborious for clinical use. Recently, 3D ETI has been developed [53] but has not yet been tested in vivo.

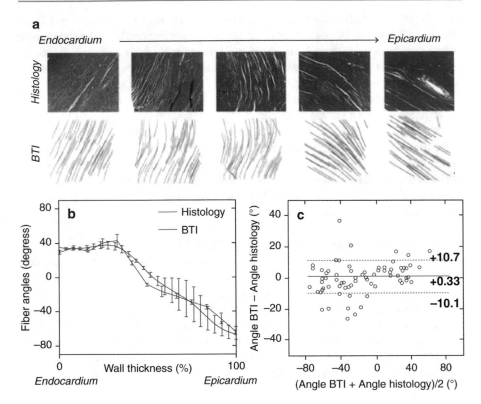

Fig. 2.8 Fiber orientation using BTI in comparison to histology. LV fiber orientation using BTI is compared with five corresponding histological slices (**a**). Fiber angle variation between BTI and histology is compared throughout myocardial layers (**b**). Bland-Altman plot of the transmural fiber angles estimated by 3D-BTI and histology (**c**). (Courtesy of Papadacci et al.: Papadacci, C., Finel, V., Provost, J. et al. Imaging the dynamics of cardiac fiber orientation in vivo using 3D Ultrasound Backscatter Tensor Imaging. *Sci Rep* **7**, 830 (2017) doi:https://doi.org/10.1038/s41598-017-00946-7)

2.5   Clinical Applications of Ultrafast Ultrasound Imaging

While the current clinical cardiovascular applications for UF ultrasound are limited, it can be expected that this technique will have major applications for patients with congenital heart disease. However, as for any novel technology, it will take many years before this technology will be fully implemented in clinical care.

2.5.1   Ventricular Function

Myocardial stiffness estimation has shown potential as a measure of contractility and in identifying subclinical abnormalities not seen using conventional methods. Studies in animal models have demonstrated MS as a noninvasive index of myocardial contractility [41, 54], while in humans, differences in end-systolic MS has been shown between healthy patients and those with amyloidosis in whom conventional measures of systolic function are normal [55]. Having more geometric and load-independent measures of systolic function would certainly be beneficial for patients with congenital heart disease, where morphology and loading are highly variable.

Myocardial stiffness assessment plays an even more important role for diastolic assessment, where stiffness and assessment of filling pressures are the main clinical questions. Current echocardiographic diastolic assessment has largely focused on early diastolic events mainly influenced by myocardial relaxation. In adults with acquired heart disease, relaxation abnormalities are an essential component of diastolic dysfunction. This is less obvious in children as diastolic dysfunction may be present without early relaxation being significantly affected [56]. The current adult paradigm of transition from early relaxation abnormalities to restrictive physiology may not be applicable for pediatric patients. Additionally, in patients with congenital heart disease mitral inflow, tissue Doppler velocities and pulmonary venous flows are often influenced by age, heart rate, loading conditions (eg. left-right shunts), valve abnormalities, and other factors, reducing their utility for diastolic assessment. Shear wave imaging, however, allows for noninvasive myocardial diastolic stiffness estimation independent of geometry and loading. Studies in animal models demonstrated that SWI is able to differentiate between stiff-infarcted myocardium and more compliant "stunned" myocardium with excellent correlation with invasive measurements of the end-diastolic strain-stress relationship [57]. In humans, myocardial diastolic stiffness has been shown to significantly increase with age [58, 59] and be abnormally high in patients with hypertrophic cardiomyopathy [60, 61], cardiac amyloidosis [55], and hypertension-induced LV hypertrophy [59]. These are the first human data demonstrating its utility for clinical use. Further validation and technical standardization will be needed before widespread clinical use will become possible, but the initial findings are promising.

Blood speckle-tracking technology will also add novel information for both systolic and diastolic function assessment. Better visualization of complex flow patterns has been demonstrated to be potentially clinically useful in the assessment of ventricular function in different diseases [36]. However, there is no good standardization of vector flow acquisition methods, analysis, or interpretation as it is still unclear which flow parameters are clinically relevant. Applications have been suggested but so far have not reached routine clinical practice. For instance, flow analysis could help in better positioning of mechanical mitral valves during surgical implantation as more physiological orientation of the valve leaflets determines vortex direction and is associated with variable systolic energy losses [62, 63]. In animal models, significant correlations have been reported between the systolic vorticity/energy losses and load-independent measures of systolic function like end-systolic elastance and stroke work [64].

Blood flow imaging also adds to diastolic assessment. Abnormalities in valve structure and function result in abnormal intraventricular flow profiles with increased systolic and diastolic energy losses contributing to hemodynamic inefficiencies. For example, severe aortic regurgitation is associated with increased diastolic energy losses contributing to abnormal filling characteristics [65]. Patients with dilated cardiomyopathies (DCM) have larger vortices, with increased diastolic energy losses and vorticity index [66, 67]. Conversely, patients with nonobstructive hypertrophic cardiomyopathies have increased energy losses with smaller vortices [68]. Intraventricular pressure gradients during early filling allow to evaluate the contribution of diastolic suction to ventricular filling. In hypertrophic cardiomyopathy patients, this has been shown to correlate with invasively measured LV end-diastolic pressure [68].

In congenital heart disease, flow dynamics have been investigated in patients with single ventricle physiology [69], after tetralogy of Fallot repair [70], and in patients with transposition of the great arteries (TGA), after the arterial switch operation [71] however current studies are small and use diverse methodologies. More studies are clearly needed.

2.5.2 Evaluating Coronary Perfusion and Cardiac Structure in CHD

CUDA has not yet been explored in patients with congenital heart disease however assessment of coronary microperfusion may be extremely relevant for certain congenital defects. Patients post Fontan procedure for pulmonary atresia intact ventricular septum (PAIVS) with right ventricular-dependent coronary circulation (RVDCC) are at increased risk of sudden death and have a significantly reduced survival rate post Fontan than those without RVDCC [72]. Identifying patients earlier with reduced coronary perfusion and flow reserve could help risk stratify these patients and reduce the risk of sudden death. Patients requiring coronary manipulation such as patients with transposition of the great arteries undergoing an arterial switch represent another important group. Currently risk for ischemic events is based on postoperative coronary artery Doppler patterns [73]; however, CUDA could replace this method by evaluating postrepair coronary flow in 2D and assessing coronary flow reserve prior to the patient leaving the operating room.

Myocardial fiber orientation plays an important role in the mechanics of cardiac function [74]. The LV and RV architecture differ in normal hearts with three layers being present in the high-pressure LV [75] and two main layers in the low-pressure RV. Patients with congenital heart disease and cardiomyopathies may have an abnormal fiber architecture [76] which combined with abnormal loading conditions may predispose decreased function [77, 78]. BTI could help to understand the pathophysiology of CHD and offers great potential for novel insights.

2.5.3 Rhythm Abnormalities

Electromechanical wave imaging is well-suited for the assessment of arrhythmias in children. Recent work has shown its use in discriminating between an epicardial and endocardial source of ventricular ectopics [79]. This has significant clinical implications as epicardial foci are not ideally suited for catheter ablation. Electromechanical wave imaging has also been used in 3D localization of accessory pathways, a particularly useful application for catheter planning. Melki et al. demonstrated its superiority in pathway localization compared to conventional noninvasive methods. Pathways were successfully localized (with EP study/ablation used as the gold standard) in all 14 patients using EWI compared to 11 using ECG analysis (Fig. 2.9).

2.5.4   Future Directions

Echocardiographic imaging for a "complete study" of both anatomy and functional assessment may take up to an hour or longer. Structures are imaged from multiple angles with hemodynamic and tissue motion measurements performed using multiple methods. UF ultrasound imaging using simultaneous 4D image acquisition could improve this, where color doppler, tissue doppler, chamber volumes, blood flow imaging, shear wave imaging, and tissue orientation are recorded in 3D and in a single acquisition. Simultaneous acquisition of multiple functional parameters would result in increased consistency between measurements and could lead to new algorithms and indices for functional assessment.

Another unexplored application of UF ultrasound is during fetal life. Fetal mapping of myocardial development using BTI/WEI could provide new insights into normal myocardial development as well as the pathogenesis and progression of congenital heart disease. Combining this method with assessment of blood flow using BSI could help to better understand the relationship between blood flow and myocardial architecture in the development and progression of congenital heart disease.

2.5.5   Current Limitation of HFRUS

Despite UF ultrasound currently being used in other specialties, it remains in the preclinical phase for cardiology. While it provides exponential improvements in framerate with acceptable spatial resolution, it remains an imperfect method. Tissue penetration, in particular, remains an important challenge, especially for teenagers and adults. Structures continue to be difficult to image due to signal attenuation and the dissipation and diffraction of ultrasound waves. Anatomical location of structures like the anteriorly positioned RV walls remains a challenge. Furthermore, although the use of plane/diverging waves has significantly reduced the influence of acquisition angle in measurements such as blood velocity, the angle of sonification remains an important factor in 2D quantification of flow. The use of newer matrix array probes will improve this and have recently been used to evaluate 3D electromechanical activation [48] and blood flow [4]. Finally, UF imaging generates very large data sets and although there has been marked improvement in graphic and data processing, this remains relatively slow, limiting current clinical utility.

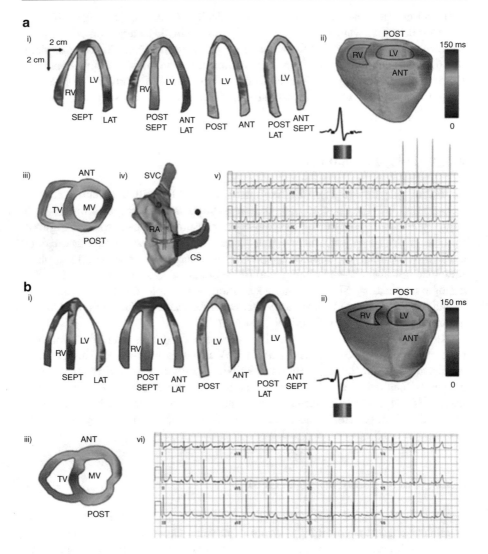

Fig. 2.9 EWI isochrones of a 7-year-old female with a left lateral pathway before and after successful radio frequency ablation. Isochrones demonstrating activation times prior to ablation (**a**) and postablation (**b**). Red indicates earliest activation and blue the latest. (**a**: i–iii) show earliest activation in the lateral LV wall; (iv) electroanatomic map (LAO view), where the yellow dot represents the HIS site and red dot the site of ablation; (v) shows resting ECG prior to ablation with evidence of preexcitation. (**b**: i–iii) show earliest activation now in the normal septal positions; (iv) resting ECG postablation without evidence of preexcitation. (Courtesy of Melki et al.: Melki L, Grubb CS, Weber R, Nauleau P, Garan H, Wan E, Silver ES, Liberman L, Konofagou EE (2019) Localization of Accessory Pathways in Pediatric Patients With Wolff-Parkinson-White Syndrome Using 3D-Rendered Electromechanical Wave Imaging. JACC Clin Electrophysiol 5:427–437)

2.6   Summary/Conclusion

UF ultrasound has the potential to revolutionize echocardiography. The applications include novel methods for imaging cardiac tissue structure, tissue motion, and blood flow. Cardiac fiber orientation has been shown feasible using BTI and ETI, providing new insights into the pathogenesis of congenital and also acquired heart disease. Noninvasive shear wave imaging and intracardiac blood flow analysis may prove to be completely new markers of cardiac function, shifting the paradigm to function being quantified for the entire cardiac cycle rather than as an averaged global marker. Furthermore, pressure gradients obtained using BSI may provide quantified estimates of filling pressures. Finally, CUDA has the potential to replace the current gold standard methods of coronary blood flow imaging reducing the use of invasive procedures.

References

1. Feigenbaum H. Role of M-mode technique in today's echocardiography. J Am Soc Echocardiogr. 2010;23:240–57.
2. Fenster A, Downey DB. 3-D ultrasound imaging: a review. IEEE Eng Med Biol Mag. 1996;15:41–51.
3. Lang RM, Badano LP, Tsang W, et al. EAE/ASE recommendations for image acquisition and display using three-dimensional echocardiography. Eur Heart J Cardiovasc Imaging. 2012;13:1–46.
4. Provost J, Papadacci C, Arango JE, Imbault M, Fink M, Gennisson J-L, Tanter M, Pernot M. 3D ultrafast ultrasound imaging in vivo. Phys Med Biol. 2014;59:L1.
5. Pearlman AS, Stevenson JG, Baker DW. Doppler echocardiography: applications, limitations and future directions. Am J Cardiol. 1980;46:1256–62.
6. Garcia MJ, Thomas JD, Klein AL. New Doppler echocardiographic applications for the study of diastolic function. J Am Coll Cardiol. 1998;32:865–75.
7. Maresca D, Correia M, Villemain O, Bizé A, Sambin L, Tanter M, Ghaleh B, Pernot M. Noninvasive imaging of the coronary vasculature using ultrafast ultrasound. JACC Cardiovasc Imaging. 2018;11:798–808.
8. Kanai H, Hasegawa H, Chubachi N, Koiwa Y, Tanaka M. Noninvasive evaluation of local myocardial thickening and its color-coded imaging. IEEE Trans Ultrason Ferroelectr Freq Control. 1997;44:752–68.
9. D'hooge J, Bijnens B, Thoen J, Van de Werf F, Sutherland GR, Suetens P. Echocardiographic strain and strain-rate imaging: a new tool to study regional myocardial function. IEEE Trans Med Imaging. 2002;21:1022–30.
10. Bijnens BH, Cikes M, Claus P, Sutherland GR. Velocity and deformation imaging for the assessment of myocardial dysfunction. Eur J Echocardiogr. 2008;10:216–26.
11. Lai WW, Mertens LL, Cohen MS, Geva T. Echocardiography in pediatric and congenital heart disease: from fetus to adult: second edition. Hoboken, NJ: Wiley Blackwell; 2016. https://doi.org/10.1002/9781118742440.
12. Cikes M, Tong L, Sutherland GR, D'Hooge J. Ultrafast cardiac ultrasound imaging: technical principles, applications, and clinical benefits. JACC Cardiovasc Imaging. 2014;7:812–23.
13. Tanter M, Fink M. Ultrafast imaging in biomedical ultrasound. IEEE Trans Ultrason Ferroelectr Freq Control. 2014;61:102–19.

14. Montaldo G, Tanter M, Bercoff J, Benech N, Fink M. Coherent plane-wave compounding for very high frame rate ultrasonography and transient elastography. IEEE Trans Ultrason Ferroelectr Freq Control. 2009;56:489–506.

15. Papadacci C, Pernot M, Couade M, Fink M, Tanter M. High-contrast ultrafast imaging of the heart. IEEE Trans Ultrason Ferroelectr Freq Control. 2014;61:288–301.

16. Yamakoshi Y, Nakajima T, Kasahara T, Yamazaki M, Koda R, Sunaguchi N. Shear wave imaging of breast tissue by color doppler shear wave elastography. IEEE Trans Ultrason Ferroelectr Freq Control. 2017;64:340–8.

17. Curiel L, Souchon R, Rouvière O, Gelet A, Chapelon JY. Elastography for the follow-up of high-intensity focused ultrasound prostate cancer treatment: initial comparison with MRI. Ultrasound Med Biol. 2005;31:1461–8.

18. Demené C, Pernot M, Biran V, Alison M, Fink M, Baud O, Tanter M. Ultrafast Doppler reveals the mapping of cerebral vascular resistivity in neonates. J Cereb Blood Flow Metab. 2014;34:1009–17.

19. Frulio N, Trillaud H. Ultrasound elastography in liver. Diagn Interv Imaging. 2013;94:515–34.

20. Tanaka M, Sakamoto T, Saijo Y, Katahira Y, Sugawara S, Nakajima H, Kurokawa T, Kanai H. Role of intra-ventricular vortex in left ventricular ejection elucidated by echo-dynamography. J Med Ultrason. 2019;46:413. https://doi.org/10.1007/s10396-019-00943-5.

21. Soliman OII, Kirschbaum SW, van Dalen BM, van der Zwaan HB, Delavary BM, Vletter WB, van Geuns RJM, Ten Cate FJ, Geleijnse ML. Accuracy and reproducibility of quantitation of left ventricular function by real-time three-dimensional echocardiography versus cardiac magnetic resonance. Am J Cardiol. 2008;102:778–83.

22. Dragulescu A, Grosse-Wortmann L, Fackoury C, Riffle S, Waiss M, Jaeggi E, Yoo SJ, Friedberg MK, Mertens L. Echocardiographic assessment of right ventricular volumes after surgical repair of tetralogy of fallot: clinical validation of a new echocardiographic method. J Am Soc Echocardiogr. 2011;24:1191–8.

23. Panesar DK, Burch M. Assessment of diastolic function in congenital heart disease. Front Cardiovasc Med. 2017;4:1–10.

24. Mitter SS, Shah SJ, Thomas JD. A test in context: E/A and E/e' to assess diastolic dysfunction and LV filling pressure. J Am Coll Cardiol. 2017;69:1451–64.

25. Nagueh SF, Smiseth OA, Appleton CP, et al. Recommendations for the evaluation of left ventricular diastolic function by echocardiography: an update from the American Society of Echocardiography and the European Association of Cardiovascular Imaging I. General Principles for Echocardiographic Asses. J Am Soc Echocardiogr. 2016;29:277–314.

26. Bot H, Verburg J, Delemarre BJ, Strackee J. Determinants of the occurrence of vortex rings in the left ventricle during diastole. J Biomech. 1990;23:607–15.

27. Pedrizzetti G, Sengupta PP. Vortex imaging: new information gain from tracking cardiac energy loss. Eur Heart J Cardiovasc Imaging. 2015;16:719–20.

28. Kheradvar A, Houle H, Pedrizzetti G, Tonti G, Belcik T, Ashraf M, Lindner JR, Gharib M, Sahn D. Echocardiographic particle image velocimetry: a novel technique for quantification of left ventricular blood vorticity pattern. J Am Soc Echocardiogr. 2010;23:86–94.

29. Prinz C, Faludi R, Walker A, Amzulescu M, Gao H, Uejima T, Fraser AG, Voigt JU. Can echocardiographic particle image velocimetry correctly detect motion patterns as they occur in blood inside heart chambers? A validation study using moving phantoms. Cardiovasc Ultrasound. 2012;10:24.

30. Garcia D, Juan JC, Tanné D, et al. Two-dimensional intraventricular flow mapping by digital processing conventional color-doppler echocardiography images. IEEE Trans Med Imaging. 2010;29:1701–13.

31. Løvstakken L, Bærum S, Martens D, Torp H. Blood flow imaging—a new real-time, 2-D flow imaging technique. IEEE Trans Ultrason Ferroelectr Freq Control. 2006;53:289–99.

32. Sengupta PP, Pedrizzetti G, Kilner PJ, Kheradvar A, Ebbers T, Tonti G, Fraser AG, Narula J. Emerging trends in CV flow visualization. JACC Cardiovasc Imaging. 2012;5:305–16.

33. de Waal K, Crendal E, Boyle A. Left ventricular vortex formation in preterm infants assessed by blood speckle imaging. Echocardiography. 2019;36:1364. https://doi.org/10.1111/echo.14391.
34. Fadnes S, Ekroll IK, Nyrnes SA, Torp H, Lovstakken L. Robust angle-independent blood velocity estimation based on dual-angle plane wave imaging. IEEE Trans Ultrason Ferroelectr Freq Control. 2015;62:1757–67.
35. Xu L, Sun C, Zhu X, Weihua MM, Mbbs L, Ta S, Mbbs DZ, Wang F, Liwen MM. Characterization of left ventricle energy loss in healthy adults using vector flow mapping: preliminary results. Echocardiography. 2017;34:700.
36. Mele D, Smarrazzo V, Pedrizzetti G, Capasso F, Pepe M, Severino S, Luisi GA, Maglione M, Ferrari R. Intracardiac flow analysis: techniques and potential clinical applications. J Am Soc Echocardiogr. 2019;32:319–32.
37. Hansen KL, Nielsen MB, Jensen JA. Vector velocity estimation of blood flow – a new application in medical ultrasound. Ultrasound. 2017;25:189–99.
38. Fadnes S, Wigen MS, Nyrnes SA, Lovstakken L. In vivo intracardiac vector flow imaging using phased array transducers for pediatric cardiology. IEEE Trans Ultrason Ferroelectr Freq Control. 2017;64:1318–26.
39. Sarvazyan AP, Rudenko OV, Swanson SD, Fowlkes JB, Emelianov SY. Shear wave elasticity imaging: a new ultrasonic technology of medical diagnostics. Ultrasound Med Biol. 1998;24:1419–35.
40. Santos P, Petrescu AM, Pedrosa JP, Orlowska M, Komini V, Voigt JU, D'Hooge J. Natural shear wave imaging in the human heart: normal values, feasibility, and reproducibility. IEEE Trans Ultrason Ferroelectr Freq Control. 2019;66:442–52.
41. Pernot M, Couade M, Mateo P, Crozatier B, Fischmeister R, Tanter M. Real-time assessment of myocardial contractility using shear wave imaging. J Am Coll Cardiol. 2011;58:65–72.
42. Pernot M, Fujikura K, Fung-Kee-Fung SD, Konofagou EE. ECG-gated, mechanical and electromechanical wave imaging of cardiovascular tissues in vivo. Ultrasound Med Biol. 2007;33:1075–85.
43. Kanai H. Propagation of spontaneously actuated pulsive vibration in human heart wall and in vivo viscoelasticity estimation. IEEE Trans Ultrason Ferroelectr Freq Control. 2005;52:1931–42.
44. Pislaru C, Pellikka PA, Pislaru SV. Wave propagation of myocardial stretch: correlation with myocardial stiffness. Basic Res Cardiol. 2014;109:438. https://doi.org/10.1007/s00395-014-0438-5.
45. Cordeiro JM, Greene L, Heilmann C, Antzelevitch D, Antzelevitch C. Transmural heterogeneity of calcium activity and mechanical function in the canine left ventricle. Am J Physiol Heart Circ Physiol. 2004;286:F1471. https://doi.org/10.1152/ajpheart.00748.2003.
46. Provost J, Lee WN, Fujikura K, Konofagou EE. Imaging the electromechanical activity of the heart in vivo. Proc Natl Acad Sci U S A. 2011;108:8565–70.
47. Melki L, Grubb CS, Weber R, Nauleau P, Garan H, Wan E, Silver ES, Liberman L, Konofagou EE. Localization of accessory pathways in pediatric patients with wolff-parkinson-white syndrome using 3D-rendered electromechanical wave imaging. JACC Clin Electrophysiol. 2019;5:427–37.
48. Grondin J, Wang D, Grubb CS, Trayanova N, Konofagou EE. 4D cardiac electromechanical activation imaging. Comput Biol Med. 2019;113:103382.
49. Derode A, Fink M. Spatial coherence of ultrasonic speckle in composites. IEEE Trans Ultrason Ferroelectr Freq Control. 1993;40:666–75.
50. Papadacci C, Tanter M, Pernot M, Fink M. Ultrasound backscatter tensor imaging (BTI): analysis of the spatial coherence of ultrasonic speckle in anisotropic soft tissues. IEEE Trans Ultrason Ferroelectr Freq Control. 2014;61:986–96.
51. Papadacci C, Finel V, Provost J, Villemain O, Bruneval P, Gennisson JL, Tanter M, Fink M, Pernot M. Imaging the dynamics of cardiac fiber orientation in vivo using 3D Ultrasound Backscatter Tensor Imaging. Sci Rep. 2017;7:1–9.

52. Lee W-N, Pernot M, Couade M, Messas E, Bruneval P, Bel A, Hagège AA, Fink M, Tanter M. Mapping myocardial fiber orientation using echocardiography-based shear wave imaging. IEEE Trans Med Imaging. 2012;31:554–62.
53. Correia M, Deffieux T, Chatelin S, Provost J, Tanter M, Pernot M. 3D elastic tensor imaging in weakly transversely isotropic soft tissues. Phys Med Biol. 2018;63:155005.
54. Vejdani-Jahromi M, Freedman J, Nagle M, Kim Y-J, Trahey GE, Wolf PD. Quantifying myocardial contractility changes using ultrasound-based shear wave elastography. J Am Soc Echocardiogr. 2017;30:90–6.
55. Petrescu A, Santos P, Orlowska M, et al. Velocities of naturally occurring myocardial shear waves increase with age and in cardiac amyloidosis. JACC Cardiovasc Imaging. 2019;12:2389. https://doi.org/10.1016/j.jcmg.2018.11.029.
56. Dragulescu A, Mertens L, Friedberg MK. Interpretation of left ventricular diastolic dysfunction in children with cardiomyopathy by echocardiography clinical perspective. Circ Cardiovasc Imaging. 2013;6:254.
57. Pernot M, Lee WN, Bel A, Mateo P, Couade M, Tanter M, Crozatier B, Messas E. Shear wave imaging of passive diastolic myocardial stiffness: stunned versus infarcted myocardium. JACC Cardiovasc Imaging. 2016;9:1023–30.
58. Villemain O, Correia M, Mousseaux E, et al. Myocardial stiffness evaluation using noninvasive shear wave imaging in healthy and hypertrophic cardiomyopathic adults. JACC Cardiovasc Imaging. 2018;12:1135. https://doi.org/10.1016/j.jcmg.2018.02.002.
59. Cvijic M, Bézy S, Petrescu A, et al. Interplay of cardiac remodelling and myocardial stiffness in hypertensive heart disease: a shear wave imaging study using high-frame rate echocardiography. Eur Heart J Cardiovasc Imaging. 2020;21:664. https://doi.org/10.1093/ehjci/jez205.
60. Villemain O, Correia M, Khraiche D, Podetti I, Meot M, Legendre A, Tanter M, Bonnet D, Pernot M. Myocardial stiffness assessment using shear wave imaging in pediatric hypertrophic cardiomyopathy. JACC Cardiovasc Imaging. 2017;11:779. https://doi.org/10.1016/j.jcmg.2017.08.018.
61. Strachinaru M, Bosch JG, van Gils L, van Dalen BM, Schinkel AFL, van der Steen AFW, de Jong N, Michels M, Vos HJ, Geleijnse ML. Naturally occurring shear waves in healthy volunteers and hypertrophic cardiomyopathy patients. Ultrasound Med Biol. 2019;45:1977–86.
62. Nakashima K, Itatani K, Kitamura T, Oka N, Horai T, Miyazaki S, Nie M, Miyaji K. Energy dynamics of the intraventricular vortex after mitral valve surgery. Heart Vessel. 2017;32:1123–9.
63. Faludi R, Szulik M, D'hooge J, Herijgers P, Rademakers F, Pedrizzetti G, Voigt JU. Left ventricular flow patterns in healthy subjects and patients with prosthetic mitral valves: an in vivo study using echocardiographic particle image velocimetry. J Thorac Cardiovasc Surg. 2010;139:1501–10.
64. Goya S, Wada T, Shimada K, Hirao D, Tanaka R. The relationship between systolic vector flow mapping parameters and left ventricular cardiac function in healthy dogs. Heart Vessel. 2018;33:549–60.
65. Stugaard M, Koriyama H, Katsuki K, Masuda K, Asanuma T, Takeda Y, Sakata Y, Itatani K, Nakatani S. Energy loss in the left ventricle obtained by vector flow mapping as a new quantitative measure of severity of aortic regurgitation: a combined experimental and clinical study. Eur Heart J Cardiovasc Imaging. 2015;16:723–30.
66. Hong GR, Pedrizzetti G, Tonti G, et al. Characterization and quantification of vortex flow in the human left ventricle by contrast echocardiography using vector particle image velocimetry. JACC Cardiovasc Imaging. 2008;1:705–17.
67. Bermejo J, Benito Y, Alhama M, et al. Intraventricular vortex properties in nonischemic dilated cardiomyopathy. Am J Physiol Heart Circ Physiol. 2014;306:718–29.
68. Prinz C, Lehmann R, Brandao Da Silva D, Jurczak B, Bitter T, Faber L, Horstkotte D. Echocardiographic particle image velocimetry for the evaluation of diastolic function in hypertrophic nonobstructive cardiomyopathy. Echocardiography. 2014;31:886–94.
69. Amodeo A, Grigioni M, Oppido G, Daniele C, D'Avenio G, Pedrizzetti G, Giannico S, Filippelli S, Di Donato RM. The beneficial vortex and best spatial arrangement in total extracardiac cavopulmonary connection. J Thorac Cardiovasc Surg. 2002;124:471–8.

70. Kutty S, Li L, Danford DA, Houle H, Datta S, Mancina J, Xiao Y, Pedrizzetti G, Porter TR. Effects of right ventricular hemodynamic burden on Intraventricular flow in tetralogy of fallot: an echocardiographic contrast particle imaging velocimetry study. J Am Soc Echocardiogr. 2014;27:1311–8.
71. Riesenkampff E, Nordmeyer S, Al-Wakeel N, Kropf S, Kutty S, Berger F, Kuehne T. Flow-sensitive four-dimensional velocity-encoded magnetic resonance imaging reveals abnormal blood flow patterns in the aorta and pulmonary trunk of patients with transposition. Cardiol Young. 2014;24:47–53.
72. Elias P, Poh CL, du Plessis K, Zannino D, Rice K, Radford DJ, Bullock AR, Wheaton G, Celermajer DS, d'Udekem Y. Long-term outcomes of single-ventricle palliation for pulmonary atresia with intact ventricular septum: fontan survivors remain at risk of late myocardial ischaemia and death. Eur J Cardiothorac Surg. 2018;53:1230–6.
73. Nield LE, Dragulescu A, MacColl C, Manlhiot C, Brun H, McCrindle BW, Kuipers B, Caldarone CA, Miner SES, Mertens L. Coronary artery Doppler patterns are associated with clinical outcomes post-arterial switch operation for transposition of the great arteries. Eur Heart J Cardiovasc Imaging. 2018;19:461–8.
74. Buckberg G, Hoffman JIE, Mahajan A, Saleh S, Coghlan C. Cardiac mechanics revisited: the relationship of cardiac architecture to ventricular function. Circulation. 2008;118:2571–87.
75. Ho SY. Anatomy and myoarchitecture of the left ventricular wall in normal and in disease. Eur J Echocardiogr. 2009;10:3–7.
76. Sanchez-Quintana D, Anderson RH, Ho SY. Ventricular myoarchitecture in tetralogy of Fallot. Heart. 1996;76:280–6.
77. Ghonim S, Voges I, Gatehouse PD, Keegan J, Gatzoulis MA, Kilner PJ, Babu-Narayan SV. Myocardial architecture, mechanics, and fibrosis in congenital heart disease. Front Cardiovasc Med. 2017;4:1–15.
78. Ramalli A, Santos P, D'Hooge J. Ultrasound imaging of cardiac fiber orientation: what are we looking at? In: IEEE Int Ultrason Symp IUS; 2018. p. 1–9.
79. Costet A, Wan E, Melki L, Bunting E, Grondin J, Garan H, Konofagou E. Non-invasive characterization of focal arrhythmia with electromechanical wave imaging in vivo. Ultrasound Med Biol. 2018;44:2241–9.

MRI T1 Mapping: Myocardial Fibrosis

Erica Dall'Armellina, Malenka M. Bissell,
David A. Broadbent, and Sven Plein

3.1 Introduction

Compared to other non-invasive imaging tools, cardiac magnetic resonance (CMR) has superior clinical utility in that it offers (a) three-dimensional anatomical views of the heart and vascular connections, (b) superior volumetric assessment of the cardiac chambers, and most importantly, (c) myocardial tissue characterization. These advantageous properties make CMR particularly suitable for clinical applications in congenital heart disease. As in many cardiac conditions, in congenital heart disease, diffuse fibrosis is known to cause loss of myocardial function [1, 2] and may potentially be a substrate for electric instability and life-threatening ventricular arrhythmia [3]. The main determinants of diffuse fibrosis in congenital heart disease are abnormal loading conditions, cyanosis, and genetic predisposition.

It has been demonstrated that interstitial myocardial fibrosis is a reversible process and as such a potential target for treatment. CMR techniques allowing for quantification of diffuse fibrosis could play a key role in the longitudinal monitoring of the effects of treatments. Standard late gadolinium techniques are excellent in detecting regional scarring and focal fibrosis, but less so when it comes to diffuse fibrosis. Recently validated T1 mapping techniques have been demonstrated to have incremental clinical utility by allowing for voxel-wise quantification of variations of

E. Dall'Armellina (✉) · M. M. Bissell · S. Plein
Department of Biomedical Imaging Science, Leeds Institute of Cardiovascular and Metabolic Medicine, University of Leeds, Leeds, UK
e-mail: E.DallArmellina@leeds.ac.uk; M.M.Bissell@leeds.ac.uk; S.Plein@leeds.ac.uk

D. A. Broadbent
Medical Physics and Engineering, Leeds Teaching Hospitals NHS Trust, Leeds, UK
e-mail: d.broadbent@nhs.net

© Springer Nature Switzerland AG 2021
P. Gallego, I. Valverde (eds.), *Multimodality Imaging Innovations In Adult Congenital Heart Disease*, Congenital Heart Disease in Adolescents and Adults,
https://doi.org/10.1007/978-3-030-61927-5_3

T1 values as markers of diffuse fibrosis. Two main imaging biomarkers derived from T1 mapping methods have been validated against histology in the LV [4] and can be used clinically: native T1 values and extracellular volume (ECV) derived from pre- and post-contrast T1 mapping.

A prolongation in pre-contrast or native T1 values can be due to different factors such as increased water content due to oedema [5, 6], deposition of proteins (such as amyloid) [7], or increased fibrosis. In adults with severe aortic stenosis, native T1 values correlate with the degree of biopsy-quantified diffuse fibrosis [8]. Native T1 times are longer in patients with hypertrophic and dilated cardiomyopathy than in normal controls. However, the significant overlap between native T1 in health and disease prohibits its use in differentiating normal from abnormal in most conditions.

ECV maps are derived from both pre-contrast T1 maps and post-contrast T1 maps and represent a robust quantitative measure of collagen deposition and myocardial fibrosis [9]. Normal ECV values have been established to be on the order of $25.3 \pm 3.5\%$ at 1.5 T [10].

This chapter will describe the fundamental physical principles of T1 mapping techniques and the clinical applicability of mapping imaging biomarkers in congenital heart disease.

3.2 Physics Principles

3.2.1 What Is T1, Native vs Post-contrast

MRI is unique in its ability to characterize soft tissue composition by quantifying how rapidly excited magnetization returns to its equilibrium state after the application of RF pulses. T1 or longitudinal relaxation is a measure of the recovery of magnetization parallel to the externally applied magnetic field. The rate of this recovery depends on mechanisms that allow the spins to exchange energy with their surroundings, including interactions with magnetic moments from neighbouring molecules [11].

In the heart, there are three key tissue types with substantially different native T1, depending on the tissue composition and the proportion of water versus other components: blood has a relatively long T1 albeit not as long as pure water or some other biological liquids such as cerebrospinal fluid; myocardium has intermediate T1, similar to skeletal muscle and other soft tissues, while fat has shorter T1 [12]. Table 3.1 provides an example of T1 values acquired in normal volunteers using one of the available T1 mapping techniques called MOdified Look-Locker Inversion

Table 3.1 Normal values of T1 in myocardium, blood, and fat acquired using a MOLLI sequence on a Philips scanner

Approximate T1 values	1.5 T	3 T
Myocardium [14]	950 ms	1052 ms
Blood [14]	1551 ms	1736 ms
Fat [15]	288 ms	371 ms

recovery (MOLLI) sequence (see below for further details) on Philips scanners. As per expert recommendation [13], normal T1 values must be established in each centre with consideration of the field strength of the scanner and the acquisition method used (Table 3.1).

By using external gadolinium-based contrast agents (GBCAs) and modifying the properties of the naturally present hydrogen nuclei, T1 values can be shortened. Once injected intravenously, GBCAs are distributed throughout the body in blood plasma and leak out of the microvasculature accumulating into interstitial spaces but not in the cells. These are the physical principles based on which standard late gadolinium enhancement (LGE) techniques allow to depict focal scarring. Whilst LGE techniques are particularly suited to assess focal scarring with major accumulation of GBCA, in order to depict subtle diffuse fibrosis and/or increased ECV, post-contrast T1 mapping techniques are needed. Following the injection, over time, the contrast agent concentration in the interstitial spaces equalizes with that in the blood plasma ('contrast equilibrium phase'). For ECV quantification, a post-contrast T1 map is acquired at a sufficiently delayed phase to allow contrast equilibrium to be established in addition to a pre-contrast map. Establishing equilibrium can take several minutes [16] and will take longer if the interstitial space is large, and/or the tissue is poorly perfused. Once equilibrium is attained, the relative contrast agent concentration in myocardium and blood (the partition coefficient, λ) is equal to the ratio of extracellular volume fractions and reflected in changes in T1 [17]:

$$\lambda = \frac{ECV_{myocardium}}{ECV_{blood}} = \frac{\dfrac{1}{T1_{(post\ contrast\ myocardium)}} - \dfrac{1}{T1_{(native\ myocardium)}}}{\dfrac{1}{T1_{(post\ contrast\ blood)}} - \dfrac{1}{T1_{(native\ blood)}}}$$

The ECV in the blood is equal to the plasma volume fraction, which can be calculated from the haematocrit. In addition to the four T1 values required to calculate λ, it is, therefore, also necessary for the haematocrit to be known in order to calculate ECV.

$$ECV_{myocardium} = (1 - Hct)\lambda$$

Haematocrit can be measured independently through blood sampling close to the MR study. Alternatively, it has been suggested that native blood T1 can be used as a surrogate to estimate haematocrit, removing the need for blood sampling and analysis [18].

This new metric enables the assessment of diffuse myocardial disease previously not easily detectable by standard CMR techniques, including LGE. Validation has been performed against histology in different cardiac diseases [4].

3.2.2 T1 Mapping Sequences

Rather than containing relative signal intensity values (which depend on a range of parameters in addition to T1), T1 maps contain quantitative values in each voxel. By isolating this single parameter, it can depict small and diffuse changes in tissue composition. This can also allow objective comparison of tissues between scans or between subjects.

The general methodology behind T1 mapping starts with acquisition of multiple images with different T1 weightings. A mathematical model describing the theoretically expected signal behaviour is then fitted to the observed data in order to estimate T1 on a voxel-by-voxel basis (Fig. 3.1). In this process, T1 and other unknown model parameters are adjusted iteratively to change the shape of the mathematical model until it best matches the observed data (a perfect fit is not obtained due to limitations in the model and the presence of noise in the data).

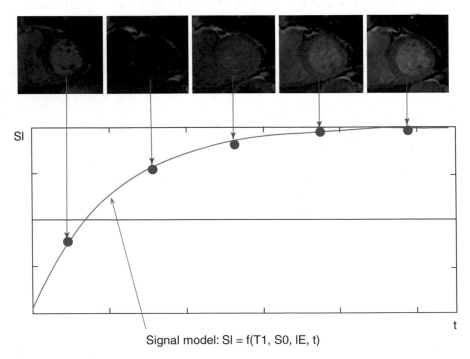

Signal model: SI = f(T1, S0, IE, t)

Fig. 3.1 Fitting process (adapted from EACVI CMR Pocket Guide (Physics for Clinicians) [19] with permission from the authors). Multiple images (top row) are generated with differing T1 contrast, for example, by different inversion recovery delays. Signal intensities are extracted from corresponding voxels from each image (middle). A mathematical model that describes the sequence signal intensities (SI) is then fitted to the observed data. This model will be a function of known (fixed) parameters (e.g. sequence timings) as well as unknown variable parameters (including T1, and in this case equilibrium signal, S0, and inversion pulse efficiency, IE). The variable parameters are adjusted iteratively until the best fit to the data is found. The T1 value from that optimum set is then inserted into the corresponding voxel of the T1 map

In general, at least as many different T1 weightings are required as there are free parameters in the model although including extra data improves precision at the expense of longer scan duration. Typically for T1 measurement, the free parameters include T1, equilibrium signal, and potentially a small number of additional parameters such as RF pulse efficiency.

If the images are acquired with the tissue in the same place, a map of T1 values can be produced. This can be achieved through combinations of physiological triggering, breath-holding, and post-acquisition motion correction. If motion prevents mapping, then T1 can instead be estimated for segmented tissue regions.

3.2.2.1 Magnetisation Preparation Based Methods

The most widely used methods for myocardial T1 mapping are based on acquisition of multiple magnetization prepared images, most commonly inversion recovery (IR) sequences, but saturation recovery (SR) may also be used.

Inversion Recovery Methods

In conventional IR-based T1 mapping, a single image would be acquired after a dedicated inversion pulse. However, after each acquisition it is necessary to allow time for near complete magnetization recovery before applying the next inversion pulse. This approach is, therefore, too slow to be compatible with the time constraints imposed on clinical myocardial T1 mapping. Instead, multiple single-shot images can be obtained following each inversion pulse.

In MOLLI T1 mapping [20], multiple images are acquired after inversion. To obtain images at the same cardiac phase, a fast single-shot imaging sequence is used, and this is repeated at the same delay after the physiological trigger (typically the R-wave of the ECG trace). The inversion pulse is performed at a prescribed time before the first image acquisition. This provides multiple images with differing TI values (Fig. 3.2). However, the spacing between TI values is equal to the cardiac cycle duration. If only a single inversion was performed, there would be insufficient sampling early in the recovery to characterize the T1 values encountered in the heart. To resolve this, multiple inversion pulses are applied, each with multiple images subsequently acquired. A different delay is used between each inversion pulse and acquisition of the following image.

Within the constraints imposed by the cardiac cycle length three inversion pulses are the realistic maximum that can be used within a breath-hold. Early MOLLI implementations used three inversion pulses with a total of 11 images acquired over 17 cardiac cycles [20]. Several strategy refinements have been proposed [21] to shorten the overall duration of the acquisition by either reducing the number of inversions or the number of images after each inversion [22]. A further refinement to reduce these effects is to specify target durations (in seconds) rather than numbers of cardiac cycles. The sequence thus adapts to maintain approximately consistent breath-hold durations regardless of heart rate and can reduce the related variability in accuracy [21].

An alternative approach is to use a fixed acquisition scheme but with a conditional fitting algorithm as proposed in the ShMOLLI (shortened MOLLI) method

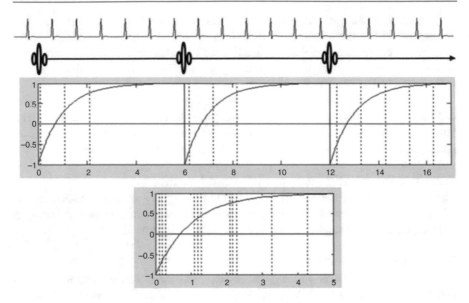

Fig. 3.2 Illustration of MOLLI acquisition using the originally proposed scheme (adapted from EACVI CMR Pocket Guide (Physics for Clinicians) [19] with permission from the authors). Inversion pulses (second row) are applied after the first, seventh, and thirteenth R-wave trigger (first row). After each, a series of images are acquired at the same phase of subsequent cardiac cycles (indicated by red-dashed lines on third row). Note that the delay between each inversion and the following image varies. A recovery period is left prior to the second and third inversion pulses. The data is collated for use in the T1 estimation process, as shown on the bottom row, where the horizontal axis represents time since most recent inversion

[23]. In this technique (three inversions for seven images over nine cardiac cycles), a conditional selective algorithm is used in the fitting process as, in all but the shortest T1 tissues, biases would be introduced due to incomplete magnetization recovery if all data were used. An initial estimate is performed using the five images acquired after the first inversion pulse, with additional data from the later inversions used only if the estimated T1 is sufficiently short. This approach has been shown to have less bias and heart rate dependence than others, although at the expense of reduced precision due to the smaller number of samples used in the fitting process.

Saturation Recovery
Similar to MOLLI, in SAturation recovery Single-sHot Acquisition (SASHA [24]), T1 mapping, multiple images are acquired at the same cardiac phase but with different delays after magnetization preparation. However, in this case, a saturation pulse is used for preparation instead of inversion.

Use of saturation preparation has a significant key benefit. With ideal saturation pulse performance, the magnetization is completely eradicated after application and with that the dependence of the signal on previous magnetization evolution is removed. Consequently, there is no need to allow (near) complete longitudinal recovery between preparation pulses. This removes a source of measurement bias and also allows shorter gaps between preparation pulses to be used, allowing more data to be acquired in the same time (without the need for recovery periods). The disadvantage of saturation preparation compared to inversion is a reduced dynamic range (half that of IR techniques, as only positive magnetization occurs after preparation, rather than any inverted values). This tends to lead to SR sequences having improved accuracy but reduced precision compared to MOLLI-based approaches [21, 25].

Image Readout, Spatial Coverage, and Resolution
Each image in MOLLI or SASHA sequences is acquired independently during the corresponding cardiac cycle. However, the full cycle is not available for each image; in order to minimize artefacts from cardiac motion, each image must be acquired rapidly. Despite optimizations and acceleration strategies, spatial resolution and coverage are limited, which can make interpretation of T1 maps in myocardium outside the left ventricle difficult. Care must always be taken to avoid misinterpretation due to blood pool contamination of myocardial voxels. Furthermore, coverage in conventional techniques is limited to a single slice per breath-hold. However, refinements of imaging techniques are promising developments such as free-breathing multi-slice [26] or 3D acquisition [27] in order to increase spatial coverage or concurrent measurement of multiple parameters such as T1 and T2 [28].

3.2.3 Interpretation

3.2.3.1 Native Tissue
As described above, T1 varies widely between different tissues, while values within individual tissue types also vary (less widely) due to physiological changes associated with disease [12]. Consequently, clinical information can be derived by measuring how changes in the composition of the myocardial tissue are reflected in the variations in native T1 values. An increase in T1 could be due to deposition of collagen or amyloid in the interstitium or presence of extra- or intra-cellular oedema, whilst a decrease in T1 happens following accumulation of lipids or iron. For an accurate interpretation of results, however, it is important to point out that the different methods or sequences used are known to be susceptible to different systematic biases [29], and even seemingly subtle differences in sequence set-up can substantially affect precision of the T1 measurements [30]. Consequently, these factors must be controlled, and care must be taken when comparing T1 values. The recommendations for clinical implementations clearly lay out the requirements each centre undertaking parametric mapping should fulfil, emphasizing that for native T1 mapping, local normal values should be established for each sequence, scanner manufacturer, field strength used, and local results should be benchmarked against published reported ranges [13, 31].

3.2.3.2 ECV Fraction
ECV fraction assessment is less susceptible to the same physiological confounders as for T1 [32], and it is independent of field strength, contrast agent choice, and

dose. It does, however, rely on the aggregation of multiple measurements (four T1 estimates from two time points as well as an independent haematocrit measurement), and errors in any of these will propagate into the final value. For voxel-wise mapping image registration between the pre- and post-contrast, T1 maps (which will have been acquired several minutes apart) are required.

3.3 Clinical Applications

T1 mapping in congenital heart disease is still very much embedded in the research arena. While it may have promise in delineating diffuse fibrosis in the myocardium, clinical usefulness is still under evaluation with no longitudinal follow-up data available to date.

Unlike most acquired heart disease, much of congenital heart disease pathology involves the right ventricle (RV). T1 mapping in the RV is more challenging due to the thinner wall structure. However, several centres have embarked on T1 mapping in the RV with interesting results, which will be highlighted below. Additional complications in operated congenital heart disease include the close proximity of the RV to artefacts from sternal wires. These factors are a hindrance to detecting more subtle diffuse fibrosis in the congenital heart disease cohorts [33]. Post-contrast T1 values are raised in a number of congenital heart disease conditions such as systemic RVs and tetralogy of Fallot (TOF) [34]. Cyanosis alone does not cause increase in ECV [34, 35].

While T1 mapping is still far away from being used in clinical practice, it is gaining momentum in the research arena, especially in TOF research, where assessment of fibrosis, especially in the left ventricle (LV), may become a useful biomarker in predicting malignant arrhythmia risk in these patients.

3.3.1 Tetralogy of Fallot

TOF includes a ventricular septal defect, overriding aorta, pulmonary stenosis, and right ventricular hypertrophy. After surgical correction, most patients are left with varying degree of pulmonary regurgitation, which causes volume loading on the RV. Fibrotic scaring is most commonly found around the area of the ventriculostomy site. Fibrosis is thought to be a contributor towards the risk factors of arrhythmia in these patients, and tissue mapping is of additional potential clinical utility. Figure 3.3 shows an example of T1 mapping acquisitions in a patient with repaired TOF.

A number of studies have assessed tissue mapping in TOF. In relatively young TOF patients (mean age 13), native T1 and ECV in the LV were still normal in two studies [36, 37] and abnormal in a third [38]. In this young cohort, the RV, however, is already showing increased native T1 values suggesting some degree of fibrosis already being present [36]. A different larger study in a cohort of 103 patients (mean age 28 years), including 36 with previous pulmonary valve replacement, demonstrated a significant

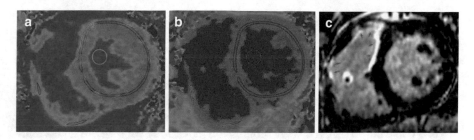

Fig. 3.3 Pre- and post-contrast T1 measurements of the LV and RV in repaired tetralogy of Fallot. In this representative image, the ROIs were drawn both on the LV and RV and showed increased values compared to normal volunteers. (**a**) pre-contrast T1 map, (**b**) post-contrast T1 map, (**c**) late gadolinium enhancement images with RV scar areas identified by yellow arrows (From Cochet H. et al. EHJCVI (2019) 20, 990–1003)

increase in LV native T1, LV ECV, RV native T1, and RV ECV compared to healthy volunteers, suggesting that fibrosis, especially in the LV, develops over time [39]. Interestingly, in patients after pulmonary valve replacement, native T1, both in the RV and LV, was shown to be lower than in patients without valve replacement despite the presence of scar in the outflow tract [39]. Such findings would be in keeping with the beneficial effect of an early pulmonary valve replacement. In addition, markers of focal and diffuse fibrosis might have a different prognostic value, especially for arrhythmogenic events. In the same study, patients with ventricular arrhythmias had higher native T1 values in both RV and LV, but these patients were also significantly older. Outcome studies are needed to delineate whether detection of fibrosis using T1 mapping could be a useful predictor of patients at risk of significant arrhythmias.

In a study of 84 patients with repaired TOF, both LV EVC and RV EVC were higher in the volume-loaded RV than the pressure-loaded RV though the number of patients in the pressure-loaded ventricle group was limited to only five subjects [40]. In this study, higher RV ECV was also associated with a lower pressure gradient in the RVOT and a lower mass-to-volume ratio in the RV. This preliminary data is inconclusive as to whether T1 mapping could be used to differentiate between a volume- or pressure-loaded ventricle. Furthermore, LV ECV in multivariate analysis was independently associated with any arrhythmia found on Holter monitor [40].

3.3.2   Ebstein Anomaly

Ebstein anomaly is an abnormality of the tricuspid valve, which is displaced towards the apex, leading to a varying degree of atrialization of the RV.

Patients with Ebstein anomaly also show increased LV ECV, especially in the septal region. An ECV higher than 30% has been shown to be associated with a worse disease status in these patients (worse NYHA classification, worse tricuspid regurgitation) [41], suggesting that progressive fibrosis is associated with worse symptoms. Whether this will be useful in clinical practice requires further longitudinal study.

3.3.3   The Systemic Right Ventricle

In the systemic RV after atrial switch procedure, the ECV has been shown to be significantly higher in the sub-pulmonary LV than the sub-aortic (systemic) RV, suggesting a higher degree of fibrosis in the detrained LV [42] (Fig. 3.4).

Increased septal EVC also correlated with increased NT-proBNT but not with VO2 max on exercise testing in patients after atrial switch [43], suggesting that fibrosis could play a part in disease progression monitoring but may not reflect clinical status and symptoms.

In contrast to these findings, children with Fontan circulation and a systemic RV had higher ECV and higher native T1 values compared to healthy volunteers and those with a systemic LV, despite being younger [44].

3.3.4   Cardiac Transplant

In cardiac transplant, fibrotic remodelling is a negative side effect and can be used for monitoring. Ide et al. [45] showed in 20 patients that areas for higher native myocardial T1 correlated to areas with histopathological signs of fibrosis. To date,

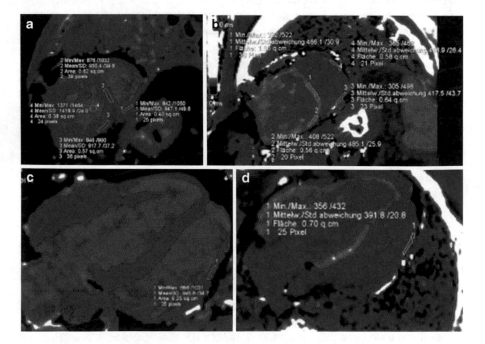

Fig. 3.4 Examples of ROI of T1 mapping in a patient with TGA after atrial switch operation without sub-pulmonary stenosis. (**a**) Native T1-mapping image in short axis. (**b**) Post-contrast T1-mapping image in short axis. (**c**) Native T1-mapping image in four chamber view. (**d**) Post-contrast T1-mapping image in four chamber view (From Shehu N. Int J Cardiovasc Imaging. 2018;34(8):1241–48

this is the most promising area in congenital heart disease, where T1 mapping can add value to clinical disease monitoring. However, no longitudinal studies are available to date to assess clinical benefits using T1 mapping for monitoring purposes.

3.3.5 Aortic Stenosis

Congenital aortic stenosis is most likely due to a bicuspid aortic valve (BAV). In a small study of 35 patients with BAV, increased ECV was associated with diastolic dysfunction and a number of aortic valve procedures [46]. But, it did not correlate with left ventricular function or mass. Further research is needed to delineate whether this has clinical implication for long-term management and could become an additional imaging biomarker for timing of valve replacement.

3.4 Summary

To date, most studies using tissue mapping in congenital heart disease are small group observational studies, which are underpowered for subgroup analysis and not yet linked to clinical outcome. However, the published evidence could indicate a potential incremental prognostic value of mapping techniques. Larger clinical outcome studies are necessary to evaluate the usefulness of tissue mapping in the clinical setting.

References

1. Cheitlin MD, et al. The distribution of fibrosis in the left ventricle in congenital aortic stenosis and coarctation of the aorta. Circulation. 1980;62(4):823–30.
2. Ho SY, et al. Fibrous matrix of ventricular myocardium in tricuspid atresia compared with normal heart. A quantitative analysis. Circulation. 1996;94(7):1642–6.
3. Vasquez C. Morley GE. The origin and arrhythmogenic potential of fibroblasts in cardiac disease. J Cardiovasc Transl Res. 2012;5(6):760–7.
4. Miller CA, et al. Comprehensive validation of cardiovascular magnetic resonance techniques for the assessment of myocardial extracellular volume. Circ Cardiovasc Imaging. 2013;6(3):373–83.
5. Mathur-De Vre R. Biomedical implications of the relaxation behaviour of water related to nmr imaging. Br J Radiol. 1984;57(683):955–76.
6. Cameron IL, Ord VA, Fullerton GD. Characterization of proton nmr relaxation times in normal and pathological tissues by correlation with other tissue parameters. Magn Reson Imaging. 1984;2(2):97–106.
7. Karamitsos TD, et al. Non-contrast T1 mapping for the diagnosis of cardiac amyloidosis. JACC: Cardiovascular Imaging. 2013;6:488. https://doi.org/10.1016/j.jcmg.2012.11.013.
8. Bull S, et al. Human non-contrast T1 values and correlation with histology in diffuse fibrosis. Heart. 2013;99(13):932–7.
9. Miller CA, et al. Comprehensive validation of cardiovascular magnetic resonance techniques for the assessment of myocardial extracellular volume. Circulation: Cardiovascular Imaging. 2013;6(3):373–83.

10. Sado DM, et al. Cardiovascular magnetic resonance measurement of myocardial extracellular volume in health and disease. Heart. 2012;98(19):1436–41.
11. Ridgway JP, Cardiovascular magnetic resonance physics for clinicians: part I. J Cardiovasc Magn Reson. 2010;12:71.
12. Haaf P, et al. Cardiac T1 Mapping and Extracellular Volume (ECV) in clinical practice: a comprehensive review. J Cardiovasc Magn Reson. 2016;18:89.
13. Moon JC, et al. Myocardial T1 mapping and extracellular volume quantification: a society for cardiovascular magnetic resonance (SCMR) and CMR working group of the european society of cardiology consensus statement. J Cardiovasc Magn Reson. 2013;15:92.
14. Dabir D, et al. Reference values for healthy human myocardium using a T1 mapping methodology: results from the International T1 Multicenter cardiovascular magnetic resonance study. Journal of Cardiovascular Magnetic Resonance. 2014;16:69.
15. Grande FD, et al. Fat-suppression techniques for 3-T MR imaging of the musculoskeletal system. Radiographics. 2014;34(1):217–33.
16. Schelbert EB, et al. Myocardial extravascular extracellular volume fraction measurement by gadolinium cardiovascular magnetic resonance in humans: slow infusion versus bolus. J Cardiovasc Magn Reson. 2011;13:16.
17. White SK, et al. T1 mapping for myocardial extracellular volume measurement by CMR: bolus only versus primed infusion technique. JACC: Cardiovascular Imaging. 2013;6(9):955–62.
18. Treibel TA, et al. Automatic measurement of the myocardial interstitium: synthetic extracellular volume quantification without hematocrit sampling. JACC Cardiovasc Imaging. 2016;9:54-63.
19. Broadbent D, Kidambi A, Biglands J. EACVI CMR pocket guides: Physics for Clinicians. 2015.
20. Messroghli DR, et al. Modified look-locker inversion recovery (MOLLI) for high-resolution T1 mapping of the heart. Magn Reson Med. 2004;52:141–46.
21. Kellman P, Hansen MS. T1-mapping in the heart: accuracy and precision. J Cardiovasc Magn Reson. 2014;16:2.
22. Messroghli DR, et al. Human myocardium: single-breath-hold MR T1 mapping with high spatial resolution—reproducibility study. Radiology. 2006;238:1004–12.
23. Piechnik SK, et al. Shortened modified look-locker inversion recovery (ShMOLLI) for clinical myocardial T1-mapping at 1.5 and 3 T within a 9 heartbeat breathhold. J Cardiovasc Magn Reson. 2010;12:69.
24. Chow K, et al. Saturation recovery single-shot acquisition (SASHA) for myocardial T(1) mapping. Magn Reson Med. 2014.71:2082–95.
25. Roujol S, et al. Accuracy, precision, and reproducibility of four T1 mapping sequences: a head-to-head comparison of MOLLI, ShMOLLI, SASHA, and SAPPHIRE. Radiology. 2014;272(3):683–89.
26. Weingartner S, et al. Free-breathing multislice native myocardial T1 mapping using the slice-interleaved T1 (STONE) sequence. Magn Reson Med. 2015;74:115–24.
27. Nordio G et al. 3D myocardial T1 mapping using saturation recovery. J Magn Reson Imaging. 2017;46:218–27.
28. Weingartner S, et al. Combined saturation/inversion recovery sequences for improved evaluation of scar and diffuse fibrosis in patients with arrhythmia or heart rate variability. Magn Reson Med. 2014;71:1024–34.
29. Roujol S, et al. Accuracy, precision, and reproducibility of four T1 mapping sequences: a head-to-head comparison of MOLLI, ShMOLLI, SASHA, and SAPPHIRE. Radiology. 2014;272:683–89.
30. Akcakaya M, et al. On the selection of sampling points for myocardial T1 mapping. Magn Reson Med. 2015;73:1741–53.
31. Messroghli DR, et al. Clinical recommendations for cardiovascular magnetic resonance mapping of T1, T2, T2* and extracellular volume: A consensus statement by the Society for Cardiovascular Magnetic Resonance (SCMR) endorsed by the European Association for Cardiovascular Imaging (EACVI). J Cardiovasc Magn Reson. 2017;19(1):75.
32. Reiter G, et al. Cardiac magnetic resonance T1 mapping. Part 1: Aspects of acquisition and evaluation. Eur J Radiol. 2018;109:223–34.

33. Ghonim S, et al. Myocardial architecture, mechanics, and fibrosis in congenital heart disease. Frontiers in Cardiovascular Medicine. 2017;4(30).
34. Broberg CS, et al. Quantification of diffuse myocardial fibrosis and its association with myocardial dysfunction in congenital heart disease. Circulation. Cardiovascular imaging. 2010;3(6):727–34.
35. Kharabish A, et al. Long-standing cyanosis in congenital heart disease does not cause diffuse myocardial fibrosis. Pediatr Cardiol. 2018;39(1):105–110.
36. Yim D, et al. Assessment of diffuse ventricular myocardial fibrosis using native t1 in children with repaired tetralogy of fallot. Circ Cardiovasc Imaging. 2017;10(3).
37. Riesenkampff E, et al. Myocardial T1 mapping in pediatric and congenital heart disease. Circ Cardiovasc Imaging. 2015.8(2):e002504.
38. Kozak MF, et al. Diffuse myocardial fibrosis following tetralogy of Fallot repair: a T1 mapping cardiac magnetic resonance study. Pediatr Radiol. 2014;44(4):403–9.
39. Cochet H, et al. Focal scar and diffuse myocardial fibrosis are independent imaging markers in repaired tetralogy of Fallot. Eur Heart J Cardiovasc Imaging. 2019;20(9):990–1003.
40. Chen CA, et al. Myocardial ECV fraction assessed by CMR is associated with type of hemodynamic load and arrhythmia in repaired tetralogy of fallot. JACC Cardiovasc Imaging. 2016;9(1):1–10.
41. Yang D, et al. Cardiovascular magnetic resonance evidence of myocardial fibrosis and its clinical significance in adolescent and adult patients with Ebstein's anomaly. Journal of cardiovascular magnetic resonance : official journal of the Society for Cardiovascular Magnetic Resonance. 2018;20(1):69.
42. Shehu N, et al. Diffuse fibrosis is common in the left, but not in the right ventricle in patients with transposition of the great arteries late after atrial switch operation. Int J Cardiovasc Imaging. 2018;34(8):1241–8.
43. Plymen CM, et al. Diffuse myocardial fibrosis in the systemic right ventricle of patients late after Mustard or Senning surgery: an equilibrium contrast cardiovascular magnetic resonance study. European Heart Journal - Cardiovascular Imaging. 2013;14(10):963–68.
44. Kato A, et al. Pediatric fontan patients are at risk for myocardial fibrotic remodeling and dysfunction. Int J Cardiol. 2017;240:172–77.
45. Ide S, et al. Histological validation of cardiovascular magnetic resonance T1 mapping markers of myocardial fibrosis in paediatric heart transplant recipients. J Cardiovasc Magn Reson. 2017;19(1):10.
46. Dusenbery SM. Myocardial extracellular remodeling is associated with ventricular diastolic dysfunction in children and young adults with congenital aortic stenosis. JACC. 2014;63:1778–85.

MR Lymphatic Imaging of Thoracic Lymphatic Disorders

4

Maxim Itkin, Paula Malagoli, and Deborah Rabinowitz

4.1 Introduction

The lymphatic system is an important part of physiologic fluid homeostasis. Approximately, 50 years ago, it was established that the lymphatics are exclusively responsible for removal of the interstitial fluid from the tissues back to the venous circulation. For that reason, the lymphatic system is extremely important in all clinical scenarios involving tissue edema, including heart failure.

The effect of congestive heart failure on the lymphatic system is profound because the elevated central venous pressure results in influx of the interstitial fluid into the tissues causing significant increase in the lymphatic flow. In spite of its significance, the lymphatic system has been largely ignored by modern medicine over the last several decades, primarily due to lack of ability to visualize the lymphatics. The lymphatics are challenging to image due to the small size of the vessels, the complexity of the lymphatic anatomy with its multiple subsystems, and the difficulty in the physical introduction of the contrast agents. Until recently, there were just two available modalities, pedal lymphangiography, and lymphoscintigraphy. However, both had significant drawbacks in terms of complexity of the examination and quality of imaging of the central lymphatic system.

Over the last decade, a new way to introduce contrast in the lymphatic system was developed by directly injecting the lymph nodes with contrast agent: intranodal

M. Itkin (✉) · P. Malagoli
HUP Center for Lymphatic Imaging, Penn Medicine, Perelman School of Medicine at the University of Pennsylvania, Hospital of the University of Pennsylvania, Philadelphia, PA, USA

D. Rabinowitz
Division of Interventional Radiology, Department of Medical Imaging, Nemours at AI Dupont Hospital for Children, Wilmington, DE, USA

Sidney Kimmel Medical College at Thomas Jefferson University, Philadelphia, PA, USA

© Springer Nature Switzerland AG 2021
P. Gallego, I. Valverde (eds.), *Multimodality Imaging Innovations In Adult Congenital Heart Disease*, Congenital Heart Disease in Adolescents and Adults, https://doi.org/10.1007/978-3-030-61927-5_4

Fig. 4.1 Schematic representation of the groin lymph node access

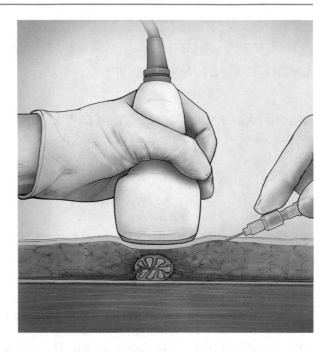

lymphangiography [1] (Fig. 4.1). This technique was initially used for fluoroscopy-guided interventional procedures in order to diagnose and treat a variety of lymphatic flow disorders. The disadvantages of the intranodal lymphangiography are poor contrast resolution of fluoroscopy and the high viscosity of the oil-based contrast Lipiodol (Guerbet Inc, Princeton, NJ) that prevents distal propagation of the contrast.

Dynamic contrast-enhanced MR lymphangiography (DCMRL) utilizes the same technique of accessing the inguinal lymph nodes with a 25 G needle (BD, Franklin Lakes, NJ); however, instead of Lipiodol, gadolinium-based contrast is injected (Fig. 4.2). The main advantages of DCMRL are significantly higher contrast resolution and 3D acquisition ability of the MRI. In addition, lower viscosity of the gadolinium-based contrast and its hydrophilic properties allow mixture of the contrast with lymph and more distal penetration into the tissues, providing much more physiological imaging of the lymphatic system. Dynamic time-resolved images also allow for more accurate physiological flow evaluation of the lymphatic system [2].

4.2   DCMRL Technique

DCMRL consists of two steps: (1) introduction of needles in the lymph nodes and (2) injection of the contrast and MR imaging acquisition.

Fig. 4.2 Position of the
25 G spinal needles in the
bilateral groin lymph nodes

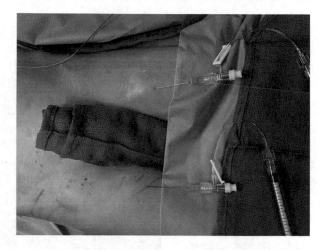

4.2.1   Placement of the Intranodal Needles

Proper placement of the injection needles in the inguinal lymph nodes under US guidance is one of the crucial parts of the procedure. Use of US machine for the placement of the needles calls for this step to be performed outside MR suite, usually in prep/waiting area. If, however, the MR suite is sufficient in size, the US machine can be positioned in the MR suite. That, however, has to be done in compliance with local MR safety policy and in consultation with the MR physicist. The two main pitfalls of this step are proper positioning of the needle in the lymph nodes to allow opacification of the efferent lymphatic vessels and the prevention of needle displacement.

Visualization of the needle in the lymph nodes on US doesn't insure that the opacification of the efferent lymphatic ducts can be achieved. The proper position of the needles has to be confirmed by injection of US-contrast (Sonovue, Bracco Diagnostic, Monroe Township, NJ) or agitated saline while observing the flow in the efferent lymphatic vessels (Fig. 4.3) [3]. In case the efferent flow is not observed, the needles need to be repositioned in a different part of the lymph node. In an awake patient, it is imperative to inject local anesthetic in the lymph node prior to injection of the gadolinium-contrast agent as it causes significant pain when injected. We usually mix the lidocaine 1% with US contrast in a 3:1 ratio. After confirmation of the correct position, the needles are then stabilized with adhesive dressing.

4.2.2   Transport of the Patient into the MR Suit

The patient is then transferred to the MRI machine, and extreme caution needs to be exercised not to dislodge the needles from the groins. Most of the newer MR machine comes with a detachable MR table that the patient can be placed on in the

Fig. 4.3 Contrast-enhanced US image demonstrating the enhancement of the lymph node (arrowhead) and afferent lymphatic vessels (arrow). (From: Nadolski GJ, Ponce-Dorrego MD, Darge K, Biko DM, Itkin M. Validation of the Position of Injection Needles with Contrast-Enhanced Ultrasound for Dynamic Contract-Enhanced MR Lymphangiography. J Vasc Interv Radiol. SIR; 2018;29(7):1028–1030)

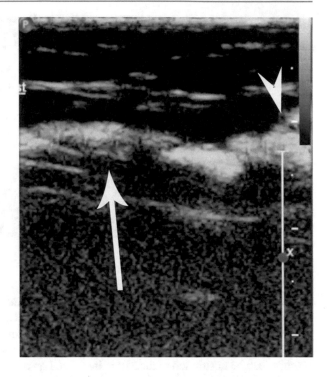

prep area before the procedure and reconnected to the MR after the needles are placed. This setup significantly minimizes the chance of needle dislodgment.

4.2.3 Coil Coverage

In the average adult, the coil coverage is limited to upper or lower part of the body (e.g., chest and upper abdomen). The coverage is usually tailored to the specific pathology, that is, the chest in case of plastic bronchitis or chylothorax and the pelvis and abdomen in chylous ascites.

4.2.4 Contrast Injection

Any standard formulation of gadolinium-based intravascular contrast can be used. In our practice, we use Dotarem (Guerbet Group, Princeton, NJ) due to its safety profile for the patient with renal insufficiency. We recommend a weight-based double dose that is split in two aliquots between the groins. The contrast can be injected manually or using automatic contrast injector. If injected manually, a 3 mL syringe is recommended to overcome the resistance of small gauge of the injection needle.

In our practice, we perform automatic injection. The advantage of the automatic injection is stability of the needle and standardization of the injection rate that allow us to potentially calculate the flow rate in the central lymphatic system. We use off-the-shelf tubing to allow splitting of the contrast from the injector into each groin. The injection parameters are as follows: injection delay 40 s, injection rate 0.15 mL/s per side.

4.2.5 MR Sequences

We utilize three types of MR sequences to image the lymphatic system:

1. T2W imaging to visualize fluid-filled objects, such as pleural effusions and lymphatic masses
2. Fast T1 angio sequence for imaging for dynamic imaging of the lymphatic system
3. High resolution-delayed angio sequence utilized for both better resolution imaging and delay imaging

MR sequences are specific to manufactures, and the specific parameters of the MR that we use in our practice (Siemens) are listed in Appendix.

4.2.6 The Contribution of Each MR Sequence

4.2.6.1 T2W Imaging

The lymphatic system consists of a network of multiple interconnected lymphatic systems. It is anatomically impossible to image the entire lymphatic system by injecting contrast in one location so the imaging territory depends on the location of the point of the injection.

The goal of DCMRL is to be able to image the central lymphatic system, primarily of the chest. Injection contrast in the inguinal lymph nodes allows for imaging of the pelvic, retroperitoneal lymphatic systems, cisterna chyli, and thoracic duct. Under normal circumstances, other parts of the lymphatic systems such as liver, kidneys, spleen, and intestine are outside of DCMRL area of imaging. However, the lymphatic system is a low pressure system and, therefore, if there is an obstruction along the typical path, contrast injected through the groin lymph nodes cannot propagate in these areas. T2W imaging is valuable in these cases, as it identifies these areas, most commonly demonstrating lymphatic masses with increased T2W signal (water) that are outside of the pathway of the contrast. T2W sequences can also demonstrate a dilated and occluded TD that is not opacified with contrast due to elevated pressure. In addition, T2W imaging of the chest can provide imaging of the lung interstitium.

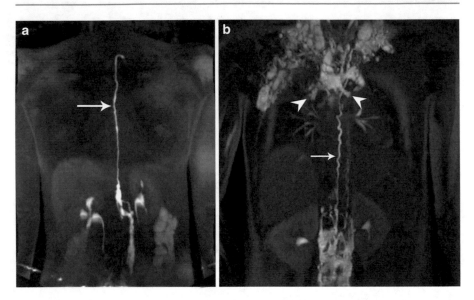

Fig. 4.4 (a) DCMRL imaging of normal TD (arrow). (b) DCMRL imaging of the patient with plastic bronchitis, demonstrating dilated and tortuous thoracic duct (arrow) and abnormal pulmonary lymphatic perfusion from the thoracic duct toward lung parenchyma (arrowheads)

4.2.6.2 Fast Acquisition T1 Angiography Imaging

The main value of DCMRL is in imaging of the central lymphatic system of the chest in patients with pulmonary lymphatic disorders, such as chylothorax, plastic bronchitis, and lymphatic malformations (LMs). In all these conditions, T1 angio (time-resolved) imaging can demonstrate a pattern of abnormal lymphatic flow from the thoracic duct and/or retroperitoneum into the lung parenchyma, recently labeled as abnormal pulmonary lymphatic perfusion (Fig. 4.4) [4]. The dynamic nature of these sequences allows the observation of the pathways of abnormal lymphatic flow over time.

Normally, most of the lymphs in the body are generated below the diaphragm, primarily in liver and intestine. The function of the thoracic duct is to collect all this lymph and deliver it back into venous circulation, typically at the junction of the left jugular and subclavian veins. In abnormal pulmonary lymphatic flow, the lymph flows into the mediastinum and lung parenchyma. It is most probably an anatomical lymphatic variant that can be asymptomatic or present clinically under certain conditions, such as increase of the lymphatic flow in patients with congenital heart disease [5]. If these collateral vessels abut the pleural surface, they result in chylothorax; if they abut the bronchial surface, patients present with plastic bronchitis; and if the flow is localized to the interstitium, they present with interstitial lung disease. In some patients, the clinical presentation can include all of these spaces.

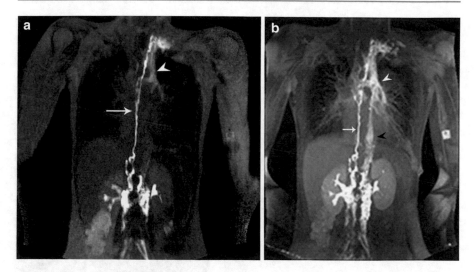

Fig. 4.5 (**a**) Dynamic angio MR imaging (TWIST) of the patient with generalized lymphatic anomaly and right chylothorax demonstrates the abnormal lymphatic flow from thoracic duct (arrow) into the mediastinum (arrowhead). (**b**) Delayed, high-resolution MR imaging (inversion recovery) demonstrates an additional pathway of the contrast from retroperitoneum into the mediastinum. (Modified from: Itkin M, Rabinowitz D, Nadolski G, Stafler P, Mascarenhas L, Adams D. Abnormal Pulmonary Lymphatic Flow in Patients with Lymphatic Anomalies and Respiratory Compromise on MR Lymphangiogram. In: *CHEST*. American College of Chest Physicians; 2019:A7386-A7386)

4.2.6.3 High-Resolution T1-Delayed Angiographic Sequences

This sequence provides high-resolution imaging of the contrast in the lymphatic system and often allows visualization of structures that are not visible on the dynamic images (Fig. 4.5).

The speed of propagation of the contrast through the lymphatic system is variable, but in most of the cases, during ~10 min of the dynamic sequences, contrast reaches the distal part of the thoracic duct. However, in some cases of slow lymphatic flow, there is a need to prolong the imaging; in these situations, the delayed T1 imaging can provide the "extended" imaging.

As a general rule, we continue to scan the patient until no further propagation of the contrast is observed.

4.2.6.4 Alternative MR Lymphangiography Imaging

Piper et al. recently described a new technique of imaging of the central lymphatic system using transpedal MR lymphangiography [6]. They reported excellent imaging of the central lymphatic system using this technique (Fig. 4.6).

The advantage of this approach is technical simplicity, no need for interventional expertise in placing the needles in the lymph nodes. In addition, this technique can

Fig. 4.6 Interstitial transpedal MR lymphangiography of the thoracic duct (arrows). (From: Pieper CC, Feisst A, Schild HH. Contrast-enhanced Interstitial Transpedal MR Lymphangiography for Thoracic Chylous Effusions. *Radiology*. 2020;295(2):458–466)

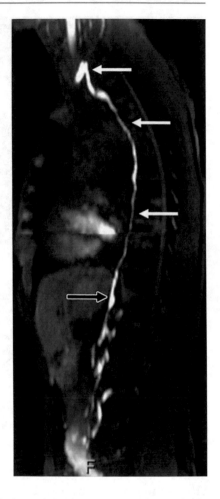

potentially provide more physiological depiction of the interstitial and lymphatic flow because the contrast is absorbed from the tissues, stimulating the transport of the interstitial fluid into initial lymphatics.

4.3   Applications of the MR Lymphangiography

As mentioned earlier, DCMRL is most informative in patient with pulmonary lymphatic disorders.

Plastic bronchitis in patients with congenital heart disease is a devastating disorder, causing severe pulmonary insufficiency. The lymphatic pathophysiology of the disorder has been suspected for a long time. DCMRL demonstrated the abnormal pulmonary lymphatic flow in these patients as the pathophysiological mechanism (Fig. 4.4) [5]. Embolization of the thoracic duct results in cure of this condition in the majority of patients. A similar pattern of abnormal pulmonary lymphatic flow

Fig. 4.7 Schematic representation of five types of abnormal pulmonary lymphatic perfusion in patients with plastic bronchitis. (From: Dori Y, Keller MS, Rome JJ, et al. Percutaneous lymphatic embolization of abnormal pulmonary lymphatic flow as treatment of plastic bronchitis in patients with congenital heart disease. *Circulation*. 2016;133(12):1160–1170)

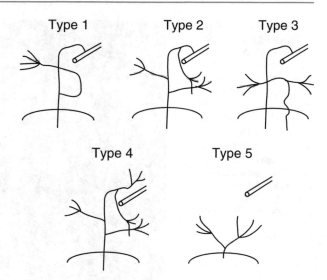

was demonstrated in noncardiac plastic bronchitis [7]. The researchers identify several patterns of abnormal pulmonary lymphatic flow (Fig. 4.7).

Postsurgical chylothorax in congenital cardiac patients is a relatively common lymphatic complication associated with significant mortality and morbidity [8]. A recent study showed that most of the time, the cause of this condition is not a trauma to the thoracic duct, but abnormal pulmonary lymphatic flow, similar to PB, raising the possibility that both conditions share the same anatomical/pathophysiological mechanism (Fig. 4.8) [9]. Indeed, it is well documented that one of the strongest predictive factors of PB in this patient population is a history of prolonged postsurgical chylothorax [10]. The same study described the third cause of chylothorax, which is called central lymphatic flow disorder (CLFD). The group defined CLFD as a condition with effusions in more than one compartment (abdomen, chest, and pericardium): abnormal central lymphatic flow and the presence of dermal backflow through lymphatic collaterals in the abdominal wall on DCMRL (Fig. 4.9). Abnormal central lymphatic flow can be caused by dysplasia and/or obstruction of the TD. Unfortunately, this condition is very difficult to treat using any type of intervention, and conservative treatment continues to be the treatment of choice. One exception to this is distal obstruction of the thoracic duct, where lymphovenous anastomosis can be attempted [9]. DCMRL is imperative in all patients with postsurgical chylothorax to identify the cause of the chylothorax and tailor an appropriate treatment.

LM is a group of lymphatic diseases that affect multiple systems in the body, including soft tissues, bones, spleen, and liver [11]. The mortality and morbidity are much higher in these patients if there is involvement of the lungs [12]. A recent study demonstrated that there is an abnormal pulmonary lymphatic flow pattern on DCMRL in LM patients with respiratory compromise [13]. This pattern is very similar to the abnormal pulmonary lymphatic flow in PB and chylothorax.

Fig. 4.8 DCMRL of the patient with postcardiac surgery chylothorax demonstrated abnormal pulmonary lymphatic flow into lung parenchyma (arrows and arrowheads). (From: Savla JJ, Itkin M, Rossano JW, Dori Y. Post-Operative Chylothorax in Patients With Congenital Heart Disease. *J Am Coll Cardiol.* 2017;69(19):2410–2422)

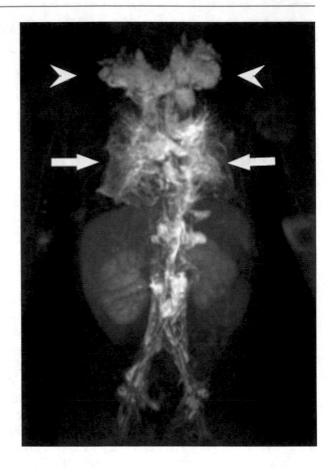

4.4 Conclusion

DCMRL is an important new imaging tool that allows demonstration of anatomical and pathological substrate of the lymphatic abnormalities of patients with pulmonary lymphatic disorders.

The discovery of the pathophysiological mechanisms allows for development of the specific treatment of these conditions.

Wide adoption of this technique depends on the development of a new set of indications for more common diseases, such as heart failure, pleural effusion of unknown etiologies, and more.

Fig. 4.9 DCMRL image of the patient with central lymphatic flow disorders demonstrates lack of propagation of the contrast in the central lymphatic system (star) and dermal collaterals in the abdominal wall (arrow) and lower extremity (arrowhead). (From: Savla JJ, Itkin M, Rossano JW, Dori Y. Post-Operative Chylothorax in Patients With Congenital Heart Disease. *J Am Coll Cardiol*. 2017;69(19):2410–2422)

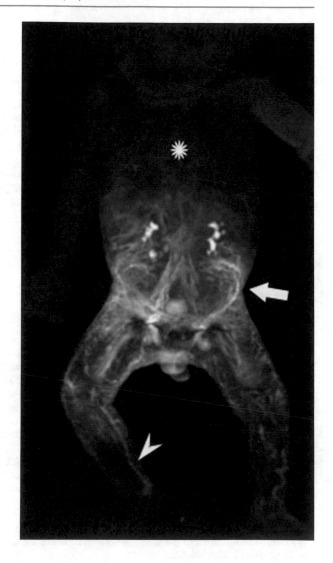

4.5 Appendix: DCMRL Technique for Chest Lymphatic Pathology

MRI sequences	Comments
Localizer	3 Plane Haste 6 mm thick 500 FOV
T2 haste coronal	T2 Haste Coronal 500 FOV, 6 mm skip 1.2 mm, 700 TR, 90 TE, 256 × 100, 2 × 2 × 6 voxel
T2 space coronal	T2W MRI lymphatic imaging is performed using a three-dimensional turbo spin echo sequence with the following parameters: matrix 256 × 256, FOV 500, TR 2500, TE 650, flip angle 140, voxel size 1.3 × 1.3 × 1.3 mm.

(continued)

MRI sequences	Comments
Flash 3D IR FatSat coronal	Scanning parameters are as follows: matrix 320 × 288, FOV 500, TR 400, TE 1.5, flip angle 15, slice thickness 1.6, isotropic voxel size 1.6 × 1.6 × 1.6
TWIST precontrast coronal	Scanning parameters are as follows: matrix 320 × 280, FOV 500, TR 3, TE 1, flip angle 25, slice thickness 1.3, isotropic voxel size 1.6 × 1.6 × 1.3. Precontrast run is one measurement: 8 s
Contrast injection	*0.2 mL/kg divided over left and right; 1 mL/minute injection. Weight-based double dose Dotarem at an injection rate of 0.15 mL/s with a 40 s delay before the start of imaging*
TWIST postcontrast coronal	The sequence parameters are adjusted with a time delay such that a complete volume was acquired approximately every 20–60 s. Total scan time was 10 min. Scan is run at 35 measurements with 13 s between each measurement
Flash 3D IR FatSat coronal	Thorax postcontrast
Reconstructions	Time-lapse subtraction of the TWIST's MIP and MPR of interest

References

1. Nadolski GJ, Itkin M. Feasibility of ultrasound-guided intranodal lymphangiogram for thoracic duct embolization. J Vasc Interv Radiol. 2012;23(5):613–6.
2. Zheng Q, Itkin M, Fan Y. Quantification of thoracic lymphatic flow patterns using dynamic contrast-enhanced MR lymphangiography. Radiology. 2020;296(1):202.
3. Nadolski GJ, Ponce-Dorrego MD, Darge K, Biko DM, Itkin M. Validation of the position of injection needles with contrast-enhanced ultrasound for dynamic contract-enhanced MR lymphangiography. J Vasc Interv Radiol. 2018;29(7):1028–30.
4. Itkin M. Interventional treatment of pulmonary lymphatic anomalies. Tech Vasc Interv Radiol. 2016;19(4):299–304.
5. Dori Y, Keller MS, Rome JJ, Gillespie MJ, Glatz AC, Dodds K, et al. Percutaneous lymphatic embolization of abnormal pulmonary lymphatic flow as treatment of plastic bronchitis in patients with congenital heart disease. Circulation. 2016;133(12):1160–70.
6. Pieper CC, Feisst A, Schild HH. Contrast-enhanced interstitial transpedal MR lymphangiography for thoracic chylous effusions. Radiology. 2020;295(2):458–66.
7. Itkin MG, McCormack FX, Dori Y. Diagnosis and treatment of lymphatic plastic bronchitis in adults using advanced lymphatic imaging and percutaneous embolization. Ann Am Thorac Soc. 2016;13(10):1689–96.
8. Zuluaga MT. Chylothorax after surgery for congenital heart disease. Curr Opin Pediatr. 2012;24:291.
9. Savla JJ, Itkin M, Rossano JW, Dori Y. Post-operative chylothorax in patients with congenital heart disease. J Am Coll Cardiol. 2017;69(19):2410–22.
10. Schumacher KR, Singh TP, Kuebler J, Aprile K, O'Brien M, Blume ED. Risk factors and outcome of Fontan-associated plastic bronchitis: a case-control study. J Am Heart Assoc. 2014;3:e000865.
11. Wassef M, Blei F, Adams D, Alomari A, Baselga E, Berenstein A, et al. Vascular anomalies classification: recommendations from the international society for the study of vascular anomalies. Pediatrics. 2015;136(1):e203–14.
12. Chen W, Adams D, Patel M, Gupta A, Dasgupta R. Generalized lymphatic malformation with chylothorax: long-term management of a highly morbid condition in a pediatric patient. J Pediatr Surg. 2013;48(3):e9–12.
13. Itkin M, Rabinowitz D, Nadolski G, Stafler P, Mascarenhas L, Adams D. Abnormal pulmonary lymphatic flow in patients with lymphatic anomalies and respiratory compromise on MR lymphangiogram. Chest. 2019:A7386.

MRI-Based Catheterization Laboratory

5

Kuberan Pushparajah

5.1 Background and Rationale

Interventional MRI (iCMR) has been available since the mid 1990s [1, 2] for use in general interventional radiology [3, 4]. Advances in real-time MRI [5, 6] paved the way for its first use in cardiology with MRI cardiac catheterisation in a cohort of patients with congenital heart disease (CHD) by Razavi et al. in 2003 [7] using a hybrid approach of X-ray fused with MRI (XMR) and solely MRI-guided catheterisation. MRI has several advantages over X-ray fluoroscopy in that there is a freedom to dynamically interrogate the heart in any plane, has excellent soft tissue visualisation, and is able to accurately provide quantitative physiological information such as flow in vessels, ventricular volumes, and function. Myocardial characterisation by MRI also allows the delineation of areas of fibrosis and scar, which can provide targets for intervention not seen on X-ray fluoroscopy. The rationale for integrating MRI to augment or replace X-ray-guided catheterisation is not just to reduce radiation burden, but to increase the accuracy of measured anatomic, physiological, and haemodynamic data and ultimately to improve outcomes for patients with CHD [8–10].

Patients with CHD are an obvious group to potentially benefit from this technology as they often require repeat diagnostic or interventional cardiac catheterisation to facilitate diagnosis, clinical decision-making, and therapy for their underlying condition. In North America alone, the IMPACT registry, which is a multi-centre registry of several large tertiary cardiac surgical centres, identified 19,608 cardiac catheterizations performed between January 2011 and March 2013 for patients with

K. Pushparajah (✉)
School of Biomedical Engineering and Imaging Sciences, King's College London, London, UK

Department of Paediatric Cardiology, Evelina London Children's Hospital, London, UK
e-mail: kuberan.pushparajah@kcl.ac.uk

© Springer Nature Switzerland AG 2021
P. Gallego, I. Valverde (eds.), *Multimodality Imaging Innovations In Adult Congenital Heart Disease*, Congenital Heart Disease in Adolescents and Adults,
https://doi.org/10.1007/978-3-030-61927-5_5

CHD [11]. In the UK, there were a total of 15,217 diagnostic and interventional procedures performed in patients with CHD between 2015 and 2018, with 5307 of these categorised as diagnostic cardiac catheters [12]. This number is likely to rise as it is recognised that not only are the proportion of adult survivors of CHD increasing, but the prevalence of those with severe disease is also on the rise as shown in population-based studies in Quebec, Canada [13, 14]. Although radiation doses are falling with the advent of new generation fluoroscopic laboratories [15], the risks of radiation from X-ray-guided procedures are well established in patients, particularly in children [16] and in staff [17].

The benefits of iCMR, as will be expanded on later in the chapter, are now recognised and have entered international guidelines and recommendations for the multi-modality imaging of adults with CHD (ACHD), acknowledging that hybrid measurements from MRI catheterisation provide a more accurate and comprehensive haemodynamic assessment than other traditional techniques [18]. There is a move to include patients with medical devices who were previously excluded from MRI scans with the introduction of clear safety guidelines and scan protocols [19–21], while newer generation of medical implants are increasingly being considered for patients with CHD who will likely require repeat MRI scans in the future, thus broadening the scope to offer iCMR to most patients with CHD. However, there remain several barriers to iCMR that need to be overcome before we see a wider dissemination of this application to meet the needs of patients.

5.2   MRI Catheter Laboratories in Practice

Since the beginning of this application, there have been a variety of combinations of interventional MRI setups over the years. The early experience for general radiology was with a 0.5 T mid-field open system scanner (Signa SP; G.E Medical Systems, Milwaukee, Wisc., USA) and biplane MRI stems such as a C-shaped magnet with one supporting pillar, allowing access from the contralateral side, head, and foot ends of the magnet (Magnetom Open T; Siemens, Erlangen, Germany), and Panorama 0.23 T (Philips Medical Systems MR Technologies Finland, Vantaa, Finland). Most of these scanners were low field strength ranging up to 0.7 T [22]. Access to patients with biplane systems did limit some vertical approaches to procedures although horizontal access was good.

Conventional 1.5 T cylindrical horizontal bore MRI scanners have the advantage of higher field strengths and gradient slew rates needed for high resolution images, higher signal-to-noise ratios, and faster scan times needed for iCMR. There are some limitations to access in small babies due to distance of the baby in the scanner from the bore edge, but this is not the case for adults and older children. The options for movable MRI scanner systems as used in hybrid neurosurgical labs [23] do not fit into the clinical pathway of clinical cardiac imaging infrastructure. The integration of X-ray with a C-arm brought in the concept of a hybrid lab for MRI-augmented catheterisation first used in general interventional radiology [24]. This type of setup allowed for the integration of X-ray and catheterisation capabilities into an MRI environment while the patient is still able to be moved swiftly from the scanner to the X-ray table within a minute [25, 26]. This then led to the development of bespoke hybrid MRI catheter systems being produced by industry, which include biplane X-ray fluoroscopy. These typically incorporate a 1.5 T magnet.

However, in facilities that do not have a hybrid XMR facility, MRI-augmented catheterisation can still be performed in one of two ways. Firstly, the previously obtained MRI images from the MRI scanner can be exported and fused onto X-ray fluoroscopic imaging to help provide a road map for the interventional cardiologist. X-ray fused with MRI techniques has been used for over 15 years [27–29] and been successfully used in a fluoroscopic catheterisation laboratory with image overlay for CHD interventions such as stenting and balloon angioplasty [30–32]. The overlay technology now incorporates respiratory motion compensation [33] to improve the registration of images. Image registration and overlay of this type has also been used to successfully perform myocardial biopsies using X-ray fused with MRI [34] as shown in Fig. 5.1.

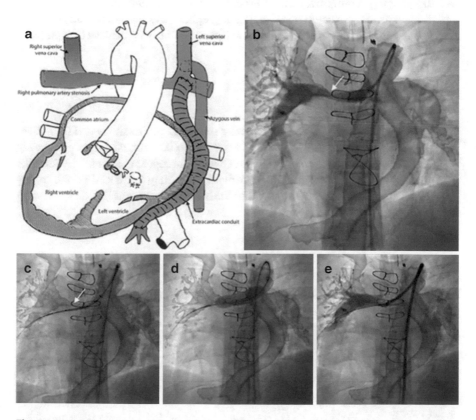

Fig. 5.1 (a–e) X-ray fused with pre-acquired MRI images to guide fluoroscopic cardiac catheter interventions. Image courtesy of Dr Kanishka Ratnayaka and Dr Robert Lederman NIH, Bethesda, USA

The second approach is to perform the X-ray-guided cardiac catherisation in a standard cardiac catheter laboratory, and then leaving an MRI safe catheter in situ in a relevant vessel such as the pulmonary artery, the patient is moved to the MRI scanner for flow and function assessments with the catheter remaining safely secured. This allows for comprehensive haemodynamic assessments, such as quantification of pulmonary vascular resistance, which is described in the section on clinical applications.

5.2.1 Practical Considerations

The procedures of iCMR are well described by the leading centres in the literature reporting the highest volumes [35, 36]. A standard hybrid X-ray and MRI laboratory at our unit as shown in Fig. 5.2 has been previously described by White et al. [37]. Conventionally, the MRI scan is driven from the control room. In cases for iCMR, the operator preforming the cardiac catheter procedure must have the ability to control the imaging required for the intervention while maintaining communication with their assistant, the scrub nurse, the radiographers, the cardiac physiologist performing haemodynamic measurements, and the patient. In anaesthetised patients, this will also include the anaesthetist.

5.2.2 Safety

Given the number of staff involved in these cases and equipment needed for a diagnostic or interventional cardiac catheter, there has to be a robust safety protocol in place, which includes staff and equipment checks and repeat counts of any metallic instruments, needles, wires, or braided catheters that may be placed on the trolley for cases using X-ray prior to moving into the MRI environment [36, 37].

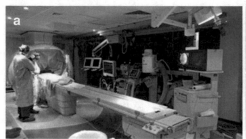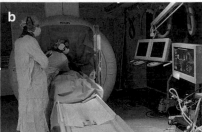

Fig. 5.2 (**a**) Hybrid X-ray and MRI suite demonstrating X-ray C-arm and MRI bore in the same facility. (**b**) MRI-guided cardiac catheterisation in action within the same facility

5.2.3 Communication

The MRI scanner is noisy and can interfere with communication within the team and with the patient. There are several verbal communication systems that can be utilised, with the most effective to date, being one using infrared technology with a wireless headphone and microphone system in the room that reduces the noise, but allows staff to communicate with each other in both the scanner and control rooms with the use of multiple headsets (Opto-acoustics, Clear-com, Gaven).

5.2.4 ECG

Reliable and accurate ECG synchronisation is essential for CMR and in particular CMR-guided cardiac catheterization. When catheters are manipulated in the heart, there is the potential to cause arrhythmias. Vector electrocardiogram (VCG) is a QRS detection algorithm that automatically adjusts to the actual electrical axis of the patient's heart and the specific multidimensional QRS waveform. In our experience, this greatly improves the reliability of R-wave detection to nearly 100%. The surface ECG can also be obtained from the patients from four surface adhesive electrodes (Expression, Invivo Medical, Gainesville, FL, USA), allowing for good R-wave detection, but identification of the ST-segment and P-wave can be obscured. Development of better ECG techniques is still being explored, driven by work in MRI-guided electrophysiology (EP).

5.2.5 Haemodynamic Monitoring

Haemodynamic monitoring is key in these environments and should have compatible connections for the MRI environment. Mostly, units have employed individual adaptations to existing systems to facilitate high-fidelity haemodynamic measurements during catheter procedures. There are new MRI compatible systems being developed for haemodynamic assessments without interference from the system [38].

5.2.6 X-ray Coils

Some CMR coils have X-ray-visible components and would need to be removed between X-ray imaging and the CMR component of the investigation. These are demonstrated in Fig. 5.3. It is, therefore, necessary to consider this during hybrid X-ray and MRI-guided procedures to minimise movement of the patient and avoid displacement of catheters. Specifically designed coils that are sufficiently radiotranslucent have been designed [39] but do not appear to have penetrated the market.

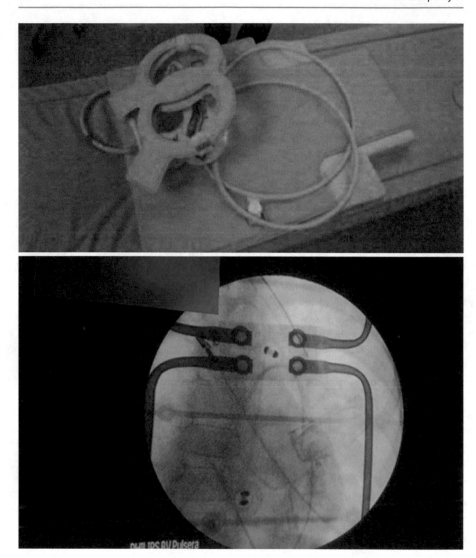

Fig. 5.3 MRI coils with corresponding views on X-ray fluoroscopy demonstrating the radiopaque components affecting imaging for cardiac catheterisation

5.3 Visualisation and Image Interrogation

Real-time imaging is key to the advancement of MRI-guided catheterisation as it requires good spatial and temporal resolution to allow catheter manipulation. Developments in real-time imaging have facilitated the progression of MRI-guided catheterisation [40–42]. Better imaging protocols including faster imaging sequences to allow for rapid scanning needed for interventions [43–45].

Catheter visualisation in the early stages included manual control of the imaging planes by someone in the control room or interventional suite, other than the primary catheter operator. There is a manual manipulation of the visualisation planes using off-the-shelf interactive modes on the scanner platform. This approach relies heavily on good communication between the primary operator and the team, manipulating the imaging planes. Adaptations to this system with a foot pedal allow the primary operator instead to manipulate the imaging planes in the interactive mode, but this is limited to single imaging planes at any one time, akin to single-plane fluoroscopy.

There are now purpose-built interactive platforms such as (Interactive Front End, Siemens; RTHawk, HeartVista; Cleartrace, MRI Interventions; iSuite, Philips), which allow for the integration of semi-automated 3D-segmented images [46, 47] into a platform which allows the user to track multiple 2D planes simultaneously, mapped against a segmented 3D geometry. This is primarily for EP but is being extended to other applications. The primary operator is able to manipulate the imaging planes independently through the use of integrated foot pedals. The user then need to be able to visualise and track the catheter during a procedure. Catheter tracking techniques are largely split into two groups – active and passive catheter tracking.

5.4   Passive Visualisation

Passive tracking is the most commonly employed method and is based on susceptibility artefacts or signal voids caused by the interventional device during CMR imaging. It is attractive as it does not require any additional hardware and can be performed on existing commercially available systems without additional modifications.

The signal voids needed can be created with relative ease, such as the use of carbon dioxide to inflate balloon angiographic catheters, thus creating a signal void to permit visualisation of the catheter tip (Fig. 5.4). This method, where catheter the tip appears black, is referred to as 'negative-contrast' imaging is widely used in clinical practice [7, 36, 48, 49]. An alternative approach is 'positive-contrast' imaging created by inflating a balloon angiographic catheter with a 1% concentration of gadolinium contrast agent [50] (Fig. 5.5). The major limitation of both methods is that the catheter shaft is not visualised, creating the potential for looping and knotting of the catheter if the operator is not vigilant. Attempts at creating better shaft visualisation by using gadolinium contrast agents in varying concentrations within catheter lumens [51] or gadolinium-like coatings over the catheter [52] have not been successful.

Dedicated scan sequences are needed to optimise passive catheter tracking. A dynamic gradient echo sequence, such as SSFP, has been shown to be ideal for passive catheter tracking, especially when signal voids or susceptibility artefacts are used for visualisation. Imaging in a standard cardiac catheterization lab has a frame rate of 25–30 frames/s. The frame rates available for CMR-guided interventions are

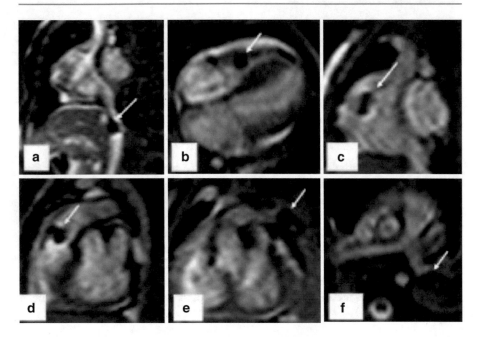

Fig. 5.4 Sequential images of the carbon dioxide-filled balloon at the tip of the angiographic catheter, appearing black, as it is guided serially from the inferior vena cava (**a**), right ventricle (**b**, **c**), right ventricular outflow tract (**d**), and left pulmonary artery (**e**, **f**)

typically limited to 10–14 frames/s. Positive contrast visualisation was conventionally utilised 'on/off' saturation pulses combining black blood imaging, where the interventional cardiologist visualises either the soft tissue or catheter tip between rapidly changing image frames [53]. At our institution, we utilise a partial saturation pulse (pSAT) using a real-time single-shot acquisition with bssfp read-out developed in-house, where each image is acquired immediately after a saturation prepulse with a reduced saturation angle to achieve partial saturation with a temporal resolution of ~7 images/s. The pSAT sequence offers real-time simultaneous high-contrast visualization of the catheter balloon and blood (Fig. 5.5). This technique provides excellent passive tracking capabilities during MR-guided catheterization in patients [54] and is now utilised in other units.

The use of passive tracking requires significant input from a skilled CMR operator in order to manipulate the imaging plane to keep the device within slice. This is relatively easily achieved in narrow tubular structures lying within a single plane, such as the aorta, but is much more difficult when there is a greater degree of three-dimensional movement as is the case for an EP study or ablation within larger cardiac chambers. Thicker imaging slices (>10 mm) improve the ability to keep the device within plane, but contrast to noise may be impaired to such a degree that the device may not be identifiable. These are all factors being considered for improvement in ongoing developments.

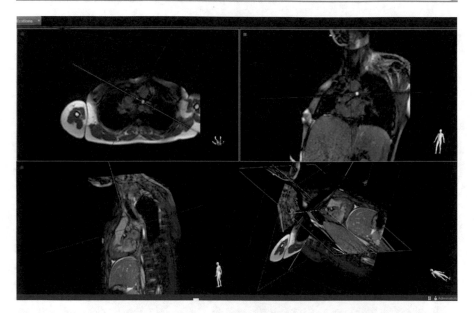

Fig. 5.5 Live multi-planar image projection of MRI-guided cardiac catheterisation using the partial saturation pulse to simultaneously visualise the soft tissue and dilute gadolinium-filled balloon tip of the angiographic catheter seen here as a white ball in the left pulmonary artery

5.5   Active Catheter Tracking and Visualization

Active catheter tracking and visualisation methods utilise an electrical connection to the MRI scanner, where the device is equipped with a coil or an antenna that functions in either receive-only mode or transmit/receive mode. Active catheters that are used as receivers have a coil or an antenna that receives signal from tissue in its immediate vicinity [55]. These devices rely on the body coil to transmit into the patient. The signal received by these coils is used to pinpoint their position. There are two main types of active catheters: those based on small coils positioned, for example, at the end of a catheter and those based on a loopless antenna that can run along a catheter or can be made into a guidewire [56]. A small resonant coil at the tip of a catheter can be identified by a series of three one-dimensional projections along each axis [55]. Real-time catheter tracking is possible if the transmit and receive can be done quickly and repeatedly for very fast updates of the catheter position, which is projected over a previously acquired road map.

Active visualisation has great potential because it allows the whole length of the catheter or guidewire to be visualised and the imaging plane to be adapted to the moving catheter automatically. However, there are challenges as these devices use intravascular coils as RF antennas, and the connection to the external circuits via a long wire in the strong magnetic field makes induction of an electrical current and heating possible. The technical challenges include RF safety for long transmission lines, which must remain capable of conducting μV MR-receive signals. Miniature transformers in the device have been used to successfully minimise while still being able to provide both the required tracking robustness and RF safety [57, 58]. Newer approaches include active catheter tracking such as using acousto-optics to sense RF signals in MRI [59].

5.5.1 Catheters and Guidewires

The potential heating of wires, devices, implants, and other instruments is an important factor in CMR development. Intravascular guidewires or device delivery systems with a metal core are unsafe in the CMR environment, with documented heating up to 74 °C (165 °F) of the tip [60–62]. In addition to the bioeffects of CMR and heating and electrical safety of interventional devices, a significant risk to interventional procedures is magnetic force and torque exerted by the magnetic field on metallic devices [63]. Interventional devices that are ferromagnetic will be subject to both deflection force (translational movement) and torque (rotational movement); therefore, they cannot be used for procedures within a CMR scanner. Conventional guidewires made of ferromagnetic materials, such as stainless steel, and catheters with metallic braiding are inherently unsafe for use in the CMR environment. However, certain other metallic alloys, such as nitinol, are CMR-compatible and are not affected by the magnetic field in terms of deflection force and torque but can still be susceptible to heating and still be unsuitable for use in CMR procedures.

The ideal catheter or guidewire should have mechanical properties that retain torque and steerability in common with standard hardware used in a catheter laboratory without the risks of heating. Susceptibility artefacts from ferromagnetic materials should also not obscure the underlying anatomy. The polymer-based materials used for making catheters typically have low-magnetic susceptibility and, therefore, cannot be easily localised on CMR images.

Alloys, such as nitinol (nickel and titanium), have magnetic susceptibility close to that of tissue and are best suited for making guidewires and braided catheters, but these are not necessarily CMR-safe. However, there are methods to reduce heating effects with such hardware by utilising different scanning parameters such as spiral imaging [64, 65].

Guidewires with a fibreglass core and non-metallic guidewires made of resin microparticle compound covered by polytetrafluoroethylene were developed for MR-guided interventions and were attractive due to their stiffness. A clinical trial with interventions in CHD was successful [36] after pre-clinical testing [66], but the wires were difficult to steer and had to be treated with caution to avoid disruption of the wire. Polymer-based guidewires were also explored as a candidate guidewire for the MRI environment. The first MR conditional and MRI visible polymer-based endovascular guidewire (EPflex GmbH, Dettingen, Germany) received a CE Mark in 2012. Commercially available CE marked wires are now available from several companies such as EP flex (hydrophilic wire made of pebax® as polyether block amide – thermoplastic elastomer), Nano4imaging GmbH, Aachen, and Marvis (GmbH, Hannover, Germany). These wires are typically 0.035″ and come in

Fig. 5.6 Appearance of an
MRI safe guidewire
(EPFlex) in the thoracic
aorta of a child with
scoliosis. The ferrous
markers (red arrow) along
the length of the wire
provide useful markers for
wire visualisation

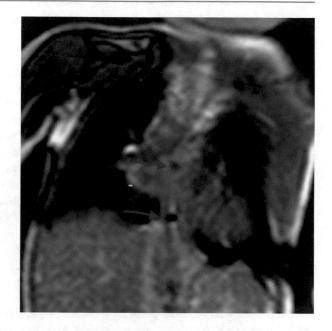

varying lengths with ferrous makers of varying positions along the wire and with
varying deposition amounts to enable visualisation of the shaft and tip (Fig. 5.6).
The challenges now are to test the mechanical and visualisation properties of these
now in a clinical environment to inform further modifications were needed to ensure
they are fit for purpose.

5.6 Clinical Applications of iCMR

5.6.1 Diagnostic MRI Catheterisation

5.6.1.1 Haemodynamic Assessments by XMR

The quantification of the degree of intracardiac shunts is key to decision-making in
CHD. The assessment of shunts by MRI was a significant first step towards a noninvasive approach to the assessment of patients with CHD, who still required invasive cardiac catheterisation with traditional Fick calculations. There is a high degree
of accuracy using phase contrast flow [67–69] by MRI-compared traditional methods. Despite this, in many parts of the world with limited access to MRI, patients
still undergo diagnostic cardiac catheterisation for a result that could be achieved
from a very simple and importantly non-invasive assessment.

This is even more relevant in the assessment of complex heart disease in ACHD
such as patients with a Fontan circulation or transposition of the great arteries post
atrial switch with baffle leaks, where there can be several sites of potential shunting.
Complex mapping of the circulation, combined with ventricular mass and function

assessments, 3D whole heart imaging, and tissue characterisation augment the hae-modynamic data and allow for better decision-making.

5.6.1.2 Pulmonary Vascular Resistance (PVR and Fick)

The assessment of pulmonary vascular resistance is a key component in CHD as it may impact on thresholds for surgical or catheter intervention or medical management based on the assessment of response to pulmonary vasodilators. It is recognised that traditional Fick methods rely on many assumptions that do not hold true for patients with CHD. A key variable is the estimation of VO_2, which is commonly calculated by formulae from Lundell, Lindahl, LaFarge, and Miettinen, each of which incorporate patients in variable ages, sizes, and states of sedation or anaesthesia. It has been further demonstrated that this error is compounded in complex CHD such as Glenn shunts, where PVR is underestimated using calculated VO_2 [70] with significant clinical implications.

Muthurangu et al. were able to demonstrate better accuracy of MRI catheterisation compared to Fick and thermodilution methods [71], particularly in the presence of pulmonary vasodilation. Since then it has been incorporated as a means of assessing PVR in many institutions worldwide [36, 48, 49, 72]. This has led to a particular focus on right heart catheterisation for the assessment of pulmonary hypertension in adults. In our own experience, we have reported on the application of this approach for the determination of pulmonary vascular resistance for surgical decision-making in patients with CHD for both single and biventricular strategies [73].

There have been several successful clinical MRI programmes reporting successful right heart catheterisation in patients with pulmonary hypertension and CHD [48, 50, 53, 74]. More recently, there have been successful clinical applications of MRI-guided catheterisation for pulmonary vascular resistance assessment in adults within a rapid clinical workflow that is acceptable to patients and fits within a deliverable clinical model [49]. The whole patient pathway for a diagnostic right heart catheter by iCMR for pulmonary vascular disease assessment in a structurally normal heart is under an hour and is now standard of care at a leading tertiary pulmonary hypertension centre.

5.6.1.3 Cardiac Performance and Output

Fenestration occlusion in MRI was first described by Tzifa et al. [75]. Test occlusion of the Fontan fenestration is always performed when fenestration occlusion is being considered. In the catheterisation laboratory, this entails measurement of the right atrial, left atrial and aortic pressures, mixed venous and aortic oxygen saturations, measurement of whole-body oxygen consumption, systemic blood flow, systemic oxygen transport, and oxygen extraction [76]. However, these measurements can be laborious and prone to errors. Fenestration occlusion in the iCMR environment (Fig. 5.7) provides an accurate and simultaneous assessment of Fontan pressures, cardiac output, and oxygen saturation.

Pressure volume (PV) loops are a powerful, load-independent measure of the ventricular performance and its relationship to the circulation it faces. PV loops derived from MRI catheterisation was first constructed in patients with pulmonary

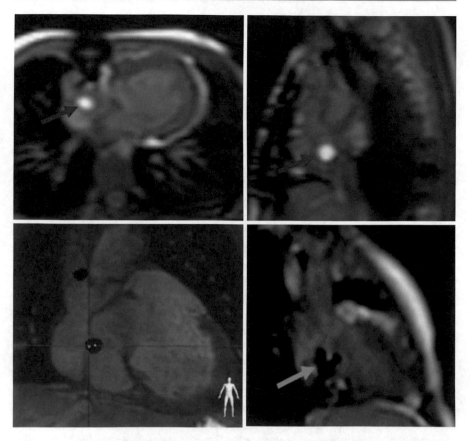

Fig. 5.7 iCMR-guided fenestration occlusion in a Fontan circulation. There is wire crossing fenestration (green arrow), balloon occlusion (red arrow), and overlay of balloon occlusion with second balloon in SVC (red balloons) to measure Fontan pressure after occlusion. (Images courtesy of Dr Tarique Hussain, UT Southwestern, Dallas, USA)

hypertension [74, 77] and are a reliable, load-independent means of assessing ventricular performance. This has also been applied to a group of Fontan patients [72] to fully map out the pulmonary vascular resistance, collateral flow, and ventricular function.

The incorporation of pharmacological stress studies using dobutamine [78] during iCMR has been helpful to assess for changes in PVR and ventricular EDP to guide management in symptomatic patients. PV loops in response to pharmacological stress have also been used to extract additional data on kinetic energy within the ventricles [79] in response to dobutamine. Pharmacological stress testing with isoprenaline in coarctation of the aorta [80] has also been used to help define changes in the aorta to help define thresholds for intervention. Dobutamine stress MRI has also been used to determine suitability for liver transplantation, for patients with

Alagille syndrome to assess RV pressures and cardiac output augmentation in the setting of right heart obstructive lesions [81].

5.6.2 MRI-Guided Interventions

There are several examples of animal models for MRI-guided catheter interventions, which include MRI-guided vascular access [82], ASD closure [83], VSD closure [84, 85], percutaneous pulmonary valve implantation [86], aortic valve implantation [87], balloon angioplasty of the aorta for aortic coarctation [88], balloon dilation of the pulmonary valve [66], coronary artery interventions [89], and formation of a superior cavopulmonary connection [90]. These experiments then led to the translation of percutaneous interventions in humans, which include with MRI-guided balloon angioplasty in aortic coarctation [88] and balloon pulmonary valvuloplasty [36, 66]. The largest successful series to date for patients with CHD had an age range of 3.5–65 years of age [36]. These methods incorporate active and passive cardiac catheter visualisation techniques.

With previous animal models of MRI-guided transcatheter superior cavopulmonary connection, there are now possible transcatheter options such as a first in human closed chest transcatheter superior cavopulmonary connection in a 35 year-old [91] with X-ray fluoroscopy. These advances open up the possibilities of MRI-guided interventions in ACHD. In the field of general radiology, breast and prostate biopsies by iCMR to detect lesions not seen on routine methods is well established [92]. Advances in real-time imaging have allowed iCMR with MRI-compatible bioptomes to improve the yield from endomyocardial biopsy [93] with tissue characterisation by MRI to define areas of myocardial fibrosis and scar and could be a significant advance in the management of patients with cardiomyopathy. Myocardial chemoablation [94] by iCMR is also now possible.

5.6.3 MRI-Guided Electrophysiology (EP)

MRI-guided EP and ablation studies are appealing as they allow for 3D morphological and tissue characterisation of the ablation substrate to enhance the functional electrophysiological data, and thus better define the target regions for ablation [95, 96]. Soft tissue visualisation from MRI also permits mapping of the effects of ablation on the tissues to immediately assess the effects and extent of ablation lesions to better treat patients (Fig. 5.8).

This has already been successfully developed and translated from animal models into in vivo studies in man for atrial flutter [97, 98]. Further work is being done in this area to now look into more complex arrhythmias such as atrial fibrillation and ventricular tachycardia [99, 100]. MR thermometry (Fig. 5.9) is means of measuring the temperature within tissues and is being studied in pre-clinical studies to potentially allow more precise means of assessing the efficacy of ablation during real-time MRI-guided EP. Several obstacles remain including accurate motion

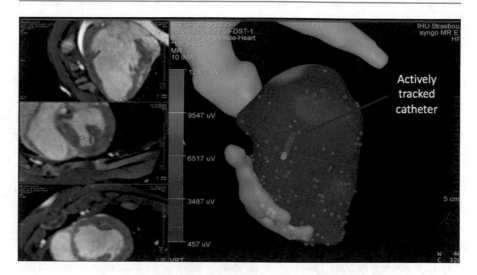

Fig. 5.8 Active catheter tracking to guide ablation catheter to region of scar segmentation on the Siemens iCMR platform (Monte-Carlo). (Image Courtesy of Dr Rahul Mukherjee, Dr Sebastien Roujol and Dr Mark O'Neil, King's College London)

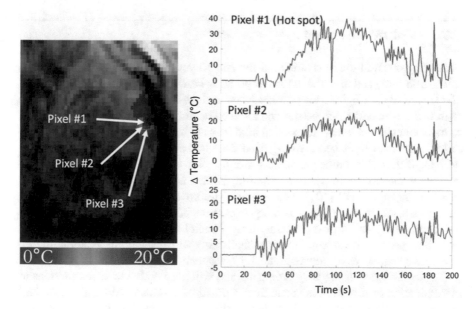

Fig. 5.9 MR thermometry showing change in temperature profiles across three pixels during MR-guided epicardial ablation in swine. (Image Courtesy of Dr Rahul Mukherjee, Dr Sebastien Roujol and Dr Mark O'Neil, King's College London)

estimation due to cardiac and respiratory motion, intra-scan motion, and inter-scan motion [96].

There are already new hardware developments of MR-EP catheters [101] and software systems, which allow for MRI-fluoroscopy-guided interventions for image-guided cardiac catheter therapy for endomyocardial interventions [102]. Additionally, there needs to be access to a working defibrillator within an MRI magnet to enable to wider human application of safe MRI-guided ablation. There is progress on this front with animal models incorporating commercial defibrillators with customised adaptations to allow for safe in-bore defibrillation and transcutaneous pacing, but there is an effect of reducing image quality, which requires further developments [103].

5.6.4   Other Applications

MRI lymphangiography [104] is an important adjunct in the assessment of lymphatic complications of CHD such as plastic bronchitis and protein-losing enteropathy, which then pave the way for treatments [105]. These are typically performed in a hybrid X-ray and MRI environment.

5.7   Future Directions

Following on from the innovations of the last 10 years, there are teams starting to think differently and move back to incorporating hardware from the traditional catheter laboratory by engineering new hardware such as braided MRI conditional wires with better mechanical properties and reduced heating [106]. Work is also ongoing to reduce heating effects with existing hardware such as recent paper using standard nitinol wires for right heart MRI-guided catheterisation with minimal heating by utilising different scanning parameters such as spiral imaging [64, 65]. A more radical step is move back to where this journey started and re-explore the potential for low field strength MRI [107]. The advent of improvements in hardware, scanning parameters, and reconstruction techniques has yielded promising results scanning at 0.5 T. Recent phantom experiments using parallel transmit radiofrequency coils also show promise for safe guidewire visualisation with capacity for integration into interactive sequences on conventional 1.5 T scanners [108].

These early results are very promising and will accelerate the development and dissemination of iCMR. In the meantime, a practical approach, combining standard catheter laboratory methods with existing MRI scanners as described, can already be utilised to provide robust haemodynamic data in the assessment of patients with ACHD to inform clinical decision-making and improve outcomes.

Acknowledgements Specific acknowledgements are to Prof Reza Razavi, Dr Aphrodite Tzifa, Dr Mari Nieves Velsaco-Forte, Dr Sebastien Roujol, Dr Torben Schneider, Dr Phuoc Duong, Dr James Wong, Dr Israel Valverde, Dr Tarique Hussain, Dr Shymala Moganasundram, Ms Tracy Moon, Mr

John Spence, the paediatric MRI radiographer and physiology teams from King's College, London, and Evelina London Children's Hospital for their contribution to the iCMR programme, which led to the developments and images used in this chapter. Many more have contributed and would have been cited within the accompanying references.

References

1. Lufkin RB. Interventional MR imaging. Radiology. 1995;197:16–8.
2. Jolesz FA, Blumenfeld SM. Interventional use of magnetic resonance imaging. Magn Reson Q. 1994;10:85–96.
3. Schenck JF, Jolesz FA, Roemer PB, Cline HE, Lorensen WE, Kikinis R, Silverman SG, Hardy CJ, Barber WD, Laskaris ET, et al. Superconducting open-configuration MR imaging system for image-guided therapy. Radiology. 1995;195:805–14.
4. Silverman SG, Collick BD, Figueira MR, Khorasani R, Adams DF, Newman RW, Topulos GP, Jolesz FA. Interactive MR-guided biopsy in an open-configuration MR imaging system. Radiology. 1995;197:175–81.
5. Gmitro AF, Ehsani AR, Berchem TA, Snell RJ. A real-time reconstruction system for magnetic resonance imaging. Magn Reson Med. 1996;35:734–40.
6. Kerr AB, Pauly JM, Hu BS, Li KC, Hardy CJ, Meyer CH, Macovski A, Nishimura DG. Real-time interactive MRI on a conventional scanner. Magn Reson Med. 1997;38:355–67.
7. Razavi R, Hill DL, Keevil SF, Miquel ME, Muthurangu V, Hegde S, Rhode K, Barnett M, van Vaals J, Hawkes DJ, Baker E. Cardiac catheterisation guided by MRI in children and adults with congenital heart disease. Lancet. 2003;362:1877–82.
8. Rogers T, Lederman RJ. Interventional CMR: clinical applications and future directions. Curr Cardiol Rep. 2015;17:31.
9. Rogers T, Ratnayaka K, Lederman RJ. MRI catheterization in cardiopulmonary disease. Chest. 2014;145:30–6.
10. Pushparajah K, Chubb H, Razavi R. MR-guided Cardiac Interventions. Top Magn Reson Imaging. 2018;27:115–28.
11. Jayaram N, Beekman RH III, Benson L, Holzer R, Jenkins K, Kennedy KF, Martin GR, Moore JW, Ringel R, Rome J, Spertus JA, Vincent R, Bergersen L. Adjusting for risk associated with pediatric and congenital cardiac catheterization: a report from the NCDR IMPACT registry. Circulation. 2015;132:1863–70.
12. National Institute for Cardiovascular Outcomes Research. National Cardiac Audit Programme (NCAP). Congenital heart disease in children and adults (congenital audit) 2015–2018 summary report. 2019. https://www.nicororguk/national-cardiac-audit-programme/congenital-heart-disease-in-children-and-adults-congenital-audit/.
13. Marelli AJ, Ionescu-Ittu R, Mackie AS, Guo L, Dendukuri N, Kaouache M. Lifetime prevalence of congenital heart disease in the general population from 2000 to 2010. Circulation. 2014;130:749–56.
14. Marelli AJ, Mackie AS, Ionescu-Ittu R, Rahme E, Pilote L. Congenital heart disease in the general population: changing prevalence and age distribution. Circulation. 2007;115:163–72.
15. Smith BG, Tibby SM, Qureshi SA, Rosenthal E, Krasemann T. Quantification of temporal, procedural, and hardware-related factors influencing radiation exposure during pediatric cardiac catheterization. Catheter Cardiovasc Interv. 2012;80:931–6.
16. Johnson JN, Hornik CP, Li JS, Benjamin DK Jr, Yoshizumi TT, Reiman RE, Frush DP, Hill KD. Cumulative radiation exposure and cancer risk estimation in children with heart disease. Circulation. 2014;130:161–7.
17. Venneri L, Rossi F, Botto N, Andreassi MG, Salcone N, Emad A, Lazzeri M, Gori C, Vano E, Picano E. Cancer risk from professional exposure in staff working in cardiac catheterization laboratory: insights from the National Research Council's Biological Effects of Ionizing Radiation VII Report. Am Heart J. 2009;157:118–24.

18. Di Salvo G, Miller O, Babu Narayan S, Li W, Budts W, Valsangiacomo Buechel ER, Frigiola A, van den Bosch AE, Bonello B, Mertens L, Hussain T, Parish V, Habib G, Edvardsen T, Geva T, Baumgartner H, Gatzoulis MA. Imaging the adult with congenital heart disease: a multimodality imaging approach-position paper from the EACVI. Eur Heart J Cardiovasc Imaging. 2018;19:1077–98.

19. Muthalaly RG, Nerlekar N, Ge Y, Kwong RY, Nasis A. MRI in patients with cardiac implantable electronic devices. Radiology. 2018;289:281–92.

20. Levine GN, Gomes AS, Arai AE, Bluemke DA, Flamm SD, Kanal E, Manning WJ, Martin ET, Smith JM, Wilke N, Shellock FS. Safety of magnetic resonance imaging in patients with cardiovascular devices: an American Heart Association scientific statement from the Committee on Diagnostic and Interventional Cardiac Catheterization, Council on Clinical Cardiology, and the Council on Cardiovascular Radiology and Intervention: endorsed by the American College of Cardiology Foundation, the North American Society for Cardiac Imaging, and the Society for Cardiovascular Magnetic Resonance. Circulation. 2007;116:2878–91.

21. Indik JH, Gimbel JR, Abe H, Alkmim-Teixeira R, Birgersdotter-Green U, Clarke GD, Dickfeld TL, Froelich JW, Grant J, Hayes DL, Heidbuchel H, Idriss SF, Kanal E, Lampert R, Machado CE, Mandrola JM, Nazarian S, Patton KK, Rozner MA, Russo RJ, Shen WK, Shinbane JS, Teo WS, Uribe W, Verma A, Wilkoff BL, Woodard PK. 2017 HRS expert consensus statement on magnetic resonance imaging and radiation exposure in patients with cardiovascular implantable electronic devices. Heart Rhythm. 2017;14:e97–e153.

22. Sequeiros RB, Ojala R, Kariniemi J, Perala J, Niinimaki J, Reinikainen H, Tervonen O. MR-guided interventional procedures: a review. Acta Radiol. 2005;46:576–86.

23. Hoult DI, Saunders JK, Sutherland GR, Sharp J, Gervin M, Kolansky HG, Kripiakevich DL, Procca A, Sebastian RA, Dombay A, Rayner DL, Roberts FA, Tomanek B. The engineering of an interventional MRI with a movable 1.5 Tesla magnet. J Magn Reson Imaging. 2001;13:78–86.

24. Adam G, Neuerburg J, Bucker A, Glowinski A, Vorwerk D, Stargardt A, Van Vaals JJ, Gunther RW. Interventional magnetic resonance. Initial clinical experience with a 1.5-tesla magnetic resonance system combined with c-arm fluoroscopy. Investig Radiol. 1997;32:191–7.

25. Fahrig R, Butts K, Rowlands JA, Saunders R, Stanton J, Stevens GM, Daniel BL, Wen Z, Ergun DL, Pelc NJ. A truly hybrid interventional MR/X-ray system: feasibility demonstration. J Magn Reson Imaging. 2001;13:294–300.

26. Fahrig R, Butts K, Wen Z, Saunders R, Kee ST, Sze DY, Daniel BL, Laerum F, Pelc NJ. Truly hybrid interventional MR/X-ray system: investigation of in vivo applications. Acad Radiol. 2001;8:1200–7.

27. Faranesh AZ, Lederman RJ. Roadmaps show the way: coregistration to enhance structural heart interventions. Catheter Cardiovasc Interv. 2013;82:443–4.

28. Rhode KS, Hill DL, Edwards PJ, Hipwell J, Rueckert D, Sanchez-Ortiz G, Hegde S, Rahunathan V, Razavi R. Registration and tracking to integrate X-ray and MR images in an XMR facility. IEEE Trans Med Imaging. 2003;22:1369–78.

29. Rhode KS, Sermesant M, Brogan D, Hegde S, Hipwell J, Lambiase P, Rosenthal E, Bucknall C, Qureshi SA, Gill JS, Razavi R, Hill DL. A system for real-time XMR guided cardiovascular intervention. IEEE Trans Med Imaging. 2005;24:1428–40.

30. Grant EK, Kanter JP, Olivieri LJ, Cross RR, Campbell-Washburn A, Faranesh AZ, Cronin I, Hamann KS, O'Byrne ML, Slack MC, Lederman RJ, Ratnayaka K. X-ray fused with MRI guidance of pre-selected transcatheter congenital heart disease interventions. Catheter Cardiovasc Interv. 2019;94:399–408.

31. Dori Y, Sarmiento M, Glatz AC, Gillespie MJ, Jones VM, Harris MA, Whitehead KK, Fogel MA, Rome JJ. X-ray magnetic resonance fusion to internal markers and utility in congenital heart disease catheterization. Circ Cardiovasc Imaging. 2011;4:415–24.

32. Abu Hazeem AA, Dori Y, Whitehead KK, Harris MA, Fogel MA, Gillespie MJ, Rome JJ, Glatz AC. X-ray magnetic resonance fusion modality may reduce radiation exposure and contrast dose in diagnostic cardiac catheterization of congenital heart disease. Catheter Cardiovasc Interv. 2014;84:795–800.

33. Faranesh AZ, Kellman P, Ratnayaka K, Lederman RJ. Integration of cardiac and respiratory motion into MRI roadmaps fused with x-ray. Med Phys. 2013;40:032302.
34. McGuirt D, Mazal J, Rogers T, Faranesh AZ, Schenke W, Stine A, Grant L, Lederman RJ. X-ray fused with magnetic resonance imaging to guide endomyocardial biopsy of a right ventricular mass. Radiol Technol. 2016;87:622–6.
35. Mazal JR, Rogers T, Schenke WH, Faranesh AZ, Hansen M, O'Brien K, Ratnayaka K, Lederman RJ. Interventional-cardiovascular MR: role of the interventional MR technologist. Radiol Technol. 2016;87:261–70.
36. Pushparajah K, Tzifa A, Razavi R. Cardiac MRI catheterisation: a 10-year single institution experience and review. Interv Cardiol. 2014;6:335–46.
37. White MJ, Thornton JS, Hawkes DJ, Hill DLG, Kitchen N, Mancini L, McEvoy AW, Razavi R, Wilson S, Yousry T, Keevil SF. Design, operation, and safety of single-room interventional MRI suites: practical experience from two centers. J Magn Reson Imaging. 2015;41:34–43.
38. Kakareka JW, Faranesh AZ, Pursley RH, Campbell-Washburn A, Herzka DA, Rogers T, Kanter J, Ratnayaka K, Lederman RJ, Pohida TJ. Physiological recording in the MRI environment (PRiME): MRI-compatible hemodynamic recording system. IEEE J Transl Eng Health Med. 2018;6:4100112.
39. Rieke V, Ganguly A, Daniel BL, Scott G, Pauly JM, Fahrig R, Pelc NJ, Butts K. X-ray compatible radiofrequency coil for magnetic resonance imaging. Magn Reson Med. 2005;53:1409–14.
40. McVeigh ER, Guttman MA, Kellman P, Raval AN, Lederman RJ. Real-time, interactive MRI for cardiovascular interventions. Acad Radiol. 2005;12:1121–7.
41. Yutzy SR, Duerk JL. Pulse sequences and system interfaces for interventional and real-time MRI. J Magn Reson Imaging. 2008;27:267–75.
42. Uecker M, Zhang S, Voit D, Karaus A, Merboldt KD, Frahm J. Real-time MRI at a resolution of 20 ms. NMR Biomed. 2010;23:986–94.
43. Campbell-Washburn AE, Faranesh AZ, Lederman RJ, Hansen MS. Magnetic resonance sequences and rapid acquisition for MR-guided interventions. Magn Reson Imaging Clin N Am. 2015;23:669–79.
44. Campbell-Washburn AE, Tavallaei MA, Pop M, Grant EK, Chubb H, Rhode K, Wright GA. Real-time MRI guidance of cardiac interventions. J Magn Reson Imaging. 2017;46:935–50.
45. Campbell-Washburn AE, Rogers T, Xue H, Hansen MS, Lederman RJ, Faranesh AZ. Dual echo positive contrast bSSFP for real-time visualization of passive devices during magnetic resonance guided cardiovascular catheterization. J Cardiovasc Magn Reson. 2014;16:88.
46. Peters J, Ecabert O, Meyer C, Schramm H, Kneser R, Groth A, Weese J. Automatic whole heart segmentation in static magnetic resonance image volumes. Med Image Comput Comput Assist Interv. 2007;10:402–10.
47. Lorenz C, et al. Interactive Frontend (IFE): a platform for graphical MR scanner control and scan automation. Proc Int Soc Mag Reson Med. 2005;13:2170.
48. Rogers T, Ratnayaka K, Khan JM, Stine A, Schenke WH, Grant LP, Mazal JR, Grant EK, Campbell-Washburn A, Hansen MS, Ramasawmy R, Herzka DA, Xue H, Kellman P, Faranesh AZ, Lederman RJ. CMR fluoroscopy right heart catheterization for cardiac output and pulmonary vascular resistance: results in 102 patients. J Cardiovasc Magn Reson. 2017;19:54.
49. Knight DS, Kotecha T, Martinez-Naharro A, Brown JT, Bertelli M, Fontana M, Muthurangu V, Coghlan JG. Cardiovascular magnetic resonance-guided right heart catheterization in a conventional CMR environment - predictors of procedure success and duration in pulmonary artery hypertension. J Cardiovasc Magn Reson. 2019;21:57.
50. Ratnayaka K, Kanter JP, Faranesh AZ, Grant EK, Olivieri LJ, Cross RR, Cronin IF, Hamann KS, Campbell-Washburn AE, O'Brien KJ, Rogers T, Hansen MS, Lederman RJ. Radiation-free CMR diagnostic heart catheterization in children. J Cardiovasc Magn Reson. 2017;19:65.

51. Omary RA, Unal O, Koscielski DS, Frayne R, Korosec FR, Mistretta CA, Strother CM, Grist TM. Real-time MR imaging-guided passive catheter tracking with use of gadolinium-filled catheters. J Vasc Interv Radiol. 2000;11:1079–85.
52. Unal O, Li J, Cheng W, Yu H, Strother CM. MR-visible coatings for endovascular device visualization. J Magn Reson Imaging. 2006;23:763–9.
53. Ratnayaka K, Faranesh AZ, Hansen MS, Stine AM, Halabi M, Barbash IM, Schenke WH, Wright VJ, Grant LP, Kellman P, Kocaturk O, Lederman RJ. Real-time MRI-guided right heart catheterization in adults using passive catheters. Eur Heart J. 2013;34:380–9.
54. Velasco Forte MN, Pushparajah K, Schaeffter T, Valverde Perez I, Rhode K, Ruijsink B, Alhrishy M, Byrne N, Chiribiri A, Ismail T, Hussain T, Razavi R, Roujol S. Improved passive catheter tracking with positive contrast for CMR-guided cardiac catheterization using partial saturation (pSAT). J Cardiovasc Magn Reson. 2017;19:60.
55. Dumoulin CL, Souza SP, Darrow RD. Real-time position monitoring of invasive devices using magnetic resonance. Magn Reson Med. 1993;29:411–5.
56. Hillenbrand CM, Elgort DR, Wong EY, Reykowski A, Wacker FK, Lewin JS, Duerk JL. Active device tracking and high-resolution intravascular MRI using a novel catheter-based, opposed-solenoid phased array coil. Magn Reson Med. 2004;51:668–75.
57. Vernickel P, Schulz V, Weiss S, Gleich B. A safe transmission line for MRI. IEEE Trans Biomed Eng. 2005;52:1094–102.
58. Weiss S, Vernickel P, Schaeffter T, Schulz V, Gleich B. Transmission line for improved RF safety of interventional devices. Magn Reson Med. 2005;54:182–9.
59. Yaras YS, Satir S, Ozsoy C, Ramasawmy R, Campbell-Washburn AE, Lederman RJ, Kocaturk O, Degertekin FL. Acousto-optic catheter tracking sensor for interventional MRI procedures. IEEE Trans Biomed Eng. 2019;66:1148–54.
60. Nitz WR, Oppelt A, Renz W, Manke C, Lenhart M, Link J. On the heating of linear conductive structures as guide wires and catheters in interventional MRI. J Magn Reson Imaging. 2001;13:105–14.
61. Konings MK, Bartels LW, Smits HF, Bakker CJ. Heating around intravascular guidewires by resonating RF waves. J Magn Reson Imaging. 2000;12:79–85.
62. Shellock FG, Shellock VJ. Cardiovascular catheters and accessories: ex vivo testing of ferromagnetism, heating, and artifacts associated with MRI. J Magn Reson Imaging. 1998;8:1338–42.
63. Luechinger R, Duru F, Scheidegger MB, Boesiger P, Candinas R. Force and torque effects of a 1.5-Tesla MRI scanner on cardiac pacemakers and ICDs. Pacing Clin Electrophysiol. 2001;24:199–205.
64. Campbell-Washburn AE, Rogers T, Stine AM, Khan JM, Ramasawmy R, Schenke WH, McGuirt DR, Mazal JR, Grant LP, Grant EK, Herzka DA, Lederman RJ. Right heart catheterization using metallic guidewires and low SAR cardiovascular magnetic resonance fluoroscopy at 1.5 Tesla: first in human experience. J Cardiovasc Magn Reson. 2018;20:41.
65. Campbell-Washburn AE, Rogers T, Basar B, Sonmez M, Kocaturk O, Lederman RJ, Hansen MS, Faranesh AZ. Positive contrast spiral imaging for visualization of commercial nitinol guidewires with reduced heating. J Cardiovasc Magn Reson. 2015;17:114.
66. Tzifa A, Krombach GA, Kramer N, Kruger S, Schutte A, von Walter M, Schaeffter T, Qureshi S, Krasemann T, Rosenthal E, Schwartz CA, Varma G, Buhl A, Kohlmeier A, Bucker A, Gunther RW, Razavi R. Magnetic resonance-guided cardiac interventions using magnetic resonance-compatible devices: a preclinical study and first-in-man congenital interventions. Circ Cardiovasc Interv. 2010;3:585–92.
67. Beerbaum P, Korperich H, Gieseke J, Barth P, Peuster M, Meyer H. Blood flow quantification in adults by phase-contrast MRI combined with SENSE--a validation study. J Cardiovasc Magn Reson. 2005;7:361–9.
68. Beerbaum P, Korperich H, Gieseke J, Barth P, Peuster M, Meyer H. Rapid left-to-right shunt quantification in children by phase-contrast magnetic resonance imaging combined with sensitivity encoding (SENSE). Circulation. 2003;108:1355–61.

69. Beerbaum P, Korperich H, Barth P, Esdorn H, Gieseke J, Meyer H. Noninvasive quantification of left-to-right shunt in pediatric patients: phase-contrast cine magnetic resonance imaging compared with invasive oximetry. Circulation. 2001;103:2476–82.
70. Shanahan CL, Wilson NJ, Gentles TL, Skinner JR. The influence of measured versus assumed uptake of oxygen in assessing pulmonary vascular resistance in patients with a bidirectional Glenn anastomosis. Cardiol Young. 2003;13:137–42.
71. Muthurangu V, Taylor A, Andriantsimiavona R, Hegde S, Miquel ME, Tulloh R, Baker E, Hill DL, Razavi RS. Novel method of quantifying pulmonary vascular resistance by use of simultaneous invasive pressure monitoring and phase-contrast magnetic resonance flow. Circulation. 2004;110:826–34.
72. Schmitt B, Steendijk P, Ovroutski S, Lunze K, Rahmanzadeh P, Maarouf N, Ewert P, Berger F, Kuehne T. Pulmonary vascular resistance, collateral flow, and ventricular function in patients with a Fontan circulation at rest and during dobutamine stress. Circ Cardiovasc Imaging. 2010;3:623–31.
73. Pushparajah K, Tzifa A, Bell A, Wong JK, Hussain T, Valverde I, Bellsham-Revell HR, Greil G, Simpson JM, Schaeffter T, Razavi R. Cardiovascular magnetic resonance catheterization derived pulmonary vascular resistance and medium-term outcomes in congenital heart disease. J Cardiovasc Magn Reson. 2015;17:28.
74. Kuehne T, Yilmaz S, Schulze-Neick I, Wellnhofer E, Ewert P, Nagel E, Lange P. Magnetic resonance imaging guided catheterisation for assessment of pulmonary vascular resistance: in vivo validation and clinical application in patients with pulmonary hypertension. Heart. 2005;91:1064–9.
75. Tzifa A, Razavi R. Test occlusion of Fontan fenestration: unique contribution of interventional MRI. Heart. 2011;97:89.
76. Hijazi ZM, Fahey JT, Kleinman CS, Kopf GS, Hellenbrand WE. Hemodynamic evaluation before and after closure of fenestrated Fontan. An acute study of changes in oxygen delivery. Circulation. 1992;86:196–202.
77. Schmitt B, Steendijk P, Lunze K, Ovroutski S, Falkenberg J, Rahmanzadeh P, Maarouf N, Ewert P, Berger F, Kuehne T. Integrated assessment of diastolic and systolic ventricular function using diagnostic cardiac magnetic resonance catheterization: validation in pigs and application in a clinical pilot study. JACC Cardiovasc Imaging. 2009;2:1271–81.
78. Pushparajah K, Wong JK, Bellsham-Revell HR, Hussain T, Valverde I, Bell A, Tzifa A, Greil G, Simpson JM, Kutty S, Razavi R. Magnetic resonance imaging catheter stress haemodynamics post-Fontan in hypoplastic left heart syndrome. Eur Heart J Cardiovasc Imaging. 2016;17:644–51.
79. Wong J, Pushparajah K, de Vecchi A, Ruijsink B, Greil GF, Hussain T, Razavi R. Pressure-volume loop-derived cardiac indices during dobutamine stress: a step towards understanding limitations in cardiac output in children with hypoplastic left heart syndrome. Int J Cardiol. 2017;230:439–46.
80. Valverde I, Staicu C, Grotenhuis H, Marzo A, Rhode K, Shi Y, Brown AG, Tzifa A, Hussain T, Greil G, Lawford P, Razavi R, Hose R, Beerbaum P. Predicting hemodynamics in native and residual coarctation: preliminary results of a Rigid-Wall Computational-Fluid-Dynamics model (RW-CFD) validated against clinically invasive pressure measures at rest and during pharmacological stress. J Cardiovasc Magn Reson. 2011;13:P49.
81. Razavi RS, Baker A, Qureshi SA, Rosenthal E, Marsh MJ, Leech SC, Rela M, Mieli-Vergani G. Hemodynamic response to continuous infusion of dobutamine in Alagille's syndrome. Transplantation. 2001;72:823–8.
82. Saikus CE, Ratnayaka K, Barbash IM, Colyer JH, Kocaturk O, Faranesh AZ, Lederman RJ. MRI-guided vascular access with an active visualization needle. J Magn Reson Imaging. 2011;34:1159–66.
83. Rickers C, Jerosch-Herold M, Hu X, Murthy N, Wang X, Kong H, Seethamraju RT, Weil J, Wilke NM. Magnetic resonance image-guided transcatheter closure of atrial septal defects. Circulation. 2003;107:132–8.

84. Ratnayaka K, Raman VK, Faranesh AZ, Sonmez M, Kim JH, Gutierrez LF, Ozturk C, McVeigh ER, Slack MC, Lederman RJ. Antegrade percutaneous closure of membranous ventricular septal defect using X-ray fused with magnetic resonance imaging. JACC Cardiovasc Interv. 2009;2:224–30.
85. Ratnayaka K, Saikus CE, Faranesh AZ, Bell JA, Barbash IM, Kocaturk O, Reyes CA, Sonmez M, Schenke WH, Wright VJ, Hansen MS, Slack MC, Lederman RJ. Closed-chest transthoracic magnetic resonance imaging-guided ventricular septal defect closure in swine. JACC Cardiovasc Interv. 2011;4:1326–34.
86. Kuehne T, Saeed M, Higgins CB, Gleason K, Krombach GA, Weber OM, Martin AJ, Turner D, Teitel D, Moore P. Endovascular stents in pulmonary valve and artery in swine: feasibility study of MR imaging-guided deployment and postinterventional assessment. Radiology. 2003;226:475–81.
87. Kuehne T, Yilmaz S, Meinus C, Moore P, Saeed M, Weber O, Higgins CB, Blank T, Elsaesser E, Schnackenburg B, Ewert P, Lange PE, Nagel E. Magnetic resonance imaging-guided transcatheter implantation of a prosthetic valve in aortic valve position: feasibility study in swine. J Am Coll Cardiol. 2004;44:2247–9.
88. Krueger JJ, Ewert P, Yilmaz S, Gelernter D, Peters B, Pietzner K, Bornstedt A, Schnackenburg B, Abdul-Khaliq H, Fleck E, Nagel E, Berger F, Kuehne T. Magnetic resonance imaging-guided balloon angioplasty of coarctation of the aorta: a pilot study. Circulation. 2006;113:1093–100.
89. Serfaty JM, Yang X, Foo TK, Kumar A, Derbyshire A, Atalar E. MRI-guided coronary catheterization and PTCA: a feasibility study on a dog model. Magn Reson Med. 2003;49:258–63.
90. Ratnayaka K, Rogers T, Schenke WH, Mazal JR, Chen MY, Sonmez M, Hansen MS, Kocaturk O, Faranesh AZ, Lederman RJ. Magnetic resonance imaging-guided transcatheter cavopulmonary shunt. JACC Cardiovasc Interv. 2016;9:959–70.
91. Ratnayaka K, Moore JW, Rios R, Lederman RJ, Hegde SR, El-Said HG. First-in-human closed-chest transcatheter superior cavopulmonary anastomosis. J Am Coll Cardiol. 2017;70:745–52.
92. Barkhausen J, Kahn T, Krombach GA, Kuhl CK, Lotz J, Maintz D, Ricke J, Schonberg SO, Vogl TJ, Wacker FK. White paper: interventional MRI: current status and potential for development considering economic perspectives, Part 1: General application. RöFo. 2017;189:611–23.
93. Rogers T, Ratnayaka K, Karmarkar P, Campbell-Washburn AE, Schenke WH, Mazal JR, Kocaturk O, Faranesh AZ, Lederman RJ. Real-time magnetic resonance imaging guidance improves the diagnostic yield of endomyocardial biopsy. JACC Basic Transl Sci. 2016;1:376–83.
94. Rogers T, Mahapatra S, Kim S, Eckhaus MA, Schenke WH, Mazal JR, Campbell-Washburn A, Sonmez M, Faranesh AZ, Ratnayaka K, Lederman RJ. Transcatheter myocardial needle chemoablation during real-time magnetic resonance imaging: a new approach to ablation therapy for rhythm disorders. Circ Arrhythm Electrophysiol. 2016;9:e003926.
95. Chubb H, Karim R, Mukherjee R, Williams SE, Whitaker J, Harrison J, Niederer SA, Staab W, Gill J, Schaeffter T, Wright M, O'Neill M, Razavi R. A comprehensive multi-index cardiac magnetic resonance-guided assessment of atrial fibrillation substrate prior to ablation: prediction of long-term outcomes. J Cardiovasc Electrophysiol. 2019;30:1894–903.
96. Mukherjee RK, Chubb H, Roujol S, Razavi R, O'Neill MD. Advances in real-time MRI-guided electrophysiology. Curr Cardiovasc Imaging Rep. 2019;12:6.
97. Chubb H, Harrison JL, Weiss S, Krueger S, Koken P, Bloch LO, Kim WY, Stenzel GS, Wedan SR, Weisz JL, Gill J, Schaeffter T, O'Neill MD, Razavi RS. Development, preclinical validation, and clinical translation of a cardiac magnetic resonance - electrophysiology system with active catheter tracking for ablation of cardiac arrhythmia. JACC Clin Electrophysiol. 2017;3:89–103.
98. Hilbert S, Sommer P, Gutberlet M, Gaspar T, Foldyna B, Piorkowski C, Weiss S, Lloyd T, Schnackenburg B, Krueger S, Fleiter C, Paetsch I, Jahnke C, Hindricks G, Grothoff M. Real-time magnetic resonance-guided ablation of typical right atrial flutter using a combination

of active catheter tracking and passive catheter visualization in man: initial results from a consecutive patient series. Europace. 2016;18:572–7.

99. Mukherjee RK, Roujol S, Chubb H, Harrison J, Williams S, Whitaker J, O'Neill L, Silberbauer J, Neji R, Schneider R, Pohl T, Lloyd T, O'Neill M, Razavi R. Epicardial electroanatomical mapping, radiofrequency ablation, and lesion imaging in the porcine left ventricle under real-time magnetic resonance imaging guidance-an in vivo feasibility study. Europace. 2018;20:f254–62.

100. Mukherjee RK, Costa CM, Neji R, Harrison JL, Sim I, Williams SE, Whitaker J, Chubb H, O'Neill L, Schneider R, Lloyd T, Pohl T, Roujol S, Niederer SA, Razavi R, O'Neill MD. Evaluation of a real-time magnetic resonance imaging-guided electrophysiology system for structural and electrophysiological ventricular tachycardia substrate assessment. Europace. 2019;21:1432–41.

101. Weiss S, Wirtz D, David B, Krueger S, Lips O, Caulfield D, Pedersen SF, Bostock J, Razavi R, Schaeffter T. In vivo evaluation and proof of radiofrequency safety of a novel diagnostic MR-electrophysiology catheter. Magn Reson Med. 2011;65:770–7.

102. van Es R, van den Broek HT, van der Naald M, de Jong L, Nieuwenhuis ER, Kraaijeveld AO, Doevendans PA, Chamuleau SAJ, van Slochteren FJ. Validation of a novel stand-alone software tool for image guided cardiac catheter therapy. Int J Card Imaging. 2019;35:225–35.

103. Shusterman V, Hodgson-Zingman D, Thedens D, Zhu X, Hoffman S, Sieren JC, Morgan GM, Faranesh A, London B. High-energy external defibrillation and transcutaneous pacing during MRI: feasibility and safety. J Cardiovasc Magn Reson. 2019;21:47.

104. Dori Y, Keller MS, Fogel MA, Rome JJ, Whitehead KK, Harris MA, Itkin M. MRI of lymphatic abnormalities after functional single-ventricle palliation surgery. Am J Roentgenol. 2014;203:426–31.

105. Dori Y, Keller MS, Rychik J, Itkin M. Successful treatment of plastic bronchitis by selective lymphatic embolization in a Fontan patient. Pediatrics. 2014;134:e590–5.

106. Yildirim KD, Basar B, Campbell-Washburn AE, Herzka DA, Kocaturk O, Lederman RJ. A cardiovascular magnetic resonance (CMR) safe metal braided catheter design for interventional CMR at 1.5 T: freedom from radiofrequency induced heating and preserved mechanical performance. J Cardiovasc Magn Reson. 2019;21:16.

107. Campbell-Washburn AE, Ramasawmy R, Restivo MC, Bhattacharya I, Basar B, Herzka DA, Hansen MS, Rogers T, Bandettini WP, McGuirt DR, Mancini C, Grodzki D, Schneider R, Majeed W, Bhat H, Xue H, Moss J, Malayeri AA, Jones EC, Koretsky AP, Kellman P, Chen MY, Lederman RJ, Balaban RS. Opportunities in interventional and diagnostic imaging by using high-performance low-field-strength MRI. Radiology. 2019;293:384–93.

108. Godinez F, Scott G, Padormo F, Hajnal JV, Malik SJ. Safe guidewire visualization using the modes of a PTx transmit array MR system. Magn Reson Med. 2020;83:2343.

Cardiac Mechanics I: 3D Speckle Tracking Echocardiography

6

Bart Bijnens, Filip Loncaric, and Silvia Montserrat

6.1 Introduction

In clinic practice, when dealing with adult CHD patients, the continuous assessment of overall cardiac pump function of how this is achieved through contraction of the individual myocardial segments is of great importance. However, quantifying cardiac pump function is not straightforward given the ambiguous definition of function and how this relates to clinical assessment and decision making. Intrinsic function quantification requires measuring true contractility of the myocardium and how this leads to pressure development and volume ejection, always in relation to potentially altered cardiac morphology, myocardial (micro-) structure and tissue properties, as well as the peripheral circulation properties. Current diagnostic tools are unable to assess all relevant aspects, but contemporary cardiac (multi-modality) imaging can contribute some of them. Especially the ability to quantify myocardial deformation can provide important information that otherwise is difficult to assess.

Echocardiography has provided an easily accessible way to measure segmental myocardial deformation by tracking the speckles (typical ultrasound interference patterns directly originating from the tissue) present in the images [1]. While 2D

B. Bijnens (✉)
ICREA, Barcelona, Spain

Institut d'Investigacions Biomèdiques August Pi i Sunyer (IDIBAPS), Barcelona, Spain
e-mail: bart.bijnens@idibaps.org

F. Loncaric
Institut d'Investigacions Biomèdiques August Pi i Sunyer (IDIBAPS), Barcelona, Spain

Cardiovascular Institute, Hospital Clinic, Universitat de Barcelona, Barcelona, Spain

S. Montserrat
Cardiovascular Institute, Hospital Clinic, Universitat de Barcelona, Barcelona, Spain
e-mail: SMONTSER@clinic.cat

© Springer Nature Switzerland AG 2021
P. Gallego, I. Valverde (eds.), *Multimodality Imaging Innovations In Adult Congenital Heart Disease*, Congenital Heart Disease in Adolescents and Adults, https://doi.org/10.1007/978-3-030-61927-5_6

deformation (strain—the relative change in dimensions of tissue segments; strain rate—the rate of deformation) is mostly used in clinical practice, 3D strain assessment has also become available. The clear advantage of 3D deformation quantification is that it can assess the full and complex 3D deformation of myocardium as it occurs during the cardiac cycle. Especially out-of-plane motion limits 2D approaches to do so. While intrinsically more suitable, current 3D imaging has the disadvantage of having less temporal resolution as compared to 2D, which is a disadvantage when quantifying cardiac deformation, especially in the time periods where fast motion occurs (especially the isovolumic periods) [2–4].

6.2   Myocardial Deformation

The heart is an intrinsic 3D object. In current clinical practice, the cardiac chambers are often simplified to (parts of) ellipsoids to quantify volume changes or deformation [5, 6]. However, understanding the 3D structure of the myocardium and how this influences deformation and how it changes with CHD is of great importance. Ventricular deformation is determined by the positioning of the cardiomyocytes with the myocardial wall. Myocytes form fibre-like aggregates that continuously and progressively change direction from the epi- to the endocardium [7]. While the endocardial direction is predominantly longitudinal (=from the valve plane towards the apex), this gradually becomes circumferential in the mid-myocardium and continues to change direction towards the endocardium, where they become longitudinal again. This arrangement determines the clinically used components of myocardial deformation: longitudinal shortening during ejection, where the atrioventricular valve plane is dragged towards the apex; circumferential shortening, where the short-axis circumference decreases; and the resulting radial thickening due to the incompressibility of tissue (Fig. 6.1). Additionally, the obliqueness of the endo- and epicardial fibres induces a rotation of the base with respect to the apex, resulting in overall torsion of the ventricles [8, 9]. The contribution of each of these components is determined by (transmural) tissue organization and properties, overall cardiac shape and morphology, perfusion and activation.

In clinic practice, most cardiac conditions are associated with a transmurally differential loss of myocardial function where the endocardium decreases first. This is related to the fact that the perfusion is supplied from epicardially positioned coronary arteries, with the endocardial tissue most distal, and thus most vulnerable, together with the fact that increased intraventricular pressure will increase the local wall stress most in the endocardially located (longitudinal) 'fibres'. This makes that, in most patients, longitudinal deformation decreases first (and can be compensated by increased circumferential deformation to maintain stroke volume and ejection fraction) [10]. Few exceptions have been suggested where circumferential deformation decreases before longitudinal and these are associated with mid-myocardial tissues damage/fibrosis, amongst others: cardiotoxicity; myocarditis; Chagas disease.

Given that longitudinal deformation is most sensitive in the majority of patients, any measure that assesses global longitudinal deformation (be it global longitudinal

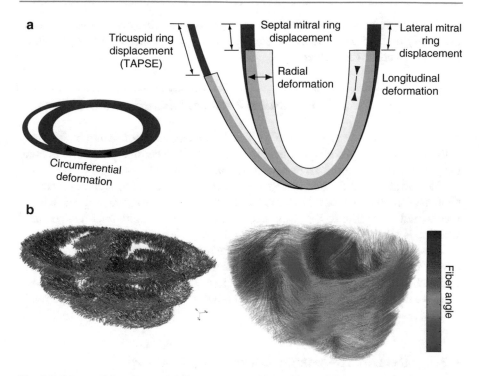

Fig. 6.1 Myocardial motion and deformation components (**a**) and fibre structure of the heart (**b**)

strain or atrioventricular valve plane displacement (MAPSE—Mitral Annular Plane Systolic Excursion; TAPSE—Tricuspid Annular Plane Systolic Excursion)) will provide a more sensitive assessment of ventricular function as compared to ejection fraction [11–14].

When quantifying deformation, both the amount of deformation (=strain (%): the change in length or thickness of segments as compared to their initial length) and the speed at which it takes place (=strain rate (1/s): the rate of deformation) are relevant. For a given ventricle, the strain at the end of ejection will determine the stroke volume, while the strain rate at each moment during ejection is related to the force development by the myocardium (working against the pressure load). Both entities are intrinsically load dependent, but strain is (by definition) very much related with volume while strain rate has shown to be more reflective of intrinsic cardiac function [15].

Specific regional changes in deformation occur in different pathologies, making the assessment of the different deformation components, and their time-course during the cardiac cycle, powerful information for diagnosis and follow-up.

Some authors have suggested that assessing regional 3D stroke volumes/ejection fraction could also assess segmental abnormalities without the need to quantify myocardial deformation [16, 17]. However, this approach is very challenging given the difficulty to assign ventricular volume regions to specific myocardial segments, especially in conditions involving shape changes, or interactions of neighbouring segments as described further.

6.3   Myocardial Deformation Patterns in Cardiac Conditions

In the past years, the assessment of (regional) myocardial deformation has dramatically increased our potential to quantify and understand cardiac mechanics in clinical practice and translate this to improved diagnosis or prognosis [18–27].

Global longitudinal strain (GLS), assessing the global deformation of a cardiac chamber (all four chambers have been studied), has shown to have prognostic information and is superior to EF given that, as stated above, longitudinal (endocardial) function is affected earlier in most conditions [28].

However, while GLS is powerful in populations and might provide some risk assessment, a more promising approach for the individual patient is to assess the regional patterns of deformation which are very specific to different conditions. Here we briefly discuss some of the most common patterns that can be observed in clinical practice.

6.3.1   Abnormal Segmental Contractility/Loading

The most common (at least in adult cardiology) condition is where regional segments have reduced contractility (e.g. due to coronary artery disease [29], or coronary anomalies [30]). This will reduce the local contractile force development in the segment while neighbouring segments remain normal. With a decrease of force development, there is a linear decrease of local systolic deformation [29]. When end-systolic deformation in a segment has reduced while it remained normal in the adjacent segment, at the moment that the pressure drops after the ventriculo-arterial valve closes, the elastic interaction forces will cause a post-systolic lengthening/thickening (PST) in the abnormal segment [31]. The presence of PST (together with a decrease in systolic deformation) is a typical segmental pattern in the presence of insufficient force development and this deformation clearly does not contribute to ejection given that it is present in the isovolumic relaxation period or even during filling. Similarly, PST will be present in regional fibrosis given that this results in decreased segmental force development/systolic deformation [32]. Keep in mind that in the presence of a transmural scar or extensive fibrosis, PST will be obliterated given that the tissue becomes too stiff for passive segment interaction [36].

Additionally, any other condition that will decrease local segmental deformation during systole, as compared to adjacent segments, will show PST. This is for example the case in regional increases in wall stress due to pressure loading (discussed more below), where more flat segments (such as the basal septum) will have a relatively larger wall stress and will show PST [33].

6.3.2   Volume Overload

Volume overload can be present due to valve leakage, shunts, anaemia …. In order for a ventricle to cope with the increased stroke volume needed, remodelling will occur. For a given ventricular size/shape, there is a fixed relation between the overall deformation and the stroke volume generated. The larger the strain, the larger the stroke volume. By dilating, but maintaining normal deformation, a ventricle can eject significantly more stroke volume, given that there is power law relation between the length change and volume [34]. However, while dilatation is efficient to cope with the need for an increased stroke volume, the disadvantage is that the increase in size results in a decrease of the sphericity (the walls get 'flatter'), which, according to Laplace's law, will increase the wall stress for a constant intraventricular pressure. Once wall stress exceeds a certain threshold, myocytes will go into apoptosis and fibrosis will occur, all leading to a local decrease in contractile force development and resulting in lower deformation. This lower deformation now needs to be compensated in order to maintain stroke volume, and the compensation mechanism is a further dilatation, thus entering a vicious circle of dilatation/damage/more dilatation/more damage/heart failure. Therefore, the assessment of deformation in volume overload is clinically useful and as long as deformation is normal (or even slightly increased) the ventricle is physiologically remodelled and coping with the load. When deformation decreases, myocardial damage is starting to occur indicating the need for urgent intervention [34].

6.3.3   Pressure Overload

Pressure overload will be present when the ventriculo-arterial valve has a (sub-) valvular obstruction, or when the compliance or overall resistance of the peripheral system connected to the ventricle is altered (such as in (pulmonary) hypertension). The increased intracavity pressure will increase the wall stress and, when loading is chronic, the myocardium will remodel to (partly) compensate for this by myocyte/wall hypertrophy (increasing the amount of contractile material and thus global force development). With acute loading, or only partial compensatory hypertrophy, deformation will change. Strain rate will decrease, given that the balance of available force versus loading force becomes disturbed; deformation will take place longer and ejection time increases; overall systolic deformation might decrease unless heart rate is very low [35]. Besides global changes, there will be specific local changes given that the ventricle is not a sphere and thus regional sphericity (determining the local increase in wall stress) changes depending on the ventricular segment [36]. Overall, the basal segments see a larger wall stress increase with increasing pressure. In the LV, the basal/inferior septum, and in the RV, the basal free wall, are mostly affected and will often show PST as well as localized hypertrophy [33]. Additionally, these are the segments where fibrosis will occur first after long-standing severe pressure loading.

Additionally, given that the endocardial wall will see the highest increase in wall stress and that the local 'fibres' are longitudinal and opposite obliquely oriented as opposed to the preserved epicardium, the overall rotation of base and apex, and the resulting twist, will increase with pressure loading given the epicardially induced rotation will not be counteracted any more by the endocardium. This paradoxical increase in torsion/twist makes this parameter rather difficult to interpret in clinical practice.

6.3.4   (Genetic) Cardiomyopathies

Cardiomyopathies are often associated with regionally decreased contractility where the typical pattern of decreased systolic deformation will be accompanied by PST. Depending on a potentially associated gene defect, this can express in different locations/patterns with different underlying myocardial/myocyte/mitochondrial changes leading to the decreased contractility. For example, in hypertrophic cardiomyopathy, resulting from sarcomere mutations, one will typically observe regions of fibre disarray (where myocytes are no longer oriented in a regular fibre-like pattern) where no coherent local deformation can be present irrespective of the viability of the tissue. Given that this location and extent of the abnormal myocardial organization is highly individual (although predominantly in the septum and more likely in the thicker segments), no standard segment changes can be described but the diagnosis can be made based on the presence of a region of virtually absent deformation, surrounded by almost normally deforming segments [37]. Many genetic cardiomyopathies such as Fabry disease [38], Duchenne muscular dystrophy or Friedreich Ataxia do not have much septal involvement but rather show decreased systolic deformation, with PST, in the (basal) free walls. Typical global storage diseases, such as amyloidosis or thalassemia, will show a uniform decrease in longitudinal deformation in all walls, with a typical strain gradient from a more or less preserved apex to a non-deforming base (apical sparing).

6.3.5   Abnormal Activation

The pump efficiency of the ventricles is very much dependent on the synchronous activation of all myocardial segments. Only when all segments start developing force at the same moment will they show full synergy resulting in uniform wall stress, fast pressure build-up and synergetic deformation, dragging the valve plane towards the apex while shortening the ventricular circumference. When a certain segment is activated before the adjacent one (as will be in the presence of a bundle branch block (BBB) or accessory pathways), it will use its contractile force development to interact with (=stretch) the neighbour rather than build up pressure or contribute to global deformation. As a result, typical deformation patterns occur such as a 'septal flash' (in the presence of LBBB) [39], an 'RV apical flash' (in RBBB) [40, 41] or a 'basal flash' (as in the presence of accessory pathways adjacent to the AV node in Ebstein anomaly) [41]. It is important to note that these abnormal deformation patterns are present in the isovolumic contraction period (as opposed to PST which is present during isovolumic relaxation) and might lead to a total non-contribution of the involved segment to the subsequent ejection, thus often leading to decreased global function or even heart failure. Given that these conditions are related to electrical abnormalities, pacing or ablation strategies could offer a useful therapeutic approach.

6.4   3D Strain

Three-dimensional echocardiography has quickly entered clinical practice in the past years. Given that the tracking of (wave interference generated) speckles is even easier in 3D as compared to 2D, since out-of-plane motion can additionally be followed during the complex segmental deformation of the myocardium, 3D strain is a logical extension of the established (2D) speckle tracking applications.

6.4.1   Advantages as Compared to 2D

- Given that myocardial deformation is intrinsically 3D (with longitudinal and circumferential shortening; radial thickening; and shearing related to base-apex rotation and endo- versus epicardial differential deformation) any 2D approximation will only partially capture this complexity.
- Speckles are only short-lived phenomena related to a specific configuration of locally present ultrasound scatterers, and any out-of-plane motion (due to for example valve to apex ring displacement in a short-axis view) would let them disappear even faster out of the 2D scan plane.
- Single volume acquisitions can be used to quantify regional deformation, thus avoiding the use of multiple 2D acquisitions with potential alignment problems as well as variations in cardiac cycle lengths.
- 3D acquisition helps avoiding apical foreshortening in apical views which would hamper true deformation quantification.

6.4.2   Current Limitations of 3D Strain

- Strain assessment, as every measurement from B-mode echocardiography, relies on as optimal as possible image quality. 3D imaging can be challenging, especially for more distal segments such as the base in apical views.
- Deformation, and especially strain rate changes, can be very fast during the cardiac cycle, especially in the isovolumic phases or in the presence of abnormal activation. To quantify these, the frame rate used has to be sufficient not to miss them. In current practice, higher frame rates can be achieved by multi-beat acquisitions, but these have the disadvantage that breathing of probe position can cause distortions.

- 3D spatial resolution is still inferior to most of the 2D acquisitions, making it more dependent on ventricular shape, size or wall thickness.
- 2D strain (especially global strain) has recently been successfully standardized amongst manufacturers of ultrasound equipment while 3D standardization is still in progress.

6.5 Changes with Congenital Heart Disease: Examples

The descriptions above clearly show that deformation is useful to assess cardiac performance in individual hearts, both when assessing global strain for risk prediction and identifying specific regional patterns for diagnosis, therapy decisions or follow-up. To illustrate these concepts in the setting of (adult) congenial heart disease, we will show some individual examples below.

6.5.1 Healthy Individual

Figures 6.2 and 6.3 show the deformation of a healthy person with no significant medical history or cardiac disease. Left ventricle is of normal dimensions, and the ejection fraction is preserved (~60%). Figure 6.2 illustrates the 2D speckle tracking

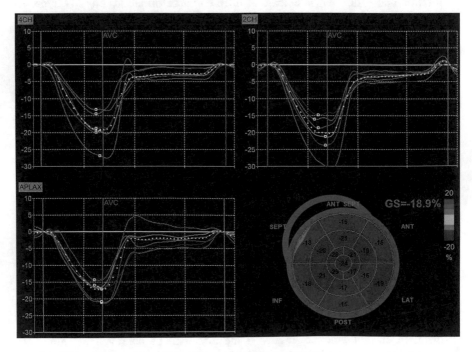

Fig. 6.2 Normal deformation: 2D strain from a healthy person

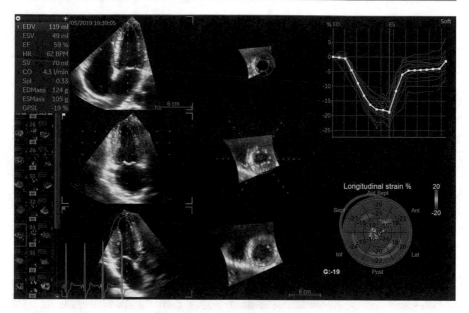

Fig. 6.3 Normal deformation: 3D strain from a healthy person

deformation analysis, performed in three apical long-axis planes: 4-chamber, 3-chamber and 2-chamber. A bullseye plot based on the 18-segment left ventricle model shows average segmental longitudinal strain values throughout the cardiac cycle, and left ventricle global longitudinal strain is calculated as an average of the segments. Global longitudinal function is in the normal range. The segmental deformation values as well as curve shapes are very uniform. Figure 6.3 shows the 4D deformation analysis which shows a similar global longitudinal function, with uniform and synchronous segmental deformation.

6.5.2   Tetralogy of Fallot (TOF)

Figures 6.4 and 6.5 show the deformation patterns of a patient with a corrected Tetralogy of Fallot. Figure 6.4 shows the 2D strain traces. While in TOF, the RV is mostly of consideration, given that in many patients, RV volume overload is present due to significant pulmonary valve regurgitation, a clear LV-RV interaction has been shown, also affecting LV function [41, 42]. This is clearly illustrated in Fig. 6.4 where in the apical 4-chamber view the GLS (−14%) is reduced (−17% is often considered a cut-off for normality). However, most obvious is the dyssynchrony present in the deformation given that none of the regional traces are similar (as compared to the above normal individual). It can be clearly seen that the apical septal segment starts deforming before the other segments while the apical lateral segments are even stretched. A little later (around the R-top in the ECG) the other segments shorten while the apical septal segment lengthens during ejection instead

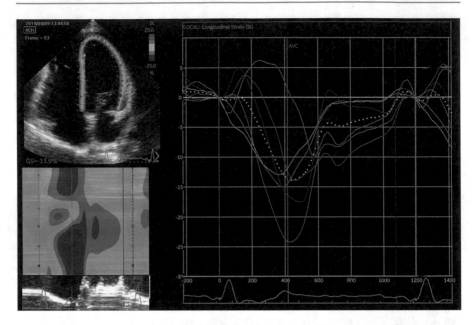

Fig. 6.4 Tetralogy of Fallot: 2D strain of a patient with a corrected Tetralogy of Fallot

of shortening. This very typical 'flash' pattern is induced by the RBBB present in this patient, where the RV base and the (joint) apex are not activated at the same time. Some authors have suggested that pacing the basal RV free wall could restore synchronicity and improve RV and thus also LV function.

Figure 6.5 shows the 3D strain traces of the same patient. When now looking at the value of global strain (−17%) it is almost normal but clearly larger as compared to 2D. The obvious reason for this is that the value in this case corresponds to the full deformation of the whole LV while in the above 2D case it only showed the 4-chamber view segments, which are clearly more affected by the dyssynchrony as compared to the other segments. Similarly to the 2D traces, the dyssynchrony can be observed from the much more divergent traces as well as from the bullseye showing the more apical septal segment to be most reduced.

6.5.3 Ebstein Anomaly (EA)

Figures 6.6 and 6.7 show the 3D deformation of a patient with an Ebstein anomaly. In Ebstein anomaly there is an abnormal deformation of the basal septum related to the fact that these segments are often located in the arterialized parts of the wall as well as the fact that in many patients accessory pathways are present short-circuiting the AV node through direct conduction from the atrial septum to the basal ventricular septum. The early activation of the basal portion of the septum results in its early deformation, before the opening of the aortic and pulmonary valves, and fast

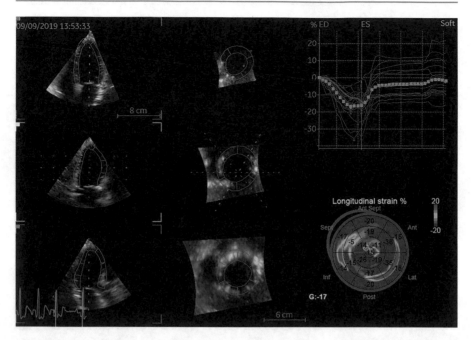

Fig. 6.5 Tetralogy of Fallot: 3D strain of the same patient with a corrected Tetralogy of Fallot

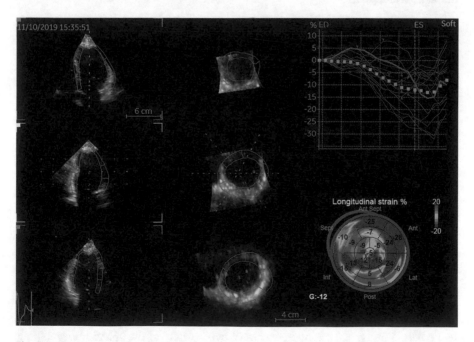

Fig. 6.6 Ebstein anomaly: 3D strain of a patient with Ebstein anomaly, highlighting the deformation of the basal septum

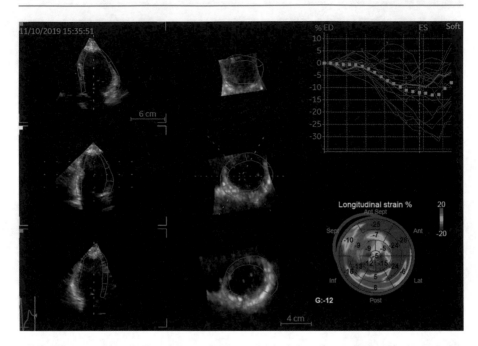

Fig. 6.7 Ebstein anomaly: 3D strain of a patient with Ebstein anomaly, highlighting the deformation of the mid-septum

lengthening during the effective ejection period, thus not contributing at all. Figure 6.6 shows the 3D deformation traces, once again illustrating the asynchronous regional deformation patterns. However, as compared to the TOF patient, where the apex is mostly involved, in EA it is predominantly the basal septum. Figure 6.6 clearly shows that the basal septum (thick yellow line amongst the traces) is being stretched throughout the ejection period and even shows prominent post-systolic shortening after aortic valve closure. This pattern originates from the accessory pathway activation and might also partly be related to some myocardial dysfunction, given that this part of the wall is atrialized at the right side. Overall, this leads to a reduced GLS of −12%.

Figure 6.7 shows the same patient but now highlighting (thick yellow line) the mid-septal deformation, showing the early 'flash' followed by clearly reduced deformation during ejection.

6.5.4 Congenitally Corrected Transposition of the Great Arteries

Figure 6.8 shows the 3D deformation of a patient with a Congenitally Corrected Transposition of the Great Arteries. There are two typical patterns present in systemic RVs. Firstly, there is often excessive hypertrophy of the apical trabeculations and moderator band (as can be seen on the apical short-axis view) which is

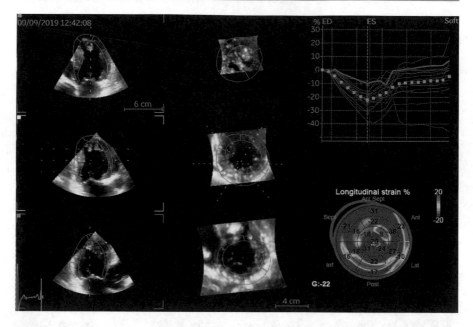

Fig. 6.8 Congenitally corrected transposition of the great arteries: 3D deformation of a patient with a CCTGA

associated with decreased deformation, not because of myocardial abnormalities but purely because of the reduced regional stroke volume associated with the full obliteration of local cavity volume in the hypertrophic trabecular region, so that no further deformation is possible. Secondly, the thereby decreased contribution to stroke volume of the apex has to be compensated by the basal segments and to maintain overall stroke volume, the base has to be dilated (as described above in volume overload). This basal dilatation results in increased wall stresses, especially in the free wall, which in turn leads to decreased deformation with PST (as seen in the basal lateral segment—thick yellow line). Note that although the basal segment is clearly abnormal, the overall GLS is still absolutely normal (−22%) in this individual.

On the longer term, this increased wall stress will lead to basal wall fibrosis and need for additional dilatation, ultimately causing the systemic RV to fail.

6.6   Conclusion

Deformation imaging, be it 2D or 3D, offers important information for the assessment of individual patients. GLS can help in risk stratification while specific regional strain patterns can help in identifying underlying aetiologies and thus aid in diagnosis and therapy planning. The temporal changes in these patterns are also ideal tools for the follow-up of patients.

Future, high frame rate 3D imaging will provide a comprehensive view on the cardiac mechanics of the whole heart.

Acknowledgements This work was partially supported by the Spanish Ministry of Economy and Competitiveness [grant TIN2014-52923-R; Maria de Maeztu Units of Excellence Programme—MDM-2015-0502] and FEDER, and the European Union H2020 programme [PIC H2020-MSCA-ITN-2017-764738].

Conflict of Interest BB received speaker fees from GE Healthcare. However, these did not influence the contents of this chapter, which was independently designed and did not involve any sponsorship.

References

1. Garcia D, Lantelme P, Saloux E. Introduction to speckle tracking in cardiac ultrasound imaging. In: Loizou CP, Pattichis CS, D'hooge J, editors. Handbook of speckle filtering and tracking in cardiovascular ultrasound imaging and video. London: Institution of Engineering and Technology; 2018.
2. Cheung YF. The role of 3D wall motion tracking in heart failure. Nat Rev Cardiol. 2012;9:644–57.
3. Jasaityte R, Heyde B, D'hooge J. Current state of three-dimensional myocardial strain estimation using echocardiography. J Am Soc Echocardiogr. 2013;26:15–28.
4. Amzulescu MS, De Craene M, Langet H, Pasquet A, Vancraeynest D, Pouleur AC, Vanoverschelde JL, Gerber BL. Myocardial strain imaging: review of general principles, validation, and sources of discrepancies. Eur Heart J Cardiovasc Imaging. 2019;20(6):605–19.
5. Bijnens B, Cikes M, Butakoff C, et al. Myocardial motion and deformation: what does it tell us and how does it relate to function? Fetal Diagn Ther. 2012;32:5–16.
6. Sengupta PP, Krishnamoorthy VK, Korinek J, Narula J, Vannan MA, Lester SJ, Tajik JA, Seward JB, Khandheria BK, Belohlavek M. Left ventricular form and function revisited: applied translational science to cardiovascular ultrasound imaging. J Am Soc Echocardiogr. 2007;20:539–51.
7. Vendelin M, Bovendeerd PH, Engelbrecht J, et al. Optimizing ventricular fibers: uniform strain or stress, but not ATP consumption, leads to high efficiency. Am J Physiol Heart Circ Physiol. 2002;283:H1072–81.
8. Ashraf M, Zhou Z, Nguyen T, et al. Apex to base left ventricular twist mechanics computed from high frame rate two-dimensional and three-dimensional echocardiography: a comparison study. J Am Soc Echocardiogr. 2012;25:121–8.
9. Henson RE, Song SK, Pastorek JS, et al. Left ventricular torsion is equal in mice and humans. Am J Physiol Heart Circ Physiol. 2000;278:H1117–23.
10. Aurigemma GP, Silver KH, Priest MA, Gaasch WH. Geometric changes allow normal ejection fraction despite depressed myocardial shortening in hypertensive left ventricular hypertrophy. J Am Coll Cardiol. 1995;26:195–202.
11. Rydman R, Söderberg M, Larsen F, Caidahl K, Alam M. Echocardiographic evaluation of right ventricular function in patients with acute pulmonary embolism: a study using tricuspid annular motion. Echocardiography. 2010;27:286–93.
12. Chrustowicz A, Gackowski A, El-Massri N, Sadowski J, Piwowarska W. Preoperative right ventricular function in patients with organic mitral regurgitation. Echocardiography. 2010;27:282–5.

13. Kjaergaard J, Iversen KK, Akkan D, Møller JE, Køber LV, Torp-Pedersen C, Hassager C. Predictors of right ventricular function as measured by tricuspid annular plane systolic excursion in heart failure. Cardiovasc Ultrasound. 2009;7:51.

14. Herrmann S, Störk S, Niemann M, Lange V, Strotmann JM, Frantz S, Beer M, Gattenlöhner S, Voelker W, Ertl G, Weidemann F. Low-gradient aortic valve stenosis myocardial fibrosis and its influence on function and outcome. J Am Coll Cardiol. 2011;58:402–4.

15. Ferferieva V, Van den Bergh A, Claus P, Jasaityte R, Veulemans P, Pellens M, La Gerche A, Rademakers F, Herijgers P, D'hooge J. The relative value of strain and strain rate for defining intrinsic myocardial function. Am J Phys Heart Circ Phys. 2012;302(1):H188–95.

16. Sonne C, Sugeng L, Takeuchi M, Weinert L, Childers R, Watanabe N, Yoshida K, Mor-Avi V, Lang RM. Real-time 3-dimensional echocardiographic assessment of left ventricular dyssynchrony: pitfalls in patients with dilated cardiomyopathy. JACC Cardiovasc Imaging. 2009;2:802–12.

17. Kapetanakis S, Kearney MT, Siva A, Gall N, Cooklin M, Monaghan MJ. Real-time three-dimensional echocardiography: a novel technique to quantify global left ventricular mechanical dyssynchrony. Circulation. 2005;112:992–1000.

18. Sutherland GR, Hatle L, Claus P, D'hooge J, Bijnens BH, editors. Doppler myocardial imaging - a textbook. Hasselt: BSWK; 2006.

19. Bijnens BH, Cikes M, Claus P, Sutherland GR. Velocity and deformation imaging for the assessment of myocardial dysfunction. Eur J Echocardiogr. 2009;10:216–26.

20. Weidemann F, Dommke C, Bijnens B, Claus P, D'hooge J, Mertens P, Verbeken E, Maes A, Van de Werf F, De Scheerder I, Sutherland GR. Defining the transmurality of a chronic myocardial infarction by ultrasonic strain rate imaging. The implications for identifying intramural viability - an experimental study. Circulation. 2003;107:883–8.

21. Kowalski M, Herbots L, Weidemann F, Breithardt O, Strotmann J, Davidavicius G, D'hooge J, Claus P, Bijnens B, Herregods MC, Sutherland GR. One-dimensional ultrasonic strain and strain rate imaging: a new approach to the quantitation of regional myocardial function in patients with aortic stenosis. Ultrasound Med Biol. 2003;29:1085–92.

22. Ishii T, McElhinney DB, Harrild DM, Marcus EN, Sahn DJ, Truong U, Tworetzky W. Circumferential and longitudinal ventricular strain in the normal human fetus. J Am Soc Echocardiogr. 2012;25:105. PubMed PMID: 22033231.

23. Van Mieghem T, Giusca S, DeKoninck P, Gucciardo L, Doné E, Hindryckx A, D'Hooge J, Deprest J. Prospective assessment of fetal cardiac function with speckle tracking in healthy fetuses and recipient fetuses of twin-to-twin transfusion syndrome. J Am Soc Echocardiogr. 2010;23:301–8.

24. Vyas HV, Eidem BW, Cetta F, Acharya G, Huhta J, Roberson D, Cuneo B. Myocardial tissue Doppler velocities in fetuses with hypoplastic left heart syndrome. Ann Pediatr Cardiol. 2011;4:129–34.

25. Comas M, Crispi F, Cruz-Martinez R, Figueras F, Gratacos E. Tissue Doppler echocardiographic markers of cardiac dysfunction in small-for-gestational age fetuses. Am J Obstet Gynecol. 2011;205:57.e1. PubMed PMID: 21620362.

26. Godfrey ME, Messing B, Cohen SM, Valsky DV, Yagel S. Functional assessment of the fetal heart: a review. Ultrasound Obstet Gynecol. 2012;39:131–44.

27. Crispi F, Bijnens B, Figueras F, Bartrons J, Eixarch E, Le Noble F, Ahmed A, Gratacós E. Fetal growth restriction results in remodeled and less efficient hearts in children. Circulation. 2010;121:2427–36.

28. Cikes M, Solomon SD. Beyond ejection fraction: an integrative approach for assessment of cardiac structure and function in heart failure. Eur Heart J. 2016;37:1642–50.

29. Bijnens B, Claus P, Weidemann F, Strotmann J, Sutherland GR. Investigating cardiac function using motion and deformation analysis in the setting of coronary artery disease. Circulation. 2007;116:2453–64.

30. Mertens L, Weidemann F, Sutherland GR. Left ventricular function before and after repair of an anomalous left coronary artery arising from the pulmonary trunk. Cardiol Young. 2001;11:79–83.

31. Claus P, Weidemann F, Dommke C, Bito V, Heinzel FR, D'hooge J, Sipido KR, Sutherland GR, Bijnens B. Mechanisms of postsystolic thickening in ischemic myocardium: mathematical modelling and comparison with experimental ischemic substrates. Ultrasound Med Biol. 2007;33:1963–70.

32. Weidemann F, Niemann M, Herrmann S, Kung M, Störk S, Waller C, Beer M, Breunig F, Wanner C, Voelker W, Ertl G, Bijnens B, Strotmann JM. A new echocardiographic approach for the detection of non-ischaemic fibrosis in hypertrophic myocardium. Eur Heart J. 2007;28(24):3020–6.

33. Baltabaeva A, Marciniak M, Bijnens B, Moggridge J, He FJ, Antonios TF, MacGregor GA, Sutherland GR. Regional left ventricular deformation and geometry analysis provides insights in myocardial remodelling in mild to moderate hyper-tension. Eur J Echocardiogr. 2008;9:501–8.

34. Marciniak A, Claus P, Sutherland GR, Marciniak M, Karu T, Baltabaeva A, Merli E, Bijnens B, Jahangiri M. Changes in systolic left ventricular function in isolated mitral regurgitation. A strain rate imaging study. Eur Heart J. 2007;28:2627–36.

35. Cikes M, Kalinic H, Hermann S, Lange V, Loncaric S, Milicic D, Beer M, Cikes I, Weidemann F, Bijnens B. Does the aortic velocity profile in aortic stenosis patients reflect more than stenosis severity? The impact of myocardial fibrosis on aortic flow symmetry. Eur Heart J. 2009;30(Suppl 1):605.

36. Choi HF, Rademakers FE, Claus P. Left-ventricular shape determines intramyocardial mechanical heterogeneity. Am J Physiol Heart Circ Physiol. 2011;301:H2351. PubMed PMID: 21949116.

37. Cikes M, Sutherland GR, Anderson LJ, Bijnens BH. The role of echocardiographic deformation imaging in hypertrophic myopathies. Nat Rev Cardiol. 2010;7:384–96.

38. Weidemann F, Breunig F, Beer M, Sandstede J, Störk S, Voelker W, Ertl G, Knoll A, Wanner C, Strotmann JM. The variation of morphological and function-al cardiac manifestation in Fabry disease: potential implications for the time course of the disease. Eur Heart J. 2005;26:1221–7.

39. Parsai C, Bijnens B, Sutherland GR, Baltabaeva A, Claus P, Marciniak M, Paul V, Scheffer M, Donal E, Derumeaux G, Anderson L. Toward understanding response to cardiac resynchronization therapy: left ventricular dyssynchrony is only one of multiple mechanisms. Eur Heart J. 2009;30:940–9.

40. Hui W, Slorach C, Dragulescu A, Mertens L, Bijnens B, Friedberg MK. Mechanisms of right ventricular electromechanical dyssynchrony and mechanical inefficiency in children after repair of tetralogy of Fallot. Circ Cardiovasc Imaging. 2014;7(4):610–8.

41. Yim D, Hui W, Larios G, Dragulescu A, Grosse-Wortmann L, Bijnens B, Mertens L, Friedberg MK. Quantification of right ventricular electromechanical dyssynchrony in relation to right ventricular function and clinical outcomes in children with repaired tetralogy of fallot. J Am Soc Echocardiogr. 2018;31(7):822–30.

42. Fujioka T, Kühn A, Sanchez-Martinez S, Bijnens BH, Hui W, Slorach C, Roehlig C, Mertens L, Vogt M, Friedberg MK. Impact of interventricular interactions on left ventricular function, stroke volume, and exercise capacity in children and adults with Ebstein's anomaly. JACC Cardiovasc Imaging. 2019;12(5):925–7.

Cardiac Mechanics II: 2D and 3D Tissue Tracking MRI

7

Andreas Schuster and Torben Lange

7.1 Introduction

Precise assessment and quantification of cardiac function is an important everyday tool in clinical routine. Cardiac magnetic resonance (CMR) imaging has emerged as a reference standard for noninvasive measurements of both myocardial morphology and functional performance [1–3]. Usually cardiac function is assessed using volumetric assessments and probably to date left ventricular ejection fraction (LV-EF) is most commonly used for cardiac performance analysis. However, LV-EF fails to describe regional changes and there is evidence to suggest that parameters that estimate myocardial deformation such as myocardial strain may be of greater value [4]. Since one of the first descriptions of CMR-based deformation analyses in 1988 by Zerhouni et al. [5], techniques have evolved considerably and CMR-based tissue tracking or feature-tracking (CMR-FT) imaging biomarkers like myocardial strain and strain rate (SR) are gaining importance and have various applications in clinical routine. Myocardial strain describes contraction and its respective direction, which provides insights into functional properties such as myofiber orientation and electrical activation patterns [6]. Theoretically, global and regional information can be obtained to describe myocardial performance in its entirety. However, since most techniques rely on two-dimensional (2D) assessments, information of features leaving the imaging space during the cardiac cycle may be lost. Notwithstanding, extensive development aims to improve MRI techniques and to advance software algorithms to achieve three-dimensional (3D) data to overcome this limitation and increase clinical use [7]. This chapter summarizes basic principles of CMR-FT, its

A. Schuster (✉) · T. Lange
Department of Cardiology and Pneumology, University Medical Center Göttingen, Georg-August University Göttingen and German Centre for Cardiovascular Research (DZHK), Partner Site Göttingen, Göttingen, Germany
e-mail: andreas.schuster@med.uni-goettingen.de; torben.lange@med.uni-goettingen.de

© Springer Nature Switzerland AG 2021
P. Gallego, I. Valverde (eds.), *Multimodality Imaging Innovations In Adult Congenital Heart Disease*, Congenital Heart Disease in Adolescents and Adults,
https://doi.org/10.1007/978-3-030-61927-5_7

current fields of application, and clinical benefits of FT-derived parameters and provides perspectives on new emerging 3D FT techniques and their future implementation in CMR post-processing.

7.2   Basic Principles

CMR-FT is performed on SSFP images that are routinely acquired during a standard CMR scan protocol and therefore do not require additional MRI sequences [8]. ECG-gated SSFP images yield high contrast between blood pool and myocardium and subsequently allow accurate assessment of ventricular myocardial function [9]. CMR-FT is based on optical flow technology, measuring motion vectors of tracked points within one or more dimensions during a cardiac cycle [10]. To ensure border tracking as precisely as possible, initial manual tracing of epi- and/or endocardial borders is usually necessary. The software's semi-automatic algorithm then tracks the border and its displacement frame by frame over the whole cardiac cycle. For this purpose, similar to echocardiographic M-mode, FT algorithms generate one-dimensional transmural cuts that are orthogonally orientated to the manual feature delineation. In this way, motion profiles of cavity-tissue interfaces can be calculated by opposing spatial movement to a timeline and subsequently tallying up several instants at once in a 2D representation by hierarchical algorithms (Fig. 7.1). For precise FT, the algorithm processes a variety of data comprising periodicity and type of motion, spatial coherence, signal/noise ratio, frame rate, temporal and spatial resolution [11]. This information is then used to flexibly adapt the size of the search window for optimal pixel/feature identification providing quantification of time-depending positional changes. These positional feature changes can then be utilized to calculate the following parameters: Left and right ventricular (LV and RV) and atrial longitudinal strains are calculated in long-axis views, while LV circumferential and radial strains are calculated in short-axis orientations. Alongside all strain parameters the respective time derivations or strain rates can be quantified. Furthermore, tissue velocity, rotational movements (angle of feature change between systole and diastole in respect to the center of gravity), and circumferential and radial uniformity ratio estimates (CURE and RURE; strain plotted against spatial position and resulting oscillations within the plots representing myocardial dyssynchrony) are typical CMR-FT-derived data that can be collected (Fig. 7.2) [11–13]. Although FT was initially developed for 2D images, new approaches using modified algorithms now allow the analysis of 3D models [14]. These ongoing developments lead to growing interest and application in clinical studies.

7.3   Established Clinical Applications

In order to establish CMR-FT-derived myocardial strain as a biomarker in clinical routine, normal values and benchmarks have been determined in the adult [15, 16] and congenital populations [17]. Since different FT algorithms are commercially

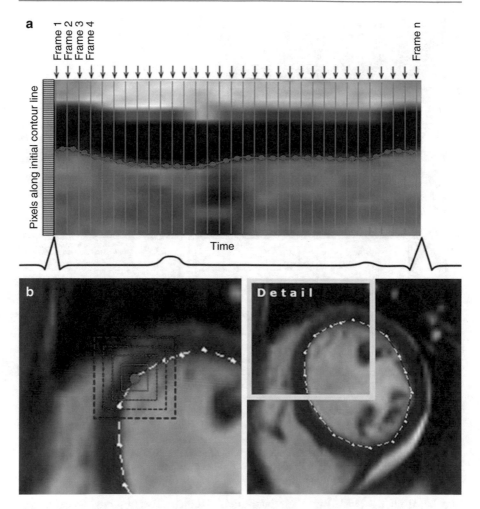

Fig. 7.1 Technical considerations of feature tracking. (**a**) Space-time presentation in one dimension. Space is displayed along a transmural cut and a single feature is one-dimensionally tracked over one cardiac cycle. (**b**) Space-time presentation in two dimensions. The search window is defined where tissue is tracked frame by frame and detection of planar motion is achieved by progressively reducing the search window in two dimensions. (Figure adapted from Schuster et al. (9) with kind permission of the copyright owner)

provided by several software developers, a variety of FT software solutions are available and numerous inter-vendor studies have been performed [18–20]. Although values partially differ between software vendors revealing limitations in inter-vendor comparability, the general and especially global reproducibility of CMR-FT-derived strain parameters within a given post-processing type is excellent [21, 22].

In addition to LV and RV strain and SR measurements, CMR-FT enables quantification of myocardial torsion and diastolic recoil. This is based on the difference in apical and basal rotation calculated from angular voxel displacement in apical

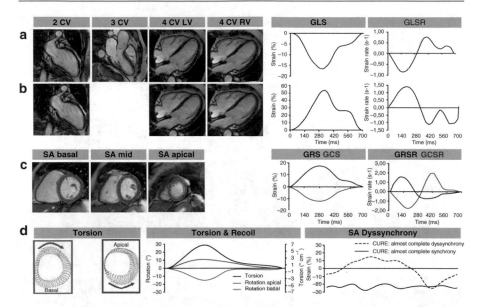

Fig. 7.2 Cardiovascular magnetic resonance-feature tracking (CMR-FT) for quantification of strain and strain rate (SR). Exemplary tracking of left ventricular long-axis views generating GLS and GLSR values (**a**) as well as left and right atrial functional strain and SR measures (**b**). Using short-axis stacks, quantification of GCS (red line)/GRS (black line) as well as GCSR and GRSR values can be performed (**c**). (**d**) SA-based myocardial torsion with clockwise basal (green) and counterclockwise apical (blue) rotation divided by the distance between both slices generates myocardial torsion. Myocardial dyssynchrony is expressed by oscillations of circumferential strain plotted against spatial positions. Values of exemplary CURE range between 0 and 1 with 0 representing complete dyssynchrony and 1 perfect synchrony. *CV* chamber view, *CURE* circumferential uniformity ratio estimate, *GCS* global circumferential strain, *GCSR* global circumferential strain rate, *GLS* global longitudinal strain, *GLSR* global longitudinal strain rate, *GRS* global radial strain, *GRSR* global radial strain rate, *SA* short axis, *SR* strain rate

and basal slices divided by their inter-slice distance. The obtained twisting and untwisting information of the myocardium allows both systolic and diastolic function evaluation [12, 23]. Further, detailed atrial function assessments by atrial longitudinal strain and SR analyses have been established [24, 25] and by applying these and the latter analyses comprehensive and contiguous deformation evaluations of all four cardiac chambers performed at rest or during different types of stress are easily obtained [26] (Fig. 7.2).

CMR-FT can be applied in a wide range of cardiac abnormalities and diseases with proven feasibility and clinical usefulness. The technique's strain analyses have been performed in different cardiomyopathies like dilated and hypertrophic cardiomyopathy (DCM and HCM) [27, 28], arrhythmogenic right ventricular cardiomyopathy (ARVC) [29], or Takotsubo cardiomyopathy [30], revealing typical deformation patterns with diagnostic and prognostic implications. Especially in ischemic cardiomyopathy and coronary artery disease (CAD), CMR-FT strain imaging was shown to hold the potential for accurate measurement of contractile reserve [31, 32]. In this way, hibernating myocardium can be detected during low-dose dobutamine stress, giving noninvasive insights with clinical relevance for further therapeutic management of CAD.

In patients with valvular heart disease and changed pre- and afterload conditions leading to fibrotic remodeling processes, CMR-FT has proven useful for analyzing myocardial remodeling [33] with FT-derived strain values showing correlation with different subtypes of aortic stenosis and predicting remodeling after valve replacement in these patients [34]. Furthermore, irrespective of symptom severity, CMR-FT strain might constitute an important parameter for selection of an optimal time point of aortic valve replacement [35]. Likewise, CMR-FT can be applied in other valvular disorders, e.g., pulmonary stenosis in tetralogy of Fallot or mitral regurgitation before and after interventional or surgical treatment for prediction and assessment of functional therapeutic success [36, 37]. Figure 7.3 demonstrates various clinical applications of CMR-FT-derived strain analyses. With a wide range of clinical patterns and unspecific symptoms, diagnosis of myocarditis is challenging and CMR imaging plays a particular role in respective diagnostic algorithms. CMR-FT-derived analysis has emerged as an appropriate tool for detection of myocarditis with exceeding accuracy compared to established parameters such as the Lake Louise Criteria (LLC) [38]. In this context, myocardial FT-derived strain analyses offer improved diagnostic performance especially when combined with LLC parameters [39–41]. Moreover, even in relatively rare diseases that can affect the myocardium like Marfan syndrome or systemic sclerosis, CMR-FT assessments have been applied and results underline the sensitivity of FT-derived strain measurements in these patient collectives. Both in Marfan syndrome [42] and in patients diagnosed with asymptomatic systemic sclerosis, impaired FT-derived strain enables identification of systolic dysfunction due to myocardial affection [43]. It is worth noting that besides the establishment of CMR-FT in adult cardiology, the scope of application also comprises pediatric and congenital assessments [44]. These include different congenital heart defects [45–48], hypertrophic cardiomyopathy [49], or other illnesses potentially affecting the myocardium, i.e., Duchenne muscular dystrophy [50] or Kawasaki disease [51].

FT-derived parameters are independent and relevant imaging biomarkers. This relevance has been determined in comparison to established CMR parameters such as LV-EF, which is still recommended by many guidelines for clinical management and treatment guidance. In ARVC early LV affection and respective changes of LV myocardial strain were documented before the presence of LV-EF reduction [52]. Likewise, reduced FT-derived strain values in patients after effective repair of aortic coarctation might indicate early LV dysfunction despite normal or preserved LV-EF [47]. Furthermore, CMR-FT-derived strain can be used as sensitive therapy monitoring parameters of cardiotoxicity during chemotherapy [53]. Left atrial (LA) strain represents a promising approach for quantifying consequences of insufficient control of blood pressure even before the occurrence of structural myocardial alterations such as left ventricular hypertrophy in patients with arterial hypertension [54]. Similar observations were made in patients with pulmonary hypertension [55]. With the rise of ventricular filling pressures, atrial function is

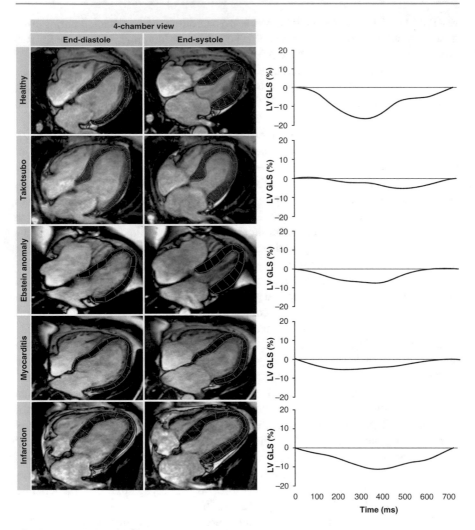

Fig. 7.3 CMR-FT in different diseases. Left ventricular (LV) epi- and endocardial borders are tracked in end-diastole and -systole; corresponding strain graphs displaying global longitudinal strain (GLS) over a whole cardiac cycle are displayed

particularly affected in patients with heart failure with preserved ejection fraction (HFpEF). In this context impaired LA strain was identified as a potential mechanism for decreased exercise capacity in these patients with functional implications independent of LV stiffness and relaxation [56]. Impaired right atrial and RV interaction was also shown to be associated with reduced exercise capacity with right atrial failure being independent of invasively measured LV stiffness and relaxation in patients with HFpEF [57].

Besides advantages over LV-EF, CMR-FT-derived strain measurements might also be superior to other diagnostic modalities in detecting myocardial abnormalities earlier. For example, FT-derived myocardial strain analysis enables detection of early impairments of systolic and diastolic function of patients suffering from amyloidosis before showing typical late gadolinium enhancement (LGE) [58, 59]. Similarly, patients with myocardial involvement in Churg-Strauss syndrome and granulomatosis with polyangiitis show distinctly decreased strain values indicating disease-specific myocardial affection despite normal ECG and inconspicuous findings on echocardiography [60].

Although FT-derived parameters can serve as (early detecting) surrogate markers for altered myocardial performance, diagnostic processes in clinical routine involve a combination of various imaging, clinical, and biochemical data. Therefore, some studies combined FT-derived strain values with other data for optimized diagnostics. The combination of native T1-mapping and FT-derived strain allows a more accurate prediction of irreversible ischemic injury in patients following ST-elevation myocardial infarction (STEMI) with higher diagnostic accuracy for prediction of final infarct size than either method alone [61]. As a result, this method might be even superseding contrast agent based LGE analyses if tissue characterization based on native technology is utilized. Another multiparametric CMR imaging model merged FT-derived strain, T2 analyses, and LGE assessment, resulting in a better diagnostic accuracy in suspected acute myocarditis compared to either imaging parameter alone [62]. By combining T1, strain, and SR as well as clinical parameters, different degrees of myocardial fibrosis were accurately predicted in patients with DCM [63]. Furthermore, FT-derived strain can be used as adjunctive parameter to imaging markers like LGE or blood biomarkers like Troponin indicating myocardial involvement in patients with myocarditis [64]. There are numerous other studies demonstrating feasibility and usefulness of FT-derived parameters with additional evidence of strong prognostic implications and clinical impact.

7.4   Prognostic Implications

Besides accurate diagnostic information mounting evidence suggests a role for prognostic stratification and clinical decision-making based on CMR-FT-derived deformation analyses. Especially LV global longitudinal strain (GLS) was found to be a powerful and independent parameter for prediction of death with superiority over established parameters like left ventricular ejection fraction (EF) [65]. In patients with DCM all strain parameters were shown to have significant associations with mortality [28]. Regardless of the underlying cause for reduced LV-EF, GLS was shown to be a powerful and independent predictor of mortality both in ischemic and non-ischemic cardiomyopathies [66]. Moreover, in patients with heart failure, FT-derived GLS as well as circumferential and radial strain values were shown to enable optimized risk stratification independently of LV-EF [67]. Not only in heart failure patients with reduced ejection fraction but also in those having HFpEF FT-derived GLS showed significant associations with adverse outcome [68]. Similar results underlining the high significance and importance of

FT-derived strain values were documented in patients following acute myocardial infarction (AMI) with global LV strain parameters emerging as important and superior measurements of LV function with potential for optimized risk stratification [4, 69]. Moreover, in patients with STEMI the extent of functional recovery can be objectified by analyzing FT-derived strain estimating infarct size without the need for contrast agent [70].

Besides a wide range of LV strain parameters carrying prognostic value, both RV and moreover LA strain alterations were also shown to have prognostic significance in patients with Takotsubo syndrome [71, 72]. Furthermore, CMR-FT-derived RV strain is independently associated with poor outcome in patients with pulmonary hypertension [73]. CMR-FT-derived LA function was identified having prognostic value in patients following AMI [74] and HCM [75]. Furthermore, FT-derived LA strain has important implications as an independent parameter for predicting the occurrence of atrial dysrhythmias and adverse outcome especially after electrophysiological ablation interventions [76–78]. This also applies to ventricular tachycardia, which can be predicted in patients with repaired tetralogy of Fallot using CMR-FT-derived SR which was also shown to predict adverse outcome independently of established risk markers [79].

Recently, strain-based alterations of myocardial uniformity were identified as novel markers for dyssynchrony (CURE and RURE). These parameters have strong implications for extended risk assessment following AMI providing additional prognostic information in patients with preserved or only moderately impaired LV-EF underlining the importance of CMR-FT-based imaging parameters beyond sole consideration of LV-EF for clinical management and medical treatment [80].

In conclusion, numerous studies investigated the prognostic implications of CMR-FT-derived parameters, which demonstrate a substantial and often superior role compared with established parameters like LV-EF. If this evidence continues to rise and these parameters will find their way into future guideline recommendations and clinical management algorithms, CMR-FT will finally be implemented in routine clinical practice.

7.5   Moving Towards 3D Applications: Future Directions of FT

Besides ongoing refinements and clinical adoption of the well-established 2D CMR-FT technique, increasing development and investigation focus on novel 3D FT techniques. This was paralleled by significant advances in CMR cine technology, which led to the introduction of 3D SSFP sequences [81, 82]. Even though the CMR-FT method was initially developed for 2D image analyses, new approaches adapt and apply this technique to extend deformation analyses by the third dimension.

Theoretical advantages of 3D analyses include tracked features, that can be simultaneously traced in all directions and therefore are less prone to through or out of plane displacements of end-diastolically tracked structures during systole [83].

Moreover, 3D assessments are independent of single image planes and therefore have a clear advantage compared to 2D approaches by depicting myocardial properties considering their anatomy and physiology in 4D [6]. Especially for the evaluation of RV deformation, that is quite challenging using 2D images due to complex morphology, 3D approaches might facilitate and optimize deformation analyses [84]. In contrast to 2D acquisitions, the shear of tracked points describing the slide between tissue layers complements the deformation analysis in 3D approaches [83]. Although similar calculations describing the shear motion as myocardial twist and torsion are established in 2D FT analyses as well [12], combining as many data as available in one single analysis clearly leads to a more precise reflection of the complex myocardial deformation. Despite the fact that 3D CMR sequences are theoretically available, CMR-FT-derived strain analyses based on true 3D SSFP images remain very challenging, mainly because of limitations in spatial and temporal resolutions and a loss of contrast between blood and myocardium [85, 86]. On the other hand, even though 2D images provide good temporal and spatial resolution for strain analyses, basic limitations of 2D imaging are present and coupled with technical constraints of CMR image acquisition [87–89]. In contrast, 3D SSFP sequences have the potential to overcome several of these 2D limitations by accelerating image acquisition time [90] or enabling image reconstruction in any orientation [91]. Nevertheless, challenges for CMR-FT applications based on true 3D datasets are apparent, and future investigations need to examine if and to what extent compromises at cost of temporal and spatial resolution are reasonable and feasible to enable 3D CMR-FT in true 3D SSFP CMR images.

Notwithstanding, efforts that aim at the computation of 3D strain representations based on conventional 2D SSFP image data have been promising. This methodology includes a preceding 2D delineation of myocardial borders to enable further software-based work steps for the calculation of a deformable 3D model. At the moment, two principal options for subsequent CMR-FT strain analysis were described using 3D models (Fig. 7.4): First, after performing CMR-FT in 2D slices, a 3D deformable model is generated by interpolation of epi- and endocardial boundaries, combining 2D-derived parameters and calculating 3D-derived GLS, global circumferential strain (GCS) and global radial strain (GRS) values as they are known from 2D analyses [14, 92]. By generating common strain parameters equally to the 2D-derived measurements, the potential of comparability is given and was shown to be accurate with no statistically significant differences between 2D and 3D strain values using the interpolation method [92]. The particular advantage over a 2D projection is accurate strain estimation because in 2D twisting of the heart results in out-of-plane rotation of a myocardial segment with subsequent false appreciation of shortening and overestimation of strain [92].

The second 3D approach estimates a principal strain component that is geometry-independent and measures the dominant direction of deformation [93]. For this method, special software generates a 3D mesh model consisting of many singular quadrangular hexahedrons. Afterwards, principal strains of three orthogonal directions can be calculated. This strain is independent of conventional directions (i.e., longitudinal, circumferential, radial). Instead, maximum (representing the

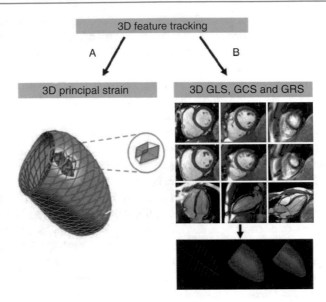

Fig. 7.4 3D-derived strain parameters. (**a**) 3D principal strain. Surface mesh models are constructed consisting of quadrangular hexahedrons enabling calculation of three orthogonally directed principal strains (this figure is modified and originally taken from Satriano et al. (91) and provided under the terms of the Creative Commons Attribution 4.0 International License (http://creativecommons.org/licenses/by/4.0/). (**b**) 3D GLS, GCS, and GRS. After defining endo- and epicardial borders in 2D short- and long-axes slices, a 3D model is generated with global longitudinal (GLS), circumferential (GCS), and radial (GRS) strain values interpolated from 2D analysis. (This figure is modified and originally taken from Liu et al. (12) and provided under the terms of the Creative Commons Attribution 4.0 International License (http://creativecommons.org/licenses/by/4.0/)

maximum of thickening/lengthening), minimum (representing maximum of shortening), and intermediate (dependent on maximum and minimum strain) principal strain values can be derived. In this way, a comprehensive 3D FT-derived strain analysis, which most likely complies with correct anatomical movement, is possible and generates data that were documented to be highly reproducible as well as shown to be strongly correlating with conventional 2D strain values [93] (Fig. 7.5). In this context, a general advantage of calculating a principal strain comprising multidirectional deformation was documented in an animal study using CMR tagging. This model allowed superior identification of infarcted myocardium compared to 2D assessments [94]. With regard to the restricted comparability of conventional FT-derived GLS, GCS, and GRS, these considerations raise a general question, whether new strain parameters, like the mentioned principal strain, are essential and more appropriate for advanced 3D methodology.

Since 2D-based 3D CMR-FT evaluation methods provide various additional information that cannot be obtained from sole 2D FT analyses, consequently first implementations of 3D CMR-FT for clinical evaluation have been performed. For example, 3D FT-derived measurements of tricuspid annular motion analysis in patients with heart failure, repaired tetralogy of Fallot, pulmonary hypertension, and

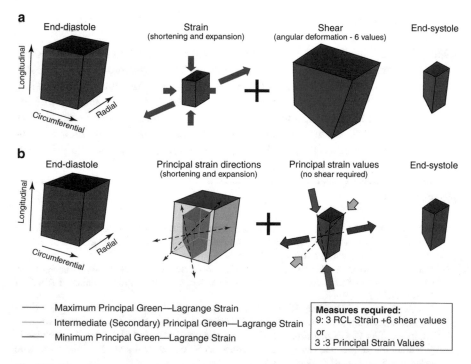

a End-diastole | Strain (shortening and expansion) | Shear (angular deformation - 6 values) | End-systole

Longitudinal / Circumferential / Radial

b End-diastole | Principal strain directions (shortening and expansion) | Principal strain values (no shear required) | End-systole

Longitudinal / Circumferential / Radial

—— Maximum Principal Green—Lagrange Strain
—— Intermediate (Secondary) Principal Green—Lagrange Strain
—— Minimum Principal Green—Lagrange Strain

Measures required:
9: 3 RCL Strain +6 shear values
or
3 :3 Principal Strain Values

Fig. 7.5 Pictorial summary of the definition of principal strain. (**a**) The deformation of a tissue element from its initial (end-diastolic) to a final (end-systolic) configuration is constituted of longitudinal and circumferential shortening, plus radial expansion (thickening) and six angular deformations (shear deformation). When using only three geometry-dependent directions (radial, circumferential, and longitudinal), strain obtained in those directions cannot account for shear and, therefore, does not offer a complete description of the strain undergone by the element. (**b**) The same deformation can be described without shear in terms of principal strain along three principal directions; these are established through a comparison of the initial and final configurations of the tissue element. (Figure by Satriano et al. (91) provided under the terms of the Creative Commons Attribution 4.0 International License http://creativecommons.org/licenses/by/4.0/)

HCM were shown to have superior diagnostic performance compared to 2D FT-derived values and showed good correlations with invasive right heart catheterization parameters [95]. In another study using new 3D-derived area strain measurements, results enabled a better assessment of treatment effects in patients with chronic thromboembolic pulmonary hypertension compared to conventional 2D FT analyses [96].

Despite these first promising examples of application, the 3D method is still going through introductory testing phases and various technical refinements are still necessary. These tasks will relate both to 3D image acquisition and to 3D FT software development to enable standardized and precise 3D deformation analyses. Thus, with a clear goal of a new powerful diagnostic and prognostic tool in sight, future efforts may enable to achieve 3D CMR-FT strain computation based on true 3D CMR datasets and establish this method in clinical practice.

7.6 Conclusion

CMR-FT techniques (mainly in 2D) are already well established in clinical routine with a wide range of applications and strong prognostic implications. At the present time, new 3D CMR-FT applications are rising and new concepts are promising. However, more adjustments and refinements are still needed to achieve full 3D CMR-FT data. If future efforts will succeed to improve the 3D technique and diagnostic as well as prognostic feasibility is demonstrated, true quantification of myocardial deformation based on 3D CMR-FT may find its way into the clinical arena.

References

1. Backhaus SJ, Staab W, Steinmetz M, et al. Fully automated quantification of biventricular volumes and function in cardiovascular magnetic resonance: applicability to clinical routine settings. J Cardiovasc Magn Reson. 2019;21:24.
2. Schuster A, Morton G, Chiribiri A, Perera D, Vanoverschelde JL, Nagel E. Imaging in the management of ischemic cardiomyopathy: special focus on magnetic resonance. J Am Coll Cardiol. 2012;59:359–70.
3. Schuster A, Lange T, Backhaus SJ, et al. Fully automated cardiac assessment for diagnostic and prognostic stratification following myocardial infarction. J Am Heart Assoc. 2020;9:e016612.
4. Reindl M, Tiller C, Holzknecht M, et al. Prognostic implications of global longitudinal strain by feature-tracking cardiac magnetic resonance in ST-elevation myocardial infarction. Circ Cardiovasc Imaging. 2019;12:e009404.
5. Zerhouni EA, Parish DM, Rogers WJ, Yang A, Shapiro EP. Human heart: tagging with MR imaging--a method for noninvasive assessment of myocardial motion. Radiology. 1988;169:59–63.
6. Hess AT, Zhong X, Spottiswoode BS, Epstein FH, Meintjes EM. Myocardial 3D strain calculation by combining cine displacement encoding with stimulated echoes (DENSE) and cine strain encoding (SENC) imaging. Magn Reson Med. 2009;62:77–84.
7. Smiseth OA, Torp H, Opdahl A, Haugaa KH, Urheim S. Myocardial strain imaging: how useful is it in clinical decision making? Eur Heart J. 2016;37:1196–207.
8. Backhaus SJ, Metschies G, Zieschang V, et al. Head-to-head comparison of cardiovascular MR feature tracking cine versus acquisition-based deformation strain imaging using myocardial tagging and strain encoding. Magn Reson Med. 2021;85:357.
9. Thiele H, Paetsch I, Schnackenburg B, et al. Improved accuracy of quantitative assessment of left ventricular volume and ejection fraction by geometric models with steady-state free precession. J Cardiovasc Magn Reson. 2002;4:327–39.
10. Dougherty L, Asmuth JC, Blom AS, Axel L, Kumar R. Validation of an optical flow method for tag displacement estimation. IEEE Trans Med Imaging. 1999;18:359–63.
11. Schuster A, Hor KN, Kowallick JT, Beerbaum P, Kutty S. Cardiovascular magnetic resonance myocardial feature tracking: concepts and clinical applications. Circ Cardiovasc Imaging. 2016;9:e004077.
12. Kowallick JT, Lamata P, Hussain ST, et al. Quantification of left ventricular torsion and diastolic recoil using cardiovascular magnetic resonance myocardial feature tracking. PLoS One. 2014;9:e109164.
13. Kowallick JT, Morton G, Lamata P, et al. Quantitative assessment of left ventricular mechanical dyssynchrony using cine cardiovascular magnetic resonance imaging: inter-study reproducibility. JRSM Cardiovasc Dis. 2017;6:2048004017710142.
14. Liu B, Dardeer AM, Moody WE, et al. Reference ranges for three-dimensional feature tracking cardiac magnetic resonance: comparison with two-dimensional methodology and relevance of age and gender. Int J Card Imaging. 2018;34:761–75.

15. Taylor RJ, Moody WE, Umar F, et al. Myocardial strain measurement with feature-tracking cardiovascular magnetic resonance: normal values. Eur Heart J Cardiovasc Imaging. 2015;16:871–81.
16. Andre F, Steen H, Matheis P, et al. Age- and gender-related normal left ventricular deformation assessed by cardiovascular magnetic resonance feature tracking. J Cardiovasc Magn Reson. 2015;17:25.
17. Shang Q, Patel S, Steinmetz M, et al. Myocardial deformation assessed by longitudinal strain: chamber specific normative data for CMR-feature tracking from the German competence network for congenital heart defects. Eur Radiol. 2018;28:1257–66.
18. Gertz RJ, Lange T, Kowallick JT, et al. Inter-vendor reproducibility of left and right ventricular cardiovascular magnetic resonance myocardial feature-tracking. PLoS One. 2018;13:e0193746.
19. Schuster A, Stahnke VC, Unterberg-Buchwald C, et al. Cardiovascular magnetic resonance feature-tracking assessment of myocardial mechanics: intervendor agreement and considerations regarding reproducibility. Clin Radiol. 2015;70:989–98.
20. Dobrovie M, Barreiro-Perez M, Curione D, et al. Inter-vendor reproducibility and accuracy of segmental left ventricular strain measurements using CMR feature tracking. Eur Radiol. 2019;29:6846.
21. Barreiro-Perez M, Curione D, Symons R, Claus P, Voigt JU, Bogaert J. Left ventricular global myocardial strain assessment comparing the reproducibility of four commercially available CMR-feature tracking algorithms. Eur Radiol. 2018;28:5137–47.
22. Morton G, Schuster A, Jogiya R, Kutty S, Beerbaum P, Nagel E. Inter-study reproducibility of cardiovascular magnetic resonance myocardial feature tracking. J Cardiovasc Magn Reson. 2012;14:43.
23. Steinmetz M, Usenbenz S, Kowallick JT, et al. Left ventricular synchrony, torsion, and recoil mechanics in Ebstein's anomaly: insights from cardiovascular magnetic resonance. J Cardiovasc Magn Reson. 2017;19:101.
24. Kowallick JT, Kutty S, Edelmann F, et al. Quantification of left atrial strain and strain rate using Cardiovascular Magnetic Resonance myocardial feature tracking: a feasibility study. J Cardiovasc Magn Reson. 2014;16:60.
25. Truong VT, Palmer C, Wolking S, et al. Normal left atrial strain and strain rate using cardiac magnetic resonance feature tracking in healthy volunteers. Eur Heart J Cardiovasc Imaging. 2020;21:446.
26. Schuster A, Kutty S, Padiyath A, et al. Cardiovascular magnetic resonance myocardial feature tracking detects quantitative wall motion during dobutamine stress. J Cardiovasc Magn Reson. 2011;13:58.
27. Neisius U, Myerson L, Fahmy AS, et al. Cardiovascular magnetic resonance feature tracking strain analysis for discrimination between hypertensive heart disease and hypertrophic cardiomyopathy. PLoS One. 2019;14:e0221061.
28. Buss SJ, Breuninger K, Lehrke S, et al. Assessment of myocardial deformation with cardiac magnetic resonance strain imaging improves risk stratification in patients with dilated cardiomyopathy. Eur Heart J Cardiovasc Imaging. 2015;16:307–15.
29. Bourfiss M, Vigneault DM, Aliyari Ghasebeh M, et al. Feature tracking CMR reveals abnormal strain in preclinical arrhythmogenic right ventricular dysplasia/cardiomyopathy: a multisoftware feasibility and clinical implementation study. J Cardiovasc Magn Reson. 2017;19:66.
30. Stiermaier T, Lange T, Chiribiri A, et al. Left ventricular myocardial deformation in Takotsubo syndrome: a cardiovascular magnetic resonance myocardial feature tracking study. Eur Radiol. 2018;28:5160–70.
31. Schuster A, Paul M, Bettencourt N, et al. Cardiovascular magnetic resonance myocardial feature tracking for quantitative viability assessment in ischemic cardiomyopathy. Int J Cardiol. 2013;166:413–20.
32. Schneeweis C, Qiu J, Schnackenburg B, et al. Value of additional strain analysis with feature tracking in dobutamine stress cardiovascular magnetic resonance for detecting coronary artery disease. J Cardiovasc Magn Reson. 2014;16:72.

33. Podlesnikar T, Delgado V, Bax JJ. Cardiovascular magnetic resonance imaging to assess myo-cardial fibrosis in valvular heart disease. Int J Card Imaging. 2018;34:97–112.
34. Buckert D, Cieslik M, Tibi R, et al. Longitudinal strain assessed by cardiac magnetic resonance correlates to hemodynamic findings in patients with severe aortic stenosis and predicts positive remodeling after transcatheter aortic valve replacement. Clin Res Cardiol. 2018;107:20–9.
35. Al Musa T, Uddin A, Swoboda PP, et al. Myocardial strain and symptom severity in severe aortic stenosis: insights from cardiovascular magnetic resonance. Quant Imaging Med Surg. 2017;7:38–47.
36. Lurz P, Serpytis R, Blazek S, et al. Assessment of acute changes in ventricular volumes, func-tion, and strain after interventional edge-to-edge repair of mitral regurgitation using cardiac magnetic resonance imaging. Eur Heart J Cardiovasc Imaging. 2015;16:1399–404.
37. Balasubramanian S, Harrild DM, Kerur B, et al. Impact of surgical pulmonary valve replace-ment on ventricular strain and synchrony in patients with repaired tetralogy of Fallot: a cardio-vascular magnetic resonance feature tracking study. J Cardiovasc Magn Reson. 2018;20:37.
38. Kotanidis CP, Bazmpani MA, Haidich AB, Karvounis C, Antoniades C, Karamitsos TD. Diagnostic accuracy of cardiovascular magnetic resonance in acute myocarditis: a sys-tematic review and meta-analysis. JACC Cardiovasc Imaging. 2018;11:1583–90.
39. Dick A, Schmidt B, Michels G, Bunck AC, Maintz D, Baessler B. Left and right atrial feature tracking in acute myocarditis: a feasibility study. Eur J Radiol. 2017;89:72–80.
40. Luetkens JA, Schlesinger-Irsch U, Kuetting DL, et al. Feature-tracking myocardial strain analysis in acute myocarditis: diagnostic value and association with myocardial oedema. Eur Radiol. 2017;27:4661–71.
41. Doerner J, Bunck AC, Michels G, Maintz D, Baessler B. Incremental value of cardiovascular magnetic resonance feature tracking derived atrial and ventricular strain parameters in a com-prehensive approach for the diagnosis of acute myocarditis. Eur J Radiol. 2018;104:120–8.
42. Winther S, Williams LK, Keir M, et al. Cardiovascular magnetic resonance provides evidence of abnormal myocardial strain and primary cardiomyopathy in Marfan syndrome. J Comput Assist Tomogr. 2019;43:410–5.
43. Bratis K, Lindholm A, Hesselstrand R, et al. CMR feature tracking in cardiac asymptomatic systemic sclerosis: clinical implications. PLoS One. 2019;14:e0221021.
44. Andre F, Robbers-Visser D, Helling-Bakki A, et al. Quantification of myocardial deformation in children by cardiovascular magnetic resonance feature tracking: determination of reference values for left ventricular strain and strain rate. J Cardiovasc Magn Reson. 2016;19:8.
45. Burkhardt BEU, Kellenberger CJ, Franzoso FD, Geiger J, Oxenius A, Valsangiacomo Buechel ER. Right and left ventricular strain patterns after the atrial switch operation for D-transposition of the great arteries-a magnetic resonance feature tracking study. Front Cardiovasc Med. 2019;6:39.
46. Steinmetz M, Broder M, Hosch O, et al. Atrio-ventricular deformation and heart failure in Ebstein's anomaly - a cardiovascular magnetic resonance study. Int J Cardiol. 2018;257:54–61.
47. Kutty S, Rangamani S, Venkataraman J, et al. Reduced global longitudinal and radial strain with normal left ventricular ejection fraction late after effective repair of aortic coarctation: a CMR feature tracking study. Int J Card Imaging. 2013;29:141–50.
48. Padiyath A, Gribben P, Abraham JR, et al. Echocardiography and cardiac magnetic resonance-based feature tracking in the assessment of myocardial mechanics in tetralogy of Fallot: an intermodality comparison. Echocardiography. 2013;30:203–10.
49. Bogarapu S, Puchalski MD, Everitt MD, Williams RV, Weng HY, Menon SC. Novel cardiac magnetic resonance feature tracking (CMR-FT) analysis for detection of myocardial fibrosis in pediatric hypertrophic cardiomyopathy. Pediatr Cardiol. 2016;37:663–73.
50. Siegel B, Olivieri L, Gordish-Dressman H, Spurney CF. Myocardial strain using cardiac MR feature tracking and speckle tracking echocardiography in Duchenne muscular dystrophy patients. Pediatr Cardiol. 2018;39:478–83.
51. Bratis K, Hachmann P, Child N, et al. Cardiac magnetic resonance feature tracking in Kawasaki disease convalescence. Ann Pediatr Cardiol. 2017;10:18–25.

52. Chen X, Li L, Cheng H, et al. Early left ventricular involvement detected by cardiovascular magnetic resonance feature tracking in arrhythmogenic right ventricular cardiomyopathy: the effects of left ventricular late gadolinium enhancement and right ventricular dysfunction. J Am Heart Assoc. 2019;8:e012989.
53. Gong IY, Ong G, Brezden-Masley C, et al. Early diastolic strain rate measurements by cardiac MRI in breast cancer patients treated with trastuzumab: a longitudinal study. Int J Card Imaging. 2019;35:653–62.
54. Li L, Chen X, Yin G, et al. Early detection of left atrial dysfunction assessed by CMR feature tracking in hypertensive patients. Eur Radiol. 2020;30:702.
55. Kallianos K, Brooks GC, Mukai K, et al. Cardiac magnetic resonance evaluation of left ventricular myocardial strain in pulmonary hypertension. Acad Radiol. 2018;25:129–35.
56. von Roeder M, Rommel KP, Kowallick JT, et al. Influence of left atrial function on exercise capacity and left ventricular function in patients with heart failure and preserved ejection fraction. Circ Cardiovasc Imaging. 2017;10:e005467.
57. von Roeder M, Kowallick JT, Rommel KP, et al. Right atrial-right ventricular coupling in heart failure with preserved ejection fraction. Clin Res Cardiol. 2020;109:54.
58. Kuetting DL, Homsi R, Sprinkart AM, et al. Quantitative assessment of systolic and diastolic function in patients with LGE negative systemic amyloidosis using CMR. Int J Cardiol. 2017;232:336–41.
59. Nucifora G, Muser D, Morocutti G, et al. Disease-specific differences of left ventricular rotational mechanics between cardiac amyloidosis and hypertrophic cardiomyopathy. Am J Physiol Heart Circ Physiol. 2014;307:H680–8.
60. Miszalski-Jamka T, Szczeklik W, Sokolowska B, et al. Standard and feature tracking magnetic resonance evidence of myocardial involvement in Churg-Strauss syndrome and granulomatosis with polyangiitis (Wegener's) in patients with normal electrocardiograms and transthoracic echocardiography. Int J Card Imaging. 2013;29:843–53.
61. Wamil M, Borlotti A, Liu D, et al. Combined T1-mapping and tissue tracking analysis predicts severity of ischemic injury following acute STEMI-an Oxford Acute Myocardial Infarction (OxAMI) study. Int J Card Imaging. 2019;35:1297–308.
62. Baessler B, Treutlein M, Schaarschmidt F, et al. A novel multiparametric imaging approach to acute myocarditis using T2-mapping and CMR feature tracking. J Cardiovasc Magn Reson. 2017;19:71.
63. Mazurkiewicz L, Petryka J, Spiewak M, et al. Biventricular mechanics in prediction of severe myocardial fibrosis in patients with dilated cardiomyopathy: CMR study. Eur J Radiol. 2017;91:71–81.
64. Weigand J, Nielsen JC, Sengupta PP, Sanz J, Srivastava S, Uppu S. Feature tracking-derived peak systolic strain compared to late gadolinium enhancement in troponin-positive myocarditis: a case-control study. Pediatr Cardiol. 2016;37:696–703.
65. Romano S, Judd RM, Kim RJ, et al. Association of feature-tracking cardiac magnetic resonance imaging left ventricular global longitudinal strain with all-cause mortality in patients with reduced left ventricular ejection fraction. Circulation. 2017;135:2313–5.
66. Romano S, Judd RM, Kim RJ, et al. Feature-tracking global longitudinal strain predicts death in a multicenter population of patients with ischemic and nonischemic dilated cardiomyopathy incremental to ejection fraction and late gadolinium enhancement. JACC Cardiovasc Imaging. 2018;11:1419–29.
67. Sardana M, Konda P, Hashmath Z, et al. Usefulness of left ventricular strain by cardiac magnetic resonance feature-tracking to predict cardiovascular events in patients with and without heart failure. Am J Cardiol. 2019;123:1301–8.
68. Kammerlander AA, Kraiger JA, Nitsche C, et al. Global longitudinal strain by CMR feature tracking is associated with outcome in HFPEF. JACC Cardiovasc Imaging. 2019;12:1585–7.
69. Eitel I, Stiermaier T, Lange T, et al. Cardiac magnetic resonance myocardial feature tracking for optimized prediction of cardiovascular events following myocardial infarction. JACC Cardiovasc Imaging. 2018;11:1433–44.

70. Buss SJ, Krautz B, Hofmann N, et al. Prediction of functional recovery by cardiac mag-
    netic resonance feature tracking imaging in first time ST-elevation myocardial infarction.
    Comparison to infarct size and transmurality by late gadolinium enhancement. Int J Cardiol.
    2015;183:162–70.
71. Stiermaier T, Lange T, Chiribiri A, et al. Right ventricular strain assessment by cardiovas-
    cular magnetic resonance myocardial feature tracking allows optimized risk stratification in
    Takotsubo syndrome. PLoS One. 2018;13:e0202146.
72. Backhaus SJ, Stiermaier T, Lange T, et al. Atrial mechanics and their prognostic impact in
    Takotsubo syndrome: a cardiovascular magnetic resonance imaging study. Eur Heart J
    Cardiovasc Imaging. 2019;20:1059–69.
73. de Siqueira ME, Pozo E, Fernandes VR, et al. Characterization and clinical significance of
    right ventricular mechanics in pulmonary hypertension evaluated with cardiovascular mag-
    netic resonance feature tracking. J Cardiovasc Magn Reson. 2016;18:39.
74. Schuster A, Backhaus SJ, Stiermaier T, et al. Left atrial function with MRI enables predic-
    tion of cardiovascular events after myocardial infarction: insights from the AIDA STEMI and
    TATORT NSTEMI trials. Radiology. 2019;293:292–302.
75. Hinojar R, Zamorano JL, Fernandez-Mendez M, et al. Prognostic value of left atrial function
    by cardiovascular magnetic resonance feature tracking in hypertrophic cardiomyopathy. Int J
    Card Imaging. 2019;35:1055–65.
76. Gucuk Ipek E, Marine JE, Habibi M, et al. Association of left atrial function with incident
    atypical atrial flutter after atrial fibrillation ablation. Heart Rhythm. 2016;13:391–8.
77. Habibi M, Lima JAC, Gucuk Ipek E, et al. The association of baseline left atrial structure and
    function measured with cardiac magnetic resonance and pulmonary vein isolation outcome in
    patients with drug-refractory atrial fibrillation. Heart Rhythm. 2016;13:1037–44.
78. Habibi M, Zareian M, Ambale Venkatesh B, et al. Left atrial mechanical function and incident
    ischemic cerebrovascular events independent of AF: insights from the MESA study. JACC
    Cardiovasc Imaging. 2019;12:2417.
79. Orwat S, Diller GP, Kempny A, et al. Myocardial deformation parameters predict outcome in
    patients with repaired tetralogy of Fallot. Heart. 2016;102:209–15.
80. Stiermaier T, Backhaus SJ, Lange T, et al. Cardiac magnetic resonance left ventricular mechan-
    ical uniformity alterations for risk assessment after acute myocardial infarction. J Am Heart
    Assoc. 2019;8:e011576.
81. Peters DC, Ennis DB, Rohatgi P, Syed MA, McVeigh ER, Arai AE. 3D breath-held cardiac
    function with projection reconstruction in steady state free precession validated using 2D cine
    MRI. J Magn Reson Imaging. 2004;20:411–6.
82. Amano Y, Suzuki Y, van Cauteren M. Evaluation of global cardiac functional parameters using
    single-breath-hold three-dimensional cine steady-state free precession MR imaging with two
    types of speed-up techniques: comparison with two-dimensional cine imaging. Comput Med
    Imaging Graph. 2008;32:61–6.
83. Pedrizzetti G, Claus P, Kilner PJ, Nagel E. Principles of cardiovascular magnetic resonance
    feature tracking and echocardiographic speckle tracking for informed clinical use. J Cardiovasc
    Magn Reson. 2016;18:51.
84. Atsumi A, Seo Y, Ishizu T, et al. Right ventricular deformation analyses using a three-
    dimensional speckle-tracking echocardiographic system specialized for the right ventricle. J
    Am Soc Echocardiogr. 2016;29:402–411.e2.
85. Nezafat R, Herzka D, Stehning C, Peters DC, Nehrke K, Manning WJ. Inflow quantification in
    three-dimensional cardiovascular MR imaging. J Magn Reson Imaging. 2008;28:1273–9.
86. Ghonim S, Voges I, Gatehouse PD, et al. Myocardial architecture, mechanics, and fibrosis in
    congenital heart disease. Front Cardiovasc Med. 2017;4:30.
87. Liu J, Spincemaille P, Codella NC, Nguyen TD, Prince MR, Wang Y. Respiratory and cardiac
    self-gated free-breathing cardiac CINE imaging with multiecho 3D hybrid radial SSFP acqui-
    sition. Magn Reson Med. 2010;63:1230–7.
88. Ferreira PF, Gatehouse PD, Mohiaddin RH, Firmin DN. Cardiovascular magnetic resonance
    artefacts. J Cardiovasc Magn Reson. 2013;15:41.

89. Greil GF, Boettger T, Germann S, et al. Quantitative assessment of ventricular function using three-dimensional SSFP magnetic resonance angiography. J Magn Reson Imaging. 2007;26:288–95.
90. Jeong D, Schiebler ML, Lai P, Wang K, Vigen KK, Francois CJ. Single breath hold 3D cardiac cine MRI using kat-ARC: preliminary results at 1.5T. Int J Card Imaging. 2015;31:851–7.
91. Atweh LA, Dodd NA, Krishnamurthy R, Pednekar A, Chu ZD, Krishnamurthy R. Comparison of two single-breath-held 3-D acquisitions with multi-breath-held 2-D cine steady-state free precession MRI acquisition in children with single ventricles. Pediatr Radiol. 2016;46:637–45.
92. Gatti M, Palmisano A, Faletti R, et al. Two-dimensional and three-dimensional cardiac magnetic resonance feature-tracking myocardial strain analysis in acute myocarditis patients with preserved ejection fraction. Int J Card Imaging. 2019;35:1101–9.
93. Satriano A, Heydari B, Narous M, et al. Clinical feasibility and validation of 3D principal strain analysis from cine MRI: comparison to 2D strain by MRI and 3D speckle tracking echocardiography. Int J Card Imaging. 2017;33:1979–92.
94. Soleimanifard S, Abd-Elmoniem KZ, Sasano T, et al. Three-dimensional regional strain analysis in porcine myocardial infarction: a 3T magnetic resonance tagging study. J Cardiovasc Magn Reson. 2012;14:85.
95. Leng S, Jiang M, Zhao XD, et al. Three-dimensional tricuspid annular motion analysis from cardiac magnetic resonance feature-tracking. Ann Biomed Eng. 2016;44:3522–38.
96. Kawakubo M, Yamasaki Y, Kamitani T, et al. Clinical usefulness of right ventricular 3D area strain in the assessment of treatment effects of balloon pulmonary angioplasty in chronic thromboembolic pulmonary hypertension: comparison with 2D feature-tracking MRI. Eur Radiol. 2019;29:4583–92.

4D Flow MRI: Flow Dynamics

8

Kelly Jarvis, Gilles Soulat, Mohammed Elbaz,
and Michael Markl

8.1 Introduction

MRI is becoming increasingly essential in the diagnosis and follow-up care of patients with adult congenital heart disease (CHD). In addition to providing anatomical insight, cardiac function, and volumetric quantification, MRI is used daily to assess blood flow using 2-dimensional cine phase-contrast MRI (2D PC-MRI), allowing quantification of cardiac output and shunt or valve regurgitation [1, 2].

In the past decade, 4D flow MRI has emerged as a cutting-edge technique, providing time-resolved visualization of 3D blood flow and quantification of a multitude of conventional and advanced hemodynamic metrics [3–9]. 4D flow MRI extends the principles of 2D PC-MRI [10], applied in all three velocity directional components to obtain three-directional velocity data through a volume of interest. Thus, 4D flow MRI is not constrained to measuring flow in only one direction (as in typical 2D PC-MR) but instead can capture complex flow changes such as eccentric regurgitation jets and vortex flow often seen in patients with CHD. Given its volumetric acquisition nature, 4D flow MRI enables full 3D coverage of the vessel or structure of interest such as the entire aorta or the whole heart and surrounding large vessels. Thus, 4D flow MRI allows for retrospective analysis of the imaged structures of interest. This is particularly useful for evaluating the unique complex geometries and flow situations of CHD. That is, rather than being limited to imaging and analyzing fixed slices prescribed during an exam, the entire imaging volume is flexibly available for post-exam analysis. This volumetric and retrospective analysis flexibility could be more effective and less time consuming than several sequential

K. Jarvis (✉) · G. Soulat · M. Elbaz · M. Markl
Department of Radiology, Feinberg School of Medicine, Northwestern University,
Chicago, IL, USA
e-mail: kelly.jarvis@northwestern.edu; gilles.soulat@northwestern.edu;
mohammed.elbaz@northwestern.edu; mmarkl@northwestern.edu

© Springer Nature Switzerland AG 2021
P. Gallego, I. Valverde (eds.), *Multimodality Imaging Innovations In Adult
Congenital Heart Disease*, Congenital Heart Disease in Adolescents and Adults,
https://doi.org/10.1007/978-3-030-61927-5_8

2D PC-MRI slices in the setting of CHD [11]. Measurements of velocities and flow rates in 4D flow MRI were validated in CHD against 2D flow and echo [12–16]. In addition to the benefit from this full volumetric coverage, the amount of information provided by the 3-directional velocity encoding can be readily used to compute advanced flow metrics such as energy-derived parameters, flow patterns, or pressure fields [17–20]. However, as with many advanced new techniques, there are several pitfalls and drawbacks of 4D flow MRI that should be considered and handled efficiently for best utilization of 4D flow MRI towards clinical translation.

8.2 Imaging Methods

8.2.1 Acquisition

Time to acquire a 4D flow MRI protocol is dependent on several factors (mainly temporal and spatial resolution, imaging coverage, and acceleration factor) and is usually set to be completed within 10 min for patient tolerance [7]. 4D flow MRI is acquired during free-breathing and gated to the cardiac cycle using an electrocardiogram with prospective or ideally (if available) retrospective gating (Fig. 8.1: left). Retrospective gating allows for the acquisition of the entire cardiac cycle, including the late atrial diastolic filling phase not acquired in prospective gating, and is thus ideal for intracardiac applications when full diastolic evaluation is

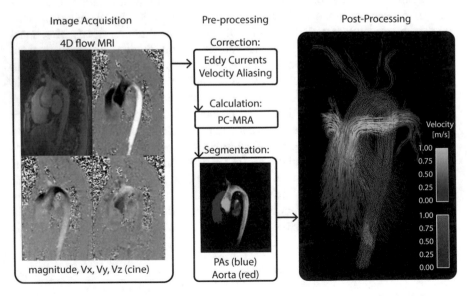

Fig. 8.1 Example of 4D flow MRI workflow in a patient with TGA treated by ASO. Here, a PC-MRA was calculated from the 4D flow MRI data to provide a 3D segmentation for separating the aorta and pulmonary arteries. The segmentation method could vary depending on the application (e.g., using steady-state free-precession cine or directly from the magnitude images of 4D flow MRI). *PAs* pulmonary arteries, *PC-MRA* phase-contrast MR angiogram

generally needed. To minimize the effects of respiratory motion, the sequence can be navigator gated to monitor the position of the diaphragm and only allow a specified acceptance window. The protocol does not require the use of contrast agents but can be acquired post-contrast (i.e., if already on board from earlier in the MRI exam) to maximize velocity-to-noise ratio. The imaging volume can be set to focus on a region of interest (such as the aorta) or to acquire the entire heart and large vessels (known as "whole heart" imaging). Regardless of the application, typical imaging parameters are as follows: temporal resolution = 40 ms, flip angle = 7–15° (non-contrast and post-contrast, respectively), $R = 5$ for k-t acceleration [21–23] and higher using compress sensing [24]. Application-specific imaging parameters are summarized in Table 8.1.

Imaging considerations include the inherent trade-off between imaging time and resolution (both temporal and spatial), as is typical for MRI techniques. See Table 8.2. Parallel imaging and more recently compressed sensing techniques have been developed to speed up acquisition with comparable resolution [26–30]. Specific to phase-contrast MRI, velocity encoding (*venc*) is a setting which should be chosen carefully depending on the disease and the clinical question, because velocity aliasing occurs when blood velocity is higher than the *venc*. However, increasing the *venc* will increase velocity noise; thus correction techniques have been developed to allow for at least some velocity aliasing [31, 32].

8.2.2   Processing

For every voxel in the imaging volume, 4D flow MRI measures velocity in the x, y, and z directions at each point in time along the cardiac cycle. These data should be corrected for Maxwell terms and eddy currents, while denoising and velocity aliasing correction could be also added in the processing [6, 31–35]. See Fig. 8.2. After the mandatory preprocessing steps, a segmentation step is often performed to depict vessel anatomy and mask velocity data (Fig. 8.1: middle). This segmentation could rely for example on the phase-contrast MR angiogram (PC-MRA) that can be calculated from 4D flow MRI [36], but also on steady-state free-precession cine [37] or directly from the magnitude images of 4D flow MRI [38]. Then, dynamic visualization of blood flow can be generated as well as quantification of key hemodynamic metrics. Example flow visualizations include velocity maximum intensity projection (MIP), streamlines, vector fields, or time-resolved pathlines (Fig. 8.1: right). Moreover, advanced hemodynamic flow metrics and maps can be processed, mostly using in-house software such as helical flow [39, 40], vortex flow [41–44], wall shear stress (WSS) [45–48], pressure mapping [49–51], energy loss [44, 52], and turbulent kinetic energy [53–55]. See Fig. 8.3.

Table 8.1 Typical 4D flow MRI scan parameters

Acquisition type	Imaging volume	Spatial resolution	Scan time	Venc	Standard evaluation	Advanced parameters, acquisitions
Guidelines:	*Cover region of interest*	*Isotropic, at least 5–6 voxels[a] across vessel of interest*	*Manage with coverage, resolution, acceleration factor*	*10% above maximum expected velocity*	*Visualize with streamlines or pathlines, quantify at multiple locations*	*Utilize 3D volumetric data, display in parametric maps*
Aorta	Thoracic aorta	$<2.5 \times 2.5 \times 2.5$ mm^3	5–8 min	150 cm/s	Flow visualization, net flow volume, regurgitation flow volume, and peak velocity in multiple analysis planes along vessel	Peak velocity in volumes of interest, wall shear stress, viscous energy losses
Intracardiac	Whole heart and aortic root	$<2.5 \times 2.5 \times 2.5$ mm^3	<10 min	120–150 cm/s	Right heart peak velocities and flow volumes, shunt flow volume, collateral flow volume, Qp/Qs	Kinetic energy, vorticity, helicity, flow eccentricity, turbulent energy losses
Whole heart and great vessels	Whole heart and large thoracic vessels	$<3.0 \times 3.0 \times 3.0$ mm^3	<10 min	100–150 cm/s	Flow visualization and analysis planes in major vessels (AAO, arch, DAO, MPA, RPA, LPA, IVC, SVC, RPV, LPV)	Peak velocity in multiple volumes/ vessels of interest, flow distribution, dual-venc, 5D flow

Note, the sequence parameters represent typically used protocols but could vary in individual cases depending on anatomy

Parameters would have to be adapted to differences in body habitus/heart size for pediatric applications

Venc settings need to be adjusted in the presence of stenosis

Scan times are for typical protocol using navigator gating and $R \sim 5$. Acquisition times could be further reduced by using compressed sensing

Aortic analysis is typically included for intracardiac (aortic valve only) and whole heart

Guidelines and typical values from 4D flow MRI consensus statement and review papers [3, 6, 7].

AAO ascending aorta, *DAO* descending aorta, *IVC* inferior vena cava, *LPA* left pulmonary artery, *LPV* left pulmonary vein, *MPA* main pulmonary artery, *QP/QS* pulmonary-to-systemic blood flow ratio, *R* acceleration factor, *RPA* right pulmonary artery, *RPV* right pulmonary vein, *SVC* superior vena cava

[a]Based on previous results [25]

Table 8.2 Imaging pitfalls

Potential pitfall	Especially when	Current solutions	Advanced, emerging, and in-development solutions
Velocity aliasing	Systemic flow in univentricular heart when *venc* is set to evaluate venous flow stenosis: coarctation, Fallot	• Anti-aliasing preprocessing • V*enc* scout to avoid aliasing	• Improve anti-aliasing post-processing • Dual-*venc*
Low VNR	Venous flow when *venc* is set to analyze systemic flow	Careful adjustment of the *venc* according to maximum velocity in the main region of interest	Dual-*venc*
Phase offset due to eddy current	• Flow analysis in regions away from the isocenter • Non-Cartesian acquisition	Polynomial fit of stationary tissue	Develop and improve automated preprocessing techniques
Coverage issue	Whole heart 4D flow	Trade-off in spatial and temporal resolution to cover the structure of interest while attaining a reasonable acquisition time	Highly accelerated 4D flow
Patient movement	Syndromic CHD with mental disorder	Decrease coverage and/or spatial resolution and/or temporal resolution to speed up acquisition	Highly accelerated 4D flow
Discomfort			
Effect of respiration on flow	Especially for venous flow in diastolic function studies	–	5D flow

VNR velocity-to-noise ratio

8.3   Applications

Several 4D flow MRI metrics have been applied to analyze various cardiac abnormalities encountered in CHD, often combined in complex cases.

8.3.1   Shunt or Leak

The ability of 4D flow MRI to allow retrospective plane placement makes it a useful tool to assess data consistency and shunting along cardiac structures. Thus, pulmonary-to-systemic blood flow ratio (QP/QS) estimation has been validated either using flow consistency on patients without cardiac shunts or compared to 2D PC-MRI in the case of a shunt, with good reproducibility [56–58]. Moreover, a multicenter study emphasized the good multilevel and interobserver reproducibility of 4D flow MRI to evaluate shunts in atrial septal defects [59]. 4D flow MRI was

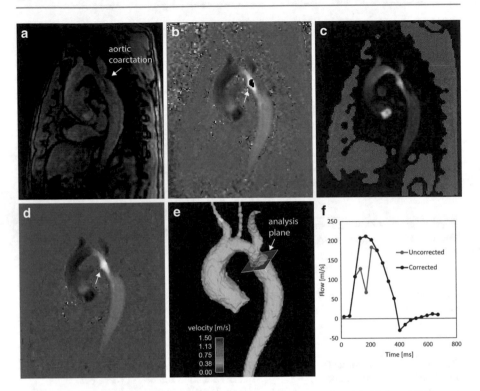

Fig. 8.2 4D flow MRI processing for a patient with aortic coarctation. (**a**) 4D flow MRI magnitude image. (**b**) 4D flow MRI velocity encoded (flow) image showing aliasing in the location of the coarctation (white arrow). (**c**) Selection of static tissue for eddy current correction. (**d**) Velocity encoded image after corrections (eddy current, noise masking, and anti-aliasing). The anti-aliasing algorithm has corrected the velocity aliasing (white arrow). (**e**) Analysis plane placement on aortic segmentation (which has been separated from the PC-MRA calculated from 4D flow MRI data). (**f**) Flow waveforms for data processed with (black) and without (blue) anti-aliasing algorithm. The scan was acquired with *venc* of 150 cm/s; however velocities near the coarctation reached almost 230 cm/s. The aliasing correction has unwrapped these voxels enabling the quantification of the flow profile

also used to assess systemic-to-pulmonary collateral blood flow in patients with univentricular heart [11] in a faster way than with 2D PC-MRI.

In addition, the use of 4D flow MRI improves the sensitivity of CMR to detect small intracardiac shunts or leaks against conventional MR imaging [27], making it clinically useful to better understand the origin of shunts and to better understand complex cases (Fig. 8.4).

8.3.2 Vascular or Valve Stenosis

The location and severity of vascular stenosis can be monitored using 4D flow MRI [60]. Thanks to the full volumetric coverage, vessels can be queried for locations of

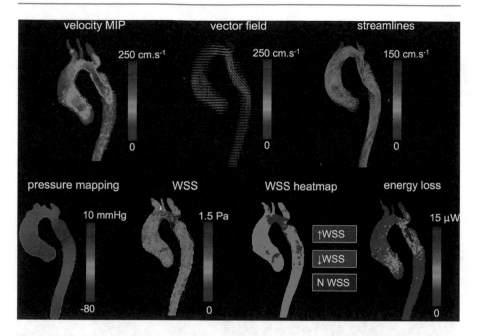

Fig. 8.3 Example of post-processing in a re-coarctation case. Above, from left to right: velocity MIP, systolic vector field, and streamlines projected in a sagittal oblique view. Below, from left to right: pressure difference mapping with a reference plane at the level of the aortic valve; wall shear stress at peak systole; heat map showing area of increase (>95 percentile, in red), decrease (<95 percentile, in blue), or normal WSS based on an age-matched control atlas; and energy loss mapping with a net energy loss of 21 mW. *MIP* maximum intensity projection, *WSS* wall shear stress

peak velocity to assess stenosis using peak velocity maps, as it was done in transposition of the great arteries (TGA) treated by the arterial switch operation (ASO) [61] (Figs. 8.5 and 8.6). Beyond peak velocity, a more precise evaluation of transvalvular gradient than the simplified Bernoulli equation (assumes steady flow) can be obtained from 4D flow MRI [62]. In addition, to characterize temporal and spatial pressure gradient variations (e.g., in the case of long stenosis), 4D flow MRI-derived pressure maps [49, 51] have been proposed and validated against invasive catheterization [50]. Of note, *venc* should be adapted to match maximum velocities, and potential measurement errors can occur in areas of turbulent flow due to intravoxel dephasing [63]. Nevertheless, further information can be derived in these regions in the form of turbulent kinetic energy [53, 54, 64], offering another tool for assessing stenosis severity.

8.3.3   Valvular Flow and Regurgitation

Thanks to time-resolved volumetric coverage, the retrospective plane placement allowed by 4D flow MRI enables the use of valve tracking [37, 65] to quantify inflow and outflow throughout the four valves simultaneously, or through

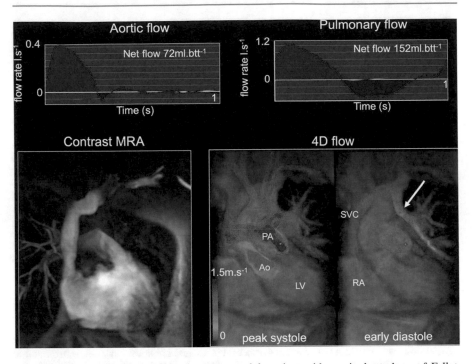

Fig. 8.4 Assessment of a cardiac shunt in an adult patient with repaired tetralogy of Fallot. Beyond a significant pulmonary regurgitation, 2D PC-MRI showed an elevated QP/QS at 2.11. Etiology of shunt was challenging to determine from conventional contrast MRA sequence while it was clear using whole heart 4D flow MRI (coronal view). This patient had pulmonary venous return anomaly of the left superior pulmonary vein in the left brachiocephalic vein (arrow, better seen in early diastole). *Ao* aorta, *LV* left ventricle, *PA* pulmonary artery, *QP/QS* pulmonary-to-systemic blood flow ratio, *RA* right atrium, *SVC* superior vena cava

atrioventricular valves in case of atrioventricular septal defects (AVSD) [66]. Particularly in the setting of AVSD correction (i.e., can lead to a complex eccentric jet), valve or jet tracking has been successfully applied to quantify atrioventricular valve regurgitations [67]. See Figs. 8.7, 8.8, and 8.9, Table 8.3.

8.3.4 Vessel Flow Patterns and Distribution

Evaluation of blood flow in Fontan circulation can provide insights into the development of complications like arteriovenous fistulae or thrombosis. Specifically, parameters such as blood flow distribution, kinetic energy, and energy loss have been studied [68–72]. See Figs. 8.10 and 8.11 for an example of blood flow distribution analysis. On a technical note, in the setting of venous blood flow with low velocities, *venc* should be carefully adapted, and eddy current correction and vessel segmentation require particular attention [73].

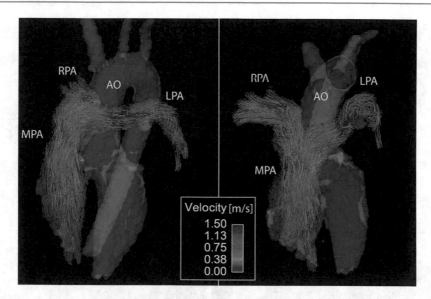

Fig. 8.5 Example of 4D flow MRI evaluation after surgical repair for TGA. Flow visualization is shown for a 24-year-old male with TGA after arterial switch operation. The left panel shows sagittal view and the right panel shows the view shifted (in the anterior and superior direction) to better visualize the pulmonary arteries. *AO* aorta, *LPA* left pulmonary artery, *MPA* main pulmonary artery, *RPA* right pulmonary artery

Fig. 8.6 Quantification of peak velocity to assess stenosis in regions of interest in the TGA-repaired patient in Fig. 8.5. A maximum intensity projection is shown. High velocities in the region of the LPA can be appreciated. *AO* aorta, *LPA* left pulmonary artery, *MPA* main pulmonary artery, *RPA* right pulmonary artery

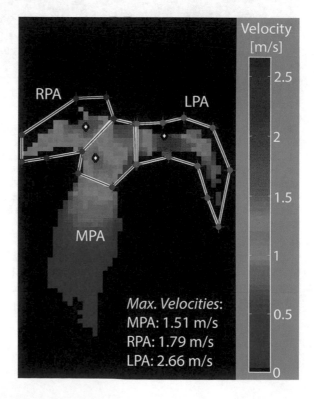

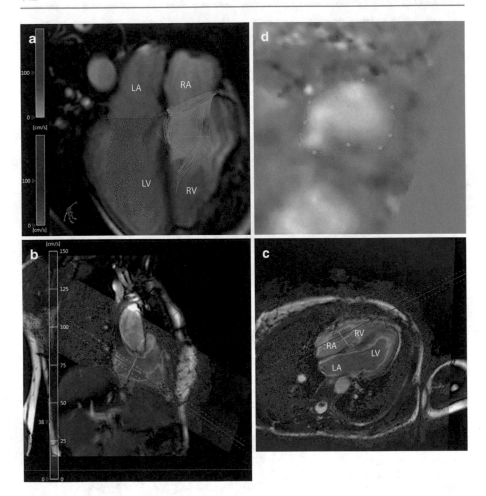

Fig. 8.7 Example of intracardiac *inflow* visualization and analysis in a 42-year-old female patient who was corrected for AVSD when she was 14 years old. (**a**) RAVV inflow streamlines are shown in blue and LAVV inflow streamlines are shown in yellow. (**b, c**) show the RAVV plane planning on two perpendicular views: (**b**) two-chamber right ventricular view, and (**c**) the four-chamber view. (**d**) shows the flow (phase) reformatting through the plane shown in (**b, c**). *LA* left atrium, *LAVV* left atrioventricular valve, *LV* left ventricle, *RA* right atrium, *RV* right ventricle, *RAVV* right atrioventricular valve. (Courtesy of Jos Westenberg, PhD, Leiden University Medical Center, Leiden, the Netherlands)

As for other cardiovascular diseases, arterial assessment of flow patterns from streamlines or pathlines could help to better understand the impact of congenital anomalies such as Fallot repair, TGA treated by ASO, BAV, or coarctation [39, 60, 74–76].

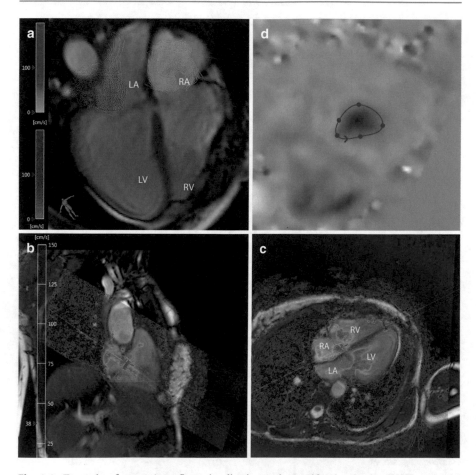

Fig. 8.8 Example of *regurgitant* flow visualization and quantification in the AVSD-corrected patient in Fig. 8.7. This patient suffers from regurgitant flow across both the RAVV and LAVV. (**a**) streamline visualization of regurgitant flow through the LAVV (yellow) and the RAVV (in blue color). (**b, c**) show the RAVV regurgitation plane planning (in magenta color) on two perpendicular views: (**b**) two-chamber right ventricular view, and (**c**) the four-chamber view. Note the magenta plane tracked over the regurgitant jet level itself not at the annulus level to allow for accurate quantification in the presence of eccentric or dynamic jets. (**d**) shows the flow (phase) reformatting through the regurgitation plane shown in (**b, c**). The patient has a mild recurrent regurgitation in RAVV (shown in blue) and LAVV (shown in yellow). *LA* left atrium, *LAVV* left atrioventricular valve, *LV* left ventricle, *RA* right atrium, *RV* right ventricle, *RAVV* right atrioventricular valve. (Courtesy of Jos Westenberg, PhD, Leiden University Medical Center, Leiden, the Netherlands)

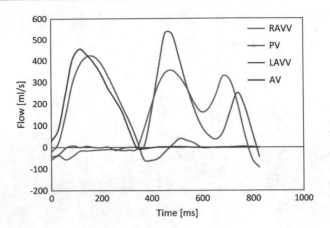

Fig. 8.9 Quantification of valvular flow across the four cardiac valves simultaneously from 4D Flow MRI in the AVSD-corrected patient presented in Figs. 8.7 and 8.8. *AV* aortic valve, *LAVV* left atrioventricular valve, *PV* pulmonary valve, *RAVV* right atrioventricular valve. (Courtesy of Jos Westenberg, PhD, Leiden University Medical Center, Leiden, the Netherlands)

Table 8.3 Flow quantifications for the AVSD-corrected patient in Figs. 8.7 and 8.9

	RAVV	PV	LAVV	AV
Forward flow [mL]	100.88	89.01	96.44	88.80
Backward flow [mL]	12.84	5.90	4.09	0.34
Net forward flow [mL]	88.04	83.11	92.35	88.47
Regurgitation fraction	0.13	0.07	0.04	0.00
Flow displacement	–	0.03	–	0.05
Heart rate [bpm]	70			
Cardiac output [L/min]	6.23			
Pulmonary shunt [%]	93.94			

LA left atrium, *LAVV* left atrioventricular valve, *LV* left ventricle, *RA* right atrium, *RV* right ventricle, *RAVV* right atrioventricular valve. (Courtesy of Jos Westenberg, PhD, Leiden University Medical Center, Leiden, the Netherlands)

8.3.5 Ventricular Hemodynamics

It is well acknowledged that our current evaluation of systolic (and even more so for diastolic) function is incomplete, especially on the right ventricle side. Energy-derived biomarkers are promising to better understand the effects of congenital abnormalities on the pulmonary or systemic ventricle. For example, kinetic energy was altered in repaired tetralogy of Fallot and related to end-diastolic volumes [77]

Fig. 8.10 Flow visualization in a 17-year-old male with Fontan circulation demonstrating complex flow in the SVC. Time-resolved pathlines were released from the IVC (yellow) and brachiocephalic veins feeding the SVC flow (blue). The PC-MRA is shown in gray to depict the surrounding vascular geometry. *IVC* inferior vena cava, *LPA* left pulmonary artery, *PC-MRA* phase-contrast magnetic resonance angiogram, *RPA* right pulmonary artery, *SVC* superior vena cava. (From Jarvis et al. [70], with permission)

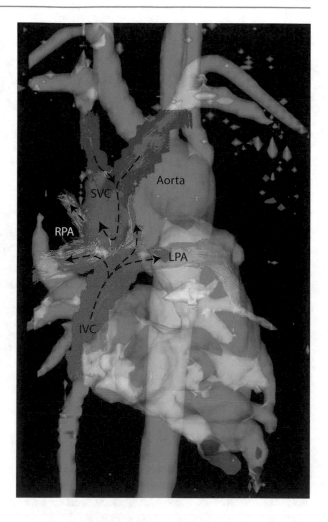

while Fontan patients showed decreased diastolic ventricular kinetic energy [78] and disproportional intraventricular energy loss [79]. Altered 3D vortex ring flow has been found in patients after correction of AVSD [42] associating with twofold to fourfold increase in diastolic viscous energy loss [44]. Recently, it has been shown that pharmacologic stress increases hemodynamic kinetic energy, viscous energy loss, and vorticity in Fontan patients. Such elevation in these advanced energetic and flow pattern hemodynamic metrics was found to be inversely correlated to exercise capacity as measured by VO_2 max [80]. Other techniques like particle tracing can also be useful to analyze distribution and stasis of ventricle flow [81].

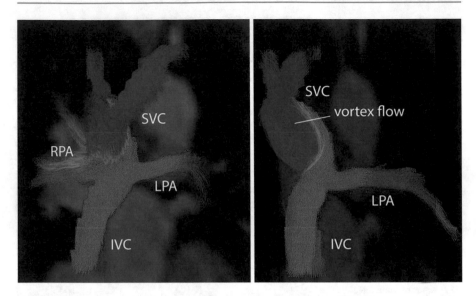

Fig. 8.11 Flow visualization of Fontan pathway for the patient in Fig. 8.10, demonstrating vortex flow in the SVC, shown in two close-up views (left, right) to appreciate flow patterns (SVC flow = blue, IVC flow = yellow). Using time-resolved pathlines, flow distribution to the LPA and RPA was quantified (IVC flow: 64% to LPA, 36% to RPA. SVC flow: 0% to LPA, 100% to RPA). *IVC* inferior vena cava, *LPA* left pulmonary artery, *RPA* right pulmonary artery, *SVC* superior vena cava. (From Jarvis et al. [70], with permission)

8.4   Challenges and Outlook

4D flow MRI is becoming more and more available in specialized cardiac imaging centers that are likely to manage complex adult CHD patients. The ability of 4D flow MRI to provide the direct visualization of complex flow is unique and well adapted for the individual assessment of adult CHD patients (who may have undergone several palliative surgeries). However, several challenges remain to increase the adoption of this tool into everyday use and research is ongoing to overcome these limits. To manage the amount of data and complexity of post-processing, deep learning techniques (which have already shown achievements in helping the workflow in the CMR field) [82–84] may help by improving, automating, and accelerating data processing. At the same time, compressed sensing techniques, eventually combined with non-cartesian acquisition, will also help to either speed up acquisition time or (using the same acquisition time) increase the information provided [27–30]. See Fig. 8.12, Table 8.4. This enables scanning with dual- or multi-*venc* [85–88] (e.g., recording within the same acquisition, venous and arterial components with equal quality) or respiratory resolved acquisition (5D whole heart MRI, 5D flow MRI) [89–91] allowing the analysis of respiratory driven changes.

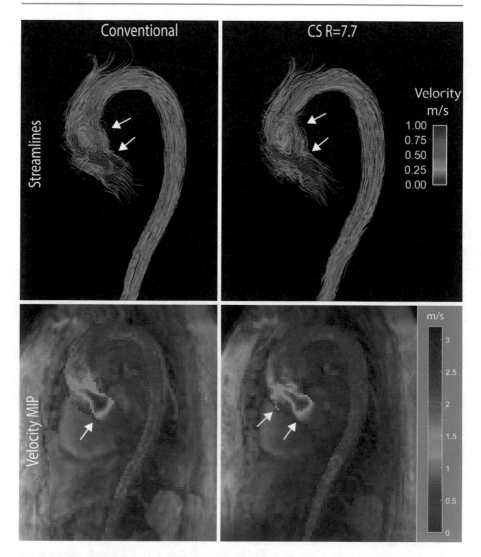

Fig. 8.12 Compressed sensing (CS) accelerated acquisition. Flow visualization and quantification in a 71-year-old patient with BAV. The CS acquisition had a 73% reduction in scan time (i.e., conventional = 7.3 min, CS (R = 7.7) = 2.0 min). The top row shows flow visualization by streamlines at peak systole for both acquisitions. Note, the CS acquisition captured the complex flow patterns in the ascending aorta (arrows at jet and vortex) although some of the definition was reduced (e.g., center of vortex). The bottom row shows a peak systolic velocity MIP for both acquisitions. The CS acquisition underestimated flow parameters (see results for peak velocity, peak flow, and net flow in Table 8.4) but the values were within 10–15% of the conventional method. The compressed sensing also detected a similar flow jet pattern (arrow) but appears to have introduced a few noisy voxels close to the vessel wall (second arrow in CS image). *BAV* bicuspid aortic valve, *MIP* maximum intensity projection, *R* acceleration factor. (Courtesy of Liliana Ma and Ashitha Pathrose, MD, Northwestern University Feinberg School of Medicine, Chicago, Illinois)

Table 8.4 Flow parameter results using conventional and CS acquisitions for the patient in Fig. 8.12

	Peak velocity [m/s]			Peak flow [mL/s]			Net flow [mL/s]		
	AAo	Arch	DAo	AAo	Arch	DAo	AAo	Arch	DAo
Conventional	3.05	0.84	0.90	310.7	170.2	164.0	78.8	38.8	31.3
CS $R = 7.7$	2.60	0.76	0.86	264.7	147.7	163.2	67.7	34.0	31.5

AAo ascending aorta, *Arch* aortic arch, *CS* compressed sensing, *DAo* descending aorta, *R* acceleration factor. (Courtesy of Liliana Ma and Ashitha Pathrose, MD, Northwestern University Feinberg School of Medicine, Chicago, Illinois)

References

1. Baumgartner H, Bonhoeffer P, De Groot NM, de Haan F, Deanfield JE, Galie N, et al. ESC Guidelines for the management of grown-up congenital heart disease (new version 2010). Eur Heart J. 2010;31(23):2915–57.
2. Stout KK, Daniels CJ, Aboulhosn JA, Bozkurt B, Broberg CS, Colman JM, et al. 2018 AHA/ACC Guideline for the management of adults with congenital heart disease: a report of the American College of Cardiology/American Heart Association Task Force on Clinical Practice Guidelines. Circulation. 2019;139(14):e698–800.
3. Markl M, Kilner PJ, Ebbers T. Comprehensive 4D velocity mapping of the heart and great vessels by cardiovascular magnetic resonance. J Cardiovasc Magn Reson. 2011;13:7.
4. Frydrychowicz A, Francois CJ, Turski PA. Four-dimensional phase contrast magnetic resonance angiography: potential clinical applications. Eur J Radiol. 2011;80(1):24–35.
5. Hope MD, Sedlic T, Dyverfeldt P. Cardiothoracic magnetic resonance flow imaging. J Thorac Imaging. 2013;28(4):217–30.
6. Dyverfeldt P, Bissell M, Barker AJ, Bolger AF, Carlhall CJ, Ebbers T, et al. 4D flow cardiovascular magnetic resonance consensus statement. J Cardiovasc Magn Reson. 2015;17(1):72.
7. Zhong L, Schrauben EM, Garcia J, Uribe S, Grieve SM, Elbaz MSM, et al. Intracardiac 4D flow MRI in congenital heart disease: recommendations on behalf of the ISMRM flow & motion study group. J Magn Reson Imaging. 2019;50(3):677–81.
8. Sierra-Galan LM, Francois CJ. Clinical applications of MRA 4D-flow. Curr Treat Opt Cardiovasc Med. 2019;21(10):58.
9. Azarine A, Garcon P, Stansal A, Canepa N, Angelopoulos G, Silvera S, et al. Four-dimensional Flow MRI: principles and cardiovascular applications. Radiographics. 2019;39(3):632–48.
10. Pelc NJ, Herfkens RJ, Shimakawa A, Enzmann DR. Phase contrast cine magnetic resonance imaging. Magn Reson Q. 1991;7(4):229–54.
11. Valverde I, Nordmeyer S, Uribe S, Greil G, Berger F, Kuehne T, et al. Systemic-to-pulmonary collateral flow in patients with palliated univentricular heart physiology: measurement using cardiovascular magnetic resonance 4D velocity acquisition. J Cardiovasc Magn Reson. 2012;14:25.
12. Nordmeyer S, Riesenkampff E, Crelier G, Khasheei A, Schnackenburg B, Berger F, et al. Flow-sensitive four-dimensional cine magnetic resonance imaging for offline blood flow quantification in multiple vessels: a validation study. J Magn Reson Imaging. 2010;32(3):677–83.
13. van der Hulst AE, Westenberg JJ, Kroft LJ, Bax JJ, Blom NA, de Roos A, et al. Tetralogy of fallot: 3D velocity-encoded MR imaging for evaluation of right ventricular valve flow and diastolic function in patients after correction. Radiology. 2010;256(3):724–34.
14. Hsiao A, Alley MT, Massaband P, Herfkens RJ, Chan FP, Vasanawala SS. Improved cardiovascular flow quantification with time-resolved volumetric phase-contrast MRI. Pediatr Radiol. 2011;41(6):711–20.

15. Gabbour M, Schnell S, Jarvis K, Robinson JD, Markl M, Rigsby CK. 4-D flow magnetic resonance imaging: blood flow quantification compared to 2-D phase-contrast magnetic resonance imaging and Doppler echocardiography. Pediatr Radiol. 2015;45(6):804–13.
16. Driessen MMP, Schings MA, Sieswerda GT, Doevendans PA, Hulzebos EH, Post MC, et al. Tricuspid flow and regurgitation in congenital heart disease and pulmonary hypertension: comparison of 4D flow cardiovascular magnetic resonance and echocardiography. J Cardiovasc Magn Reson. 2018;20(1):5.
17. Bissell MM, Hess AT, Biasiolli L, Glaze SJ, Loudon M, Pitcher A, et al. Aortic dilation in bicuspid aortic valve disease: flow pattern is a major contributor and differs with valve fusion type. Circ Cardiovasc imaging. 2013;6(4):499–507.
18. Burris NS, Hope MD. 4D flow MRI applications for aortic disease. Magn Reson Imaging Clin N Am. 2015;23(1):15–23.
19. Sjoberg P, Bidhult S, Bock J, Heiberg E, Arheden H, Gustafsson R, et al. Disturbed left and right ventricular kinetic energy in patients with repaired tetralogy of Fallot: pathophysiological insights using 4D-flow MRI. Eur Radiol. 2018;28(10):4066–76.
20. Schafer M, Barker AJ, Jaggers J, Morgan GJ, Stone ML, Truong U, et al. Abnormal aortic flow conduction is associated with increased viscous energy loss in patients with repaired tetralogy of Fallot. Eur J Cardiothorac Surg. 2020;57:588.
21. Griswold MA, Jakob PM, Heidemann RM, Nittka M, Jellus V, Wang J, et al. Generalized autocalibrating partially parallel acquisitions (GRAPPA). Magn Reson Med. 2002;47(6):1202–10.
22. Jung B, Stalder AF, Bauer S, Markl M. On the undersampling strategies to accelerate time-resolved 3D imaging using k-t-GRAPPA. Magn Reson Med. 2011;66(4):966–75.
23. Tsao J, Kozerke S. MRI temporal acceleration techniques. J Magn Reson Imaging. 2012;36(3):543–60.
24. Lustig M, Donoho D, Pauly JM. Sparse MRI: the application of compressed sensing for rapid MR imaging. Magn Reson Med. 2007;58(6):1182–95.
25. Hofman MB, Visser FC, van Rossum AC, Vink QM, Sprenger M, Westerhof N. In vivo validation of magnetic resonance blood volume flow measurements with limited spatial resolution in small vessels. Magn Reson Med. 1995;33(6):778–84.
26. Schnell S, Markl M, Entezari P, Mahadewia RJ, Semaan E, Stankovic Z, et al. k-t GRAPPA accelerated four-dimensional flow MRI in the aorta: effect on scan time, image quality, and quantification of flow and wall shear stress. Magn Reson Med. 2014;72(2):522–33.
27. Hsiao A, Lustig M, Alley MT, Murphy MJ, Vasanawala SS. Evaluation of valvular insufficiency and shunts with parallel-imaging compressed-sensing 4D phase-contrast MR imaging with stereoscopic 3D velocity-fusion volume-rendered visualization. Radiology. 2012;265(1):87–95.
28. Dyvorne H, Knight-Greenfield A, Jajamovich G, Besa C, Cui Y, Stalder A, et al. Abdominal 4D flow MR imaging in a breath hold: combination of spiral sampling and dynamic compressed sensing for highly accelerated acquisition. Radiology. 2015;275(1):245–54.
29. Cheng JY, Hanneman K, Zhang T, Alley MT, Lai P, Tamir JI, et al. Comprehensive motion-compensated highly accelerated 4D flow MRI with ferumoxytol enhancement for pediatric congenital heart disease. J Magn Reson Imaging. 2016;43(6):1355–68.
30. Ma LE, Markl M, Chow K, Huh H, Forman C, Vali A, et al. Aortic 4D flow MRI in 2 minutes using compressed sensing, respiratory controlled adaptive k-space reordering, and inline reconstruction. Magn Reson Med. 2019;81(6):3675–90.
31. Xiang QS. Temporal phase unwrapping for CINE velocity imaging. J Magn Reson Imaging. 1995;5(5):529–34.
32. Loecher M, Schrauben E, Johnson KM, Wieben O. Phase unwrapping in 4D MR flow with a 4D single-step laplacian algorithm. J Magn Reson Imaging. 2016;43(4):833–42.
33. Bernstein MA, Grgic M, Brosnan TJ, Pelc NJ. Reconstructions of phase contrast, phased array multicoil data. Magn Reson Med. 1994;32(3):330–4.
34. Walker PG, Cranney GB, Scheidegger MB, Waseleski G, Pohost GM, Yoganathan AP. Semiautomated method for noise reduction and background phase error correction in MR phase velocity data. J Magn Reson Imaging. 1993;3(3):521–30.

35. Busch J, Giese D, Kozerke S. Image-based background phase error correction in 4D flow MRI revisited. J Magn Reson Imaging. 2017;46(5):1516–25.
36. Markl M, Harloff A, Bley TA, Zaitsev M, Jung B, Weigang E, et al. Time-resolved 3D MR velocity mapping at 3T: improved navigator-gated assessment of vascular anatomy and blood flow. J Magn Reson Imaging. 2007;25(4):824–31.
37. Kamphuis VP, Rocst AAW, Ajmone Marsan N, van den Boogaard PJ, Kroft LJM, Aben JP, et al. Automated cardiac valve tracking for flow quantification with four-dimensional flow MRI. Radiology. 2019;290(1):70–8.
38. Chelu RG, Wanambiro KW, Hsiao A, Swart LE, Voogd T, van den Hoven AT, et al. Cloud-processed 4D CMR flow imaging for pulmonary flow quantification. Eur J Radiol. 2016;85(10):1849–56.
39. Bachler P, Pinochet N, Sotelo J, Crelier G, Irarrazaval P, Tejos C, et al. Assessment of normal flow patterns in the pulmonary circulation by using 4D magnetic resonance velocity mapping. Magn Reson Imaging. 2013;31(2):178–88.
40. Garcia J, Barker AJ, Collins JD, Carr JC, Markl M. Volumetric quantification of absolute local normalized helicity in patients with bicuspid aortic valve and aortic dilatation. Magn Reson Med. 2017;78(2):689–701.
41. Elbaz MS, Calkoen EE, Westenberg JJ, Lelieveldt BP, Roest AA, van der Geest RJ. Vortex flow during early and late left ventricular filling in normal subjects: quantitative characterization using retrospectively-gated 4D flow cardiovascular magnetic resonance and three-dimensional vortex core analysis. J Cardiovasc Magn Reson. 2014;16:78.
42. Calkoen EE, Elbaz MS, Westenberg JJ, Kroft LJ, Hazekamp MG, Roest AA, et al. Altered left ventricular vortex ring formation by 4-dimensional flow magnetic resonance imaging after repair of atrioventricular septal defects. J Thorac Cardiovasc Surg. 2015;150(5):1233–40.e1.
43. Hirtler D, Garcia J, Barker AJ, Geiger J. Assessment of intracardiac flow and vorticity in the right heart of patients after repair of tetralogy of Fallot by flow-sensitive 4D MRI. Eur Radiol. 2016;26(10):3598–607.
44. Elbaz MS, van der Geest RJ, Calkoen EE, de Roos A, Lelieveldt BP, Roest AA, et al. Assessment of viscous energy loss and the association with three-dimensional vortex ring formation in left ventricular inflow: in vivo evaluation using four-dimensional flow MRI. Magn Reson Med. 2017;77(2):794–805.
45. Potters WV, Ooij P, Marquering H, vanBavel E, Nederveen AJ. Volumetric arterial wall shear stress calculation based on cine phase contrast MRI. J Magn Reson Imaging. 2015;41:505–16.
46. van Ooij P, Potters WV, Collins J, Carr M, Carr J, Malaisrie SC, et al. Characterization of abnormal wall shear stress using 4D flow MRI in human bicuspid aortopathy. Ann Biomed Eng. 2015;43(6):1385–97.
47. Rizk J, Latus H, Shehu N, Mkrtchyan N, Zimmermann J, Martinoff S, et al. Elevated diastolic wall shear stress in regurgitant semilunar valvular lesions. J Magn Reson Imaging. 2019;50(3):763–70.
48. van der Palen RLF, Deurvorst QS, Kroft LJM, van den Boogaard PJ, Hazekamp MG, Blom NA, et al. Altered ascending aorta hemodynamics in patients after arterial switch operation for transposition of the great arteries. J Magn Reson Imaging. 2020;51:1105.
49. Bock J, Frydrychowicz A, Lorenz R, Hirtler D, Barker AJ, Johnson KM, et al. In vivo noninvasive 4D pressure difference mapping in the human aorta: phantom comparison and application in healthy volunteers and patients. Magn Reson Med. 2011;66(4):1079–88.
50. Riesenkampff E, Fernandes JF, Meier S, Goubergrits L, Kropf S, Schubert S, et al. Pressure fields by flow-sensitive, 4D, velocity-encoded CMR in patients with aortic coarctation. J Am Coll Cardiol Img. 2014;7(9):920–6.
51. Saitta S, Pirola S, Piatti F, Votta E, Lucherini F, Pluchinotta F, et al. Evaluation of 4D flow MRI-based non-invasive pressure assessment in aortic coarctations. J Biomech. 2019;94:13–21.
52. Barker AJ, van Ooij P, Bandi K, Garcia J, Albaghdadi M, McCarthy P, et al. Viscous energy loss in the presence of abnormal aortic flow. Magn Reson Med. 2014;72(3):620–8.

53. Dyverfeldt P, Hope MD, Tseng EE, Saloner D. Magnetic resonance measurement of turbulent kinetic energy for the estimation of irreversible pressure loss in aortic stenosis. J Am Coll Cardiol Img. 2013;6(1):64–71.
54. Binter C, Gotschy A, Sundermann SH, Frank M, Tanner FC, Luscher TF, et al. Turbulent kinetic energy assessed by multipoint 4-dimensional flow magnetic resonance imaging provides additional information relative to echocardiography for the determination of aortic stenosis severity. Circ Cardiovasc imaging. 2017;10(6):e005486.
55. Fredriksson A, Trzebiatowska-Krzynska A, Dyverfeldt P, Engvall J, Ebbers T, Carlhall CJ. Turbulent kinetic energy in the right ventricle: potential MR marker for risk stratification of adults with repaired Tetralogy of Fallot. J Magn Reson Imaging. 2018;47(4):1043–53.
56. Uribe S, Beerbaum P, Sorensen TS, Rasmusson A, Razavi R, Schaeffter T. Four-dimensional (4D) flow of the whole heart and great vessels using real-time respiratory self-gating. Magn Reson Med. 2009;62(4):984–92.
57. Tariq U, Hsiao A, Alley M, Zhang T, Lustig M, Vasanawala SS. Venous and arterial flow quantification are equally accurate and precise with parallel imaging compressed sensing 4D phase contrast MRI. J Magn Reson Imaging. 2013;37(6):1419–26.
58. Hanneman K, Sivagnanam M, Nguyen ET, Wald R, Greiser A, Crean AM, et al. Magnetic resonance assessment of pulmonary (QP) to systemic (QS) flows using 4D phase-contrast imaging: pilot study comparison with standard through-plane 2D phase-contrast imaging. Acad Radiol. 2014;21(8):1002–8.
59. Chelu RG, Horowitz M, Sucha D, Kardys I, Ingremeau D, Vasanawala S, et al. Evaluation of atrial septal defects with 4D flow MRI-multilevel and inter-reader reproducibility for quantification of shunt severity. Magma. 2019;32(2):269–79.
60. Geiger J, Hirtler D, Burk J, Stiller B, Arnold R, Jung B, et al. Postoperative pulmonary and aortic 3D haemodynamics in patients after repair of transposition of the great arteries. Eur Radiol. 2014;24(1):200–8.
61. Jarvis K, Vonder M, Barker AJ, Schnell S, Rose M, Carr J, et al. Hemodynamic evaluation in patients with transposition of the great arteries after the arterial switch operation: 4D flow and 2D phase contrast cardiovascular magnetic resonance compared with Doppler echocardiography. J Cardiovasc Magn Reson. 2016;18(1):59.
62. Falahatpisheh A, Rickers C, Gabbert D, Heng EL, Stalder A, Kramer HH, et al. Simplified Bernoulli's method significantly underestimates pulmonary transvalvular pressure drop. J Magn Reson Imaging. 2016;43(6):1313–9.
63. Garcia J, Barker AJ, Markl M. The role of imaging of flow patterns by 4D flow MRI in aortic stenosis. J Am Coll Cardiol Img. 2019;12(2):252–66.
64. Ha H, Kvitting JP, Dyverfeldt P, Ebbers T. Validation of pressure drop assessment using 4D flow MRI-based turbulence production in various shapes of aortic stenoses. Magn Reson Med. 2019;81(2):893–906.
65. Westenberg JJ, Roes SD, Ajmone Marsan N, Binnendijk NM, Doornbos J, Bax JJ, et al. Mitral valve and tricuspid valve blood flow: accurate quantification with 3D velocity-encoded MR imaging with retrospective valve tracking. Radiology. 2008;249(3):792–800.
66. Hsiao A, Tariq U, Alley MT, Lustig M, Vasanawala SS. Inlet and outlet valve flow and regurgitant volume may be directly and reliably quantified with accelerated, volumetric phase-contrast MRI. J Magn Reson Imaging. 2015;41(2):376–85.
67. Calkoen EE, Westenberg JJ, Kroft LJ, Blom NA, Hazekamp MG, Rijlaarsdam ME, et al. Characterization and quantification of dynamic eccentric regurgitation of the left atrioventricular valve after atrioventricular septal defect correction with 4D Flow cardiovascular magnetic resonance and retrospective valve tracking. J Cardiovasc Magn Reson. 2015;17:18.
68. Bachler P, Valverde I, Pinochet N, Nordmeyer S, Kuehne T, Crelier G, et al. Caval blood flow distribution in patients with Fontan circulation: quantification by using particle traces from 4D flow MR imaging. Radiology. 2013;267(1):67–75.
69. Cibis M, Jarvis K, Markl M, Rose M, Rigsby C, Barker AJ, et al. The effect of resolution on viscous dissipation measured with 4D flow MRI in patients with Fontan circulation: evaluation using computational fluid dynamics. J Biomech. 2015;48:2984.

70. Jarvis K, Schnell S, Barker AJ, Garcia J, Lorenz R, Rose M, et al. Evaluation of blood flow distribution asymmetry and vascular geometry in patients with Fontan circulation using 4-D flow MRI. Pediatr Radiol. 2016;46:1507.

71. Rijnberg FM, Elbaz MS, Westenberg JJ, Kamphuis VP, Helbing WA, Kroft LJ, et al. Four-dimensional flow magnetic resonance imaging-derived blood flow energetics of the inferior vena cava-to-extracardiac conduit junction in Fontan patients. Eur J Cardiothorac Surg. 2019;55:1202.

72. Rijnberg FM, van Assen HC, Hazekamp MG, Roest AAW. Tornado-like flow in the Fontan circulation: insights from quantification and visualization of viscous energy loss rate using 4D flow MRI. Eur Heart J. 2019;40(26):2170.

73. Jarvis K, Schnell S, Barker AJ, Rose M, Robinson JD, Rigsby CK, et al. Caval to pulmonary 3D flow distribution in patients with Fontan circulation and impact of potential 4D flow MRI error sources. Magn Reson Med. 2019;81(2):1205–18.

74. Hope MD, Meadows AK, Hope TA, Ordovas KG, Saloner D, Reddy GP, et al. Clinical evaluation of aortic coarctation with 4D flow MR imaging. J Magn Reson Imaging. 2010;31(3):711–8.

75. Frydrychowicz A, Markl M, Hirtler D, Harloff A, Schlensak C, Geiger J, et al. Aortic hemodynamics in patients with and without repair of aortic coarctation: in vivo analysis by 4D flow-sensitive magnetic resonance imaging. Investig Radiol. 2011;46(5):317–25.

76. Francois CJ, Srinivasan S, Schiebler ML, Reeder SB, Niespodzany E, Landgraf BR, et al. 4D cardiovascular magnetic resonance velocity mapping of alterations of right heart flow patterns and main pulmonary artery hemodynamics in tetralogy of Fallot. J Cardiovasc Magn Reson. 2012;14:16.

77. Robinson JD, Rose MJ, Joh M, Jarvis K, Schnell S, Barker AJ, et al. 4-D flow magnetic-resonance-imaging-derived energetic biomarkers are abnormal in children with repaired tetralogy of Fallot and associated with disease severity. Pediatr Radiol. 2019;49(3):308–17.

78. Sjoberg P, Heiberg E, Wingren P, Ramgren Johansson J, Malm T, Arheden H, et al. Decreased diastolic ventricular kinetic energy in young patients with Fontan circulation demonstrated by four-dimensional cardiac magnetic resonance imaging. Pediatr Cardiol. 2017;38(4):669–80.

79. Kamphuis VP, Elbaz MSM, van den Boogaard PJ, Kroft LJM, van der Geest RJ, de Roos A, et al. Disproportionate intraventricular viscous energy loss in Fontan patients: analysis by 4D flow MRI. Eur Heart J Cardiovasc Imaging. 2019;20(3):323–33.

80. Kamphuis VP, Elbaz MSM, van den Boogaard PJ, Kroft LJM, Lamb HJ, Hazekamp MG, et al. Stress increases intracardiac 4D flow cardiovascular magnetic resonance -derived energetics and vorticity and relates to VO2max in Fontan patients. J Cardiovasc Magn Reson. 2019;21(1):43.

81. Calkoen EE, de Koning PJ, Blom NA, Kroft LJ, de Roos A, Wolterbeek R, et al. Disturbed intracardiac flow organization after atrioventricular septal defect correction as assessed with 4D flow magnetic resonance imaging and quantitative particle tracing. Investig Radiol. 2015;50(12):850–7.

82. Retson TA, Besser AH, Sall S, Golden D, Hsiao A. Machine learning and deep neural networks in thoracic and cardiovascular imaging. J Thorac Imaging. 2019;34(3):192–201.

83. Mazurowski MA, Buda M, Saha A, Bashir MR. Deep learning in radiology: an overview of the concepts and a survey of the state of the art with focus on MRI. J Magn Reson Imaging. 2019;49(4):939–54.

84. Tao Q, Yan W, Wang Y, Paiman EHM, Shamonin DP, Garg P, et al. Deep learning-based method for fully automatic quantification of left ventricle function from cine MR images: a multivendor, multicenter study. Radiology. 2019;290(1):81–8.

85. Nett EJ, Johnson KM, Frydrychowicz A, Del Rio AM, Schrauben E, Francois CJ, et al. Four-dimensional phase contrast MRI with accelerated dual velocity encoding. J Magn Reson Imaging. 2012;35(6):1462–71.

86. Schnell S, Ansari SA, Wu C, Garcia J, Murphy IG, Rahman OA, et al. Accelerated dual-venc 4D flow MRI for neurovascular applications. J Magn Reson Imaging. 2017;46(1):102–14.

87. Zwart NR, Pipe JG. Multidirectional high-moment encoding in phase contrast MRI. Magn Reson Med. 2013;69(6):1553–64.

88. Moersdorf R, Treutlein M, Kroeger JR, Ruijsink B, Wong J, Maintz D, et al. Precision, repro-
    ducibility and applicability of an undersampled multi-venc 4D flow MRI sequence for the
    assessment of cardiac hemodynamics. Magn Reson Imaging. 2019;61:73–82.
89. Di Sopra L, Piccini D, Coppo S, Stuber M, Yerly J. An automated approach to fully self-gated
    free-running cardiac and respiratory motion-resolved 5D whole-heart MRI. Magn Reson Med.
    2019;82(6):2118–32.
90. Bastiaansen JAM, Piccini D, Di Sopra L, Roy CW, Heerfordt J, Edelman RR, et al. Natively
    fat-suppressed 5D whole-heart MRI with a radial free-running fast-interrupted steady-state
    (FISS) sequence at 1.5T and 3T. Magn Reson Med. 2020;83(1):45–55.
91. Walheim J, Dillinger H, Kozerke S. Multipoint 5D flow cardiovascular magnetic resonance -
    accelerated cardiac- and respiratory-motion resolved mapping of mean and turbulent veloci-
    ties. J Cardiovasc Magn Reson. 2019;21(1):42.

Computational Fluid Dynamics

9

Rod Hose and Francesco Migliavacca

9.1 Introduction

Computational fluid dynamics (CFD) solves a system of physics equations to evaluate fluid dynamic conditions throughout a region. The analyses might be steady-state (no variation in time), periodic (regular and repeatable changes over an interval such as a heartbeat) or fully transient. CFD analysis is a mature technology and is a standard tool in all aspects of engineering. Some of the earliest applications were in the aerospace and nuclear industries over 50 years ago. CFD is now routinely used in the design of medical devices, including stents and heart valves, and in recent times there has been a major initiative by the FDA to formalise the process for the use of simulation in medical applications [1, 2].

Most frequently the term CFD refers to the computation of pressure and velocity fields throughout a region of space, usually in 3D. There are excellent applications in cardiac and cardiovascular applications, outlined later, but in this context simpler formulations, for example one dimensional or lumped parameter (compartmental) representations, also have significant value [3, 4]. An illustration of model dimensionality and the parameter resolution at each level is presented in Fig. 9.1.

The underpinning equations ensure that the computed pressure and velocity fields are consistent with the principles of physics. Specifically they ensure that

R. Hose (✉)
Department of Infection, Immunity and Cardiovascular Disease, University of Sheffield, Sheffield, UK

Norwegian University of Science and Technology (NTNU), Trondheim, Norway
e-mail: d.r.hose@sheffield.ac.uk

F. Migliavacca
Department of Chemistry, Materials and Chemical Engineering 'Giulio Natta', Politecnico di Milano, Milan, Italy
e-mail: francesco.migliavacca@polimi.it

© Springer Nature Switzerland AG 2021
P. Gallego, I. Valverde (eds.), *Multimodality Imaging Innovations In Adult Congenital Heart Disease*, Congenital Heart Disease in Adolescents and Adults, https://doi.org/10.1007/978-3-030-61927-5_9

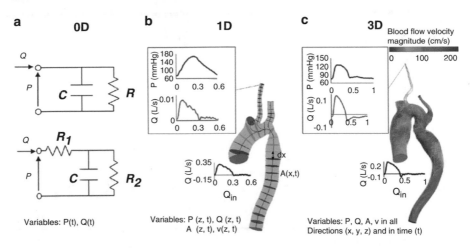

Fig. 9.1 Illustration of model scales: (**a**) 0D, (**b**) 1D, (**c**) 3D. (Courtesy of Massimilano Mercuri, PhD Thesis, University of Sheffield and published in [5])

momentum (Navier Stokes equations) and mass (continuity equation) are conserved. The equations are nonlinear, and generally there is no direct solution for any but the simplest geometrical systems. CFD produces numerical approximations that satisfy the equations within a specified error.

Once the velocity and pressure fields have been computed many other measures can be derived to characterise the solution to produce meaningful insights for clinical interpretation. Typical derived measures for cardiac and cardiovascular applications include integral measures (e.g. cardiac output), cardiac energetics parameters (e.g. ventricular work or power) and wall shear stress maps.

9.2 CFD Process for Medical Application

9.2.1 Overview

The general process for a CFD application, interpreted for medical application, is:

- Define the geometrical domain in which the analysis will be performed (anatomy)
- Define the material properties in this domain (blood rheology and wall properties)
- Define the conditions at the boundaries based on which the fluid dynamic conditions within the domain will be determined (e.g. inlet or outlet flows or pressures, distal resistances)
- Define any control parameters for the analysis, for example the details of the numerical solver and acceptable residual errors in the solution
- Solve the governing equations in the domain
- Post-process the pressure and velocity fields to extract other physical or physiological measures
- Interpret and report the results

Each of these steps has specific challenges for medical and clinical application. Steinman and Pereira [6] have published an excellent commentary on the sources of error, together with a subjective ranking of relative importance, in the context of computational analysis of cerebral aneurysms. There is increasing recognition in the biomedical modelling community of the value of benchmark problems to compare results from a range of practitioners. Examples include an FDA initiative [7] on an idealised system, and studies of a cerebral aneurysm [8] and an aortic coarctation [9].

One of the most important aspects is whether the analysis is generic, seeking insight into aspects of physiology or design that might be relevant to a population or sub-population, or personalised to an individual. The former can underpin a design process for a device or a type of surgical intervention, whilst the latter can provide diagnostic or prognostic information for an individual, as well as a prediction of how the system might respond to prospective interventions. The focus of this chapter is on personalised simulations.

9.2.2 Anatomy

A major issue for all cardiac and cardiovascular simulations is the definition of the anatomy. Unlike many other engineering applications, in which the geometry is known, for this application it is measured by a medical imaging process. Segmentation, or the labelling of regions of the image to indicate the anatomical structure, is part of the science of image processing, covered elsewhere in this book. The analyst will need to transform the segmented image into a form appropriate for CFD analysis. The details of this process depend on the underpinning mathematical formulation, but it is essential that the analyst and the clinician work together to understand any approximations in the imaging process and how they might affect the analysis. What is the spatial (and/or temporal) resolution of the image, and what are the implications for the interpretation of the analysis results? Is the anatomy actually measured under conditions that are relevant for the purpose of the analysis? For example, if the analysis is of an aortic coarctation under stress conditions, is the anatomy measured at rest an acceptable approximation? An important challenge is the determination of the extent of the domain that will be analysed. This is discussed under 'boundary conditions'.

9.2.3 Material Properties

Fundamentally the most important material properties for blood flow analysis are density and viscosity. Blood is effectively incompressible and so has a constant density, around 1060 kg/m^3. There is little variation across the population. Choice of viscosity model depends on the application. Blood is a suspension of cellular material, primarily erythrocytes, in plasma. The viscosity depends on the shear rate. At high shear rates, typical of those found in the heart and the larger vessels, the microstructure is not so important and the viscosity is approximately constant (a Newtonian fluid) and is about 3.5–4 times that of water. In the smaller vessels, less than about 1 mm in diameter, the effective viscosity increases rapidly, and in the capillaries analysis of the transport of the separate blood constituents is appropriate. Some investigators [10] use a nonlinear viscosity to capture the variation throughout the domain depending on the computed flows. The viscosity can be affected by smoking [11] but generally the variation is small compared with uncertainties in the analysis.

9.2.4 Boundary Conditions

The determination of appropriate boundary conditions is perhaps the biggest challenge facing the analyst in adding clinical value by CFD analysis.

Firstly there is the question of whether the walls of the domain are fixed or move. If they move (most cardiac and cardiovascular structures do!), how should this movement be described? The recognition of the flexibility of the structures spawned a whole academic field of application of fluid-solid interaction [12, 13]. The fluid domain is bounded by (or surrounds in the case of a heart valve analysis) a flexible structure that itself is governed by physics principles, the equations of solid mechanics. The fluid dynamic and solid mechanics equations are solved together to describe the pulsation of the walls and the pressure and flow fields in the blood. In the most sophisticated cardiac analyses [14, 15] there is further coupling of electromechanical processes so that an electrical wave passes through the walls of the cardiac chambers, stimulating a mechanical contraction of the myocardium. One of the major challenges with this type of analysis, especially in a personalised model, is that it requires definition of the material properties of the wall. The wall composition is likely to be very heterogeneous in space, especially so in pathophysiological situations in which there is scar tissue, calcification and other complications. A simpler alternative for the flow analysis, if available 4D medical imaging data supports it, is to apply measured motions at the boundaries. Often there are issues of spatial and/or temporal resolution that constrain the analysis protocol.

The next critical issue is the determination of the extent of the domain to be analysed, and the conditions that will be applied at the proximal and distal boundaries of the chambers and vessels. For a vessel, or vessel tree, analysis, where should the proximal and distal cuts be made? For a cardiac analysis, how many model chambers will be included, and what data is available to support their definition? Some combination of pressures, velocities and/or flows will be applied at the domain boundaries. It is possible to take clinical measurements of these parameters to underpin the analysis, especially of flow and/or velocity fields from exquisite modern medical imaging techniques. Pressure measurement can be extremely valuable to underpin CFD analyses, but time series pressure measurement is generally by catheter and is an invasive process. There are many traps and stumbling blocks here, and it is the responsibility of the analyst to ensure that any measurements used are consistent and appropriate for the purposes of the analysis, depending on the specific numerical formulation. It is common for clinical measurements to be mutu-ally inconsistent (e.g. measured flow into a bifurcation does not equal measured flow out of it), and this is especially so when data sources are mixed (e.g. echo with MRI data). The process of clinical data assimilation into a CFD analysis is a rich area of research in its own right, see for example [16, 17].

Seductive as the idea of use of measured individual physiological data might be, whether it is wall motion or proximal/distal conditions, it suffers from one insur-mountable flaw. Often the primary purpose of the model is to produce diagnostic or prognostic measures, and prediction of changes under prospective interventions. Manifestation of disease is usually most clearly observable in an extreme physio-logical state (e.g. stress or exercise), and it can be very challenging to make ade-quate clinical measurements in the appropriate state. Furthermore, by definition, the measurements of the effects of intervention cannot be made until the intervention is performed. The recognition of the importance of the boundary conditions has led to the development of families of systems models, typically assemblies of resistance, capacitance and inertance components in electro-hydraulic formulations to describe the conditions at proximal and distal boundaries. These models are coupled to the fluid domain at its boundaries, and the parameters can be tuned (personalised) in the measurement state and then extrapolated, based on published data, to other physi-ological states. The formal representation of the physiological envelope, or the physiological excursions that an individual makes as they live their lives, is a key challenge in the clinical translation of computational cardiovascular models [5].

9.2.5 Solver Details and Control Parameters

Systems physiology models are usually described in terms of electro-hydraulic rep-resentations. Complex physiological control systems, including the representation of major organs and sub-systems, were described by Guyton [18] half a century ago, and provided strong insight into regulation processes. Control models of this type can be very useful, for example, to understand the effects of pharmacological inter-vention. An excellent implementation of a cardiovascular systems model, targeted at medical education, is the CircAdapt software from Maastricht [19–22].

Figure 9.2 illustrates the simulation of a normal (REFERENCE) state and of an acute mitral insufficiency, both without (SNAPSHOT) and with (CURRENT) homeostatic regulation. In this example homeostatic control means that the model can vary total blood volume (i.e. preload) and systemic vascular resistance, so that mean arterial pressure and cardiac output are normalised to their default values (92 mmHg and 5.1 L/min, respectively). The resulting PV loops are also illustrated, showing very clearly the effect of the disease to reduce chamber pressures and increase stroke volume without regulation in an unregulated state and then the res-toration of pressure but further increase in stroke volume in the regulated state. Simulations of this type can greatly assist understanding of the systemic effects of disease and the likely effects of intervention both generically and, when the model parameters are personalised, for an individual case.

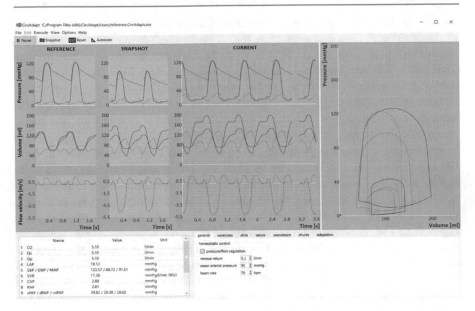

Fig. 9.2 Snapshot of system model simulation. (Courtesy Joost Lumens, University of Maastricht)

There are several numerical formulations for three-dimensional problems, and each has its merits. By far the most common numerical methods in cardiovascular application seek to solve the Navier Stokes equations using finite volume or finite element methods in an Eulerian framework, which means that the equations are solved on a fixed grid in space, or sometimes in an arbitrary Eulerian-Lagrangian framework that supports flexible geometries. Alternative approaches include Lattice Boltzmann [23] and smooth particle hydrodynamics (SPH) formulations. The former might have advantages in terms of simplicity of derivation of a model from a medical image and potentially for systems with very complex flow paths (for example a packed coil in a cerebral aneurysm or for multi-layer stents), as well as for representation of many elastic bodies (e.g. individual red cells) interacting in the flow [24]. The latter has advantages especially for free-surface or fluid mixing problems but not for most cardiovascular applications.

One important issue for transient and periodic flows is the representation of unsteady structures in the flows. The term 'turbulence' is often inappropriately used in the context of cardiovascular systems that are periodic. There might be beat-to-beat variation, and indeed more complex transient interactions with the respiratory cycle, but the flow is essentially laminar and the flow structures, like vortices, are large scale and repeatable. Turbulence refers to micro-scale flow fluctuations that are stochastic in nature. Turbulence is an important feature of many aerodynamic systems, and many models are available. Flow regimes are characterised by the Reynolds number, which describes the dominance of viscous or inertial components, and by the Strouhal number (Womersley number for cardiovascular applications) which illuminates the influence of periodicity. The onset of turbulence in steady flow in a straight tube occurs when the Reynolds number approaches 2000. Generally periodic cardiovascular flows are more stable during the accelerative phase and less stable during deceleration. Mostly throughout the cardiovascular system flow is periodic but not turbulent, with the primary exceptions being the flow in the normal aorta and sometimes in pathological situations in the regions of stenoses. Unfortunately many of the turbulence models that are used in other sectors are applicable only to high Reynolds numbers, beyond those that occur in the cardiovascular system. Low Reynolds number turbulence models and transitional models have been applied successfully. An important challenge, featuring both transitional turbulence associated with a local stenosis and blood damage elements, was issued by the FDA to the cardiovascular modelling community [7]. Most participants used a Shear Stress Transport (SST) turbulence model at appropriate Reynolds numbers: the results make interesting reading! In most commercial fluid solvers turbulence models are invoked by setting a switch in the analysis control, but this should be used with care and with the advice of an experienced CFD analyst.

Generally the CFD solver will report a residual, which is a measure of how accurately the numerical solution of the equations represents the underpinning equations. Usually the analysis either converges, by which we mean that the numerical error reduces at each iteration of the solution until in practical terms it is negligible, or it diverges and no solution is found (or the solution is absurd). The user can set an acceptable value of the residual but, especially for clinical applications, any error in the numerical solution of the equations, provided the analysis is properly prescribed, is dwarfed by the uncertainty of the patient anatomy and measured physiological parameters on which the analyses are based. It is important to note that this residual measures the accuracy of the solution of the equations, not the accuracy of the analysis including the modelling decisions that have been made!

9.2.6   Post-processing, Interpretation and Reporting

Whether the model is a lumped parameter systems model or a three-dimensional full-field analysis, generally it returns values of the parameters (pressure, flow and volume in compartments, pressure and velocity fields respectively) at the sampling points in space and time. Even for a simple lumped parameter model there might be pressure, flow and volume in ten or more compartments with results at every millisecond, so 30,000 or more computational measurements. For 3D analyses there might easily be over a billion 'measurement points' in space and time. These data cannot be interpreted without some form of post-processing. It is said that a picture is worth a thousand words, and snapshots (or indeed movies) of the flow field are routinely produced. These pictures and movies are not always easy to interpret in terms of clinical meaning, but they are always beautiful and it is not without reason that CFD has sometimes been negatively referred to as 'Colour for Doctors', or in other applications, 'Colour for Directors'. Nevertheless these images can be of immense value in communicating the structure of the flow and an important reporting tool. Almost always the data will also be post-processed to derive other, more instantly recognisable and interpretable, measures. Examples include integral measures (e.g. cardiac output, fractional flow division to multiple outlets) and extrema (e.g. maximum and minimum pressure). Furthermore many other field values, for example the distribution of wall shear stress, can be derived and similarly reported. A recent community consensus report [25] describes a formula for successful wall shear stress analysis and interpretation for a specific cardiovascular application.

One of the most successful commercialised applications of CFD in cardiovascular medicine is the computation of coronary fractional flow reserve (FFR) from CT image data, available from HeartFlow [26]. This decision support tool is approved, *inter alia*, by the FDA and by NICE in the UK. An integral part of the application is the comprehensive reporting of the analysis results, including the derived measure of FFR itself. An application also targeted at the computation of coronary FFR, but based on angiographic image data, is the VirtuHeart software [27, 28], see Fig. 9.3.

9.3   CFD for Congenital Heart Disease

Advances over the last two decades have led to successful palliation and survival of children born with cardiac defects resulting in only one functioning ventricle, such as hypoplastic left heart syndrome or tricuspid atresia. Yet, these children are still consigned to at least three surgeries, illustrated in Fig. 9.4, and a lifetime of abnormal physiology. Within a few days of life, neonates with single ventricle physiology will undergo a Stage 1 operation, which generally consists of the surgical

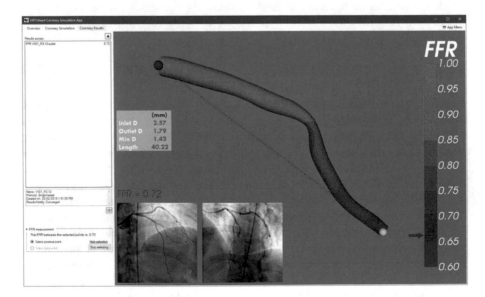

Fig. 9.3 Snapshot of output from VirtuHeart software, University of Sheffield, showing on a coloured scale the fractional flow reserve computed in a coronary artery segmented from the two angiographic projections illustrated in the main window

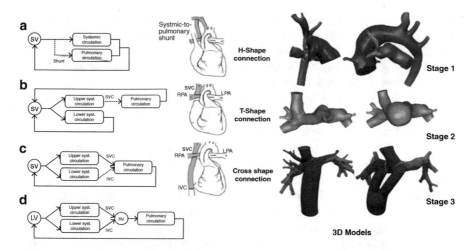

Fig. 9.4 Left: schematics of (**a**) in parallel Stage 1 circulation, with the interposition of a systemic-to-pulmonary shunt to deliver blood to the lungs; (**b**) Stage 2 circulation with upper systemic and pulmonary circulations in series; (**c**) Stage 3 or Fontan circulation, with an in-series circuit of systemic and pulmonary circulations; (**d**) physiological circulation. The three stages are illustrated on the middle. On the right, 3D reconstructed models of the three stages with surgical variants. (Image taken in part from [29] with permission)

reconstruction of univentricular outflow tract and the creation of a shunt between a systemic and a pulmonary artery, thus leading to a parallel circuit with the single ventricle pumping blood for both chambers. The shape of the connection can be seen as a 'H-type'. The Stage 2 operation is usually performed around 4–6 months of age. The shunt is excluded from the circulation and the superior vena cava is connected to the right pulmonary artery. The shape of the connection is a 'T-type'. Different variants, namely the bidirectional Glenn or the hemi-Fontan, have been proposed over the years with similar results although the haemodynamics are different [30]. At about 2 years of age, the Stage 3 operation or Fontan operation is performed, re-routing the total venous return directly to the pulmonary circulation by means of an additional anastomosis between the inferior vena cava and the right pulmonary artery, achieving a 'normal' sequence of blood flow: oxygenated blood to the body and deoxygenated blood to the lungs. The shape of the connection is a 'cross-type'.

Before reviewing more complex three-dimensional CFD models of congenital heart diseases (CHD) it is reiterated that, in common with other vascular applications, valuable insight can be gained from simpler models including zero-dimensional or lumped parameter models that do not recognise the anatomical detail. An excellent example in the context of CHD is a study [31] of pulmonary regurgitation after repair of tetralogy of Fallot. A patient with or without an effective pulmonary valve, causing pulmonary regurgitation, born with tetralogy of Fallot, palliated with a right Blalock–Taussig shunt and repaired at 8 years with a homograft right ventricle to pulmonary artery conduit and graft augmentation of the proximal left pulmonary artery was studied by means of magnetic resonance imaging. A lumped parameter model of the pulmonary circulation showed that, without the valve, there is forward flow in late diastole but a regurgitant flow in early diastole at the level of the main pulmonary artery, whilst there is no reversal of flow at capillary level. The model indicates that the regurgitant volume originates entirely from compliance of the virtual pulmonary arteries and arterioles. Thus, the amount of regurgitation, in the absence of an effective valve, depends on pulmonary arterial compliance and on the location of resistance relative to the compliance.

Because single ventricle physiology exhibits a highly variable, complex and multi-scale behaviour, advanced engineering and imaging methods hold promise to improve the care of children born with this condition.

Groundbreaking work by de Leval [32, 33], which included experimental validation, explored the utility of mathematical or computational analyses as a tool to understand single ventricle physiology and improve surgical results. These and several similar CFD models have been used to study congenital heart diseases (CHD). Although such models, using prescribed pressure or flow boundary conditions, provide a very detailed description of the local haemodynamics, they cannot describe the mutual interactions with the remainder of the circulatory system. The recognition that surgical reconstruction of the local cardiopulmonary circulation (local-scale) both affects, and is affected by, global upstream and downstream systemic dynamics (global-scale) suggests that coupled local/global (system) models are appropriate for CHD applications. In this framework 3D CFD models of the cardiac reconstruction are derived from patient-specific anatomy and physiological parameters. The computational solution is coupled to a patient-specific lumped parameter network of the entire circulatory system, where the interface conditions of flow rates and pressure feed back into the 3D model. One of the first examples of the importance of coupling models which operate at different scales is provided in [34]. Although the geometry used at that time is quite idealised, the main findings and the methodological approach are still at the state-of-the-art. Subsequent iterations of this multi-scale solution have been used to predict local cardiopulmonary pressures and flow, and global parameters such as cardiac performance, and systemic oxygen delivery [35].

In the Stage 1 operation (Fig. 9.4), two main options are available: (1) the systemic-to-pulmonary conduit connecting the innominate artery or the aorta to the right pulmonary artery and (2) the right ventricle to pulmonary artery shunt. Migliavacca et al. [34] used the coupled, multi-scale modelling approach to compare haemodynamic results for conduits of different sizes in the two anatomical configurations. The hydraulic nets (lumped resistances, compliances, inertances and elastances) which represent the systemic, coronary and pulmonary circulations and the heart were identical in the two models. Computer simulation results were compared with post-operative catheterisation data. There was a good correlation between predicted and observed data: higher aortic diastolic pressure, decreased pulmonary arterial pressure, lower pulmonary-to-systemic flow ratio and higher coronary perfusion pressure in connection with the ventricle together with a minimal regurgitant flow and a higher ejection fraction and a lower stroke work were demonstrated.

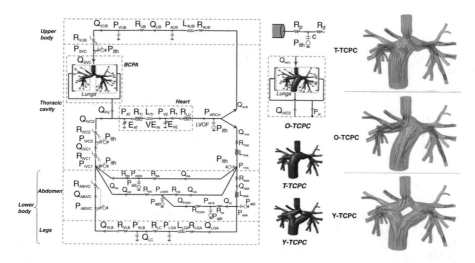

Fig. 9.5 (Left) Stage 2 coupling of the LPM with 3D model; (middle) different surgical post-operative 3D models of Stage 3. (Right) Velocity-coloured pathlines in the Stage 3 models. (Image taken from [29])

With ever-improving CT and MR imaging techniques, and increasingly powerful computational resource, multi-scale models of CHD have become more anatomically realistic and more comprehensive, see Fig. 9.5, and can be applied to a wider range of surgical options, but the adopted concepts and methods are still those described more than 10 years ago [30, 36]. The movement of the vessel boundaries based on interaction between fluid dynamics and the wall mechanics (fluid-solid interaction) and systemic regulation effects are still to be included as a standard process in these models.

As discussed previously, one of the primary advantages of the computational models lies in the fact that different pathological states can be investigated. Response to exercise is an important issue for patients with the Fontan pathology [37] because, without a reduction in the systemic resistances, it can lead to an excessive increase of central venous pressure. Figure 9.6 shows the trends in changes in cardiac output and pulmonary arterial pressure with increasing exercise state, quantified by metabolic equivalent (MET), in a Stage 3 configuration. This study investigates the effects of three functional deficiencies, namely: (1) systolic dysfunction (SysD), that is the impaired ability to increase ventricular contractility during exercise; (2) disordered respiration (DR), that is the impaired movement of the thoracic cavity caused by common or potential complications of multiple sternotomy incisions, including diaphragm plication; (3) atrial-ventricular valve insufficiency (AVVI), that is produced by a regurgitant valve. The corresponding tracings of ventricular pressure–volume loop (one cardiac cycle) and PA pressure (four cardiac cycles/one breathing cycle) at a MET of 5, representing an elevated exercise state, are also reported to illustrate how these models might be applicable in clinical routine.

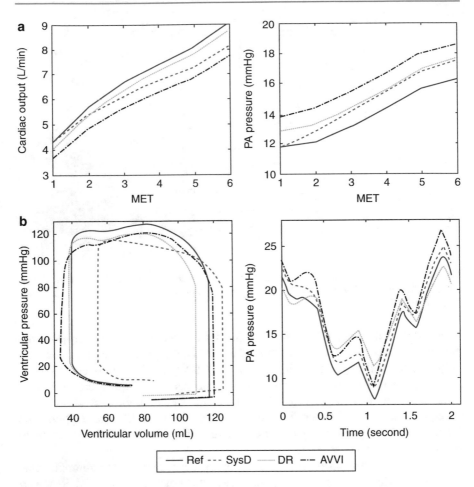

Fig. 9.6 Simulations of exercise conditions varying the exercise level, measured as metabolic equivalent (MET). (**a**). PV loop and pulmonary pressure tracings (**b**). *SysD* systolic dysfunction, *DR* disordered respiration, *AVVI* the atrial-ventricular valve insufficiency. (Figure taken from [38] with permission, Springer)

The focus in Fig. 9.6 is on the system level responses. Further important information related to the local haemodynamics can be extracted from the 3D components of the coupled model. In Stages 2 and 3 configurations, blood streamlines can give an idea on the vortices and flow disturbances created by the surgical connection. As well as increases in central venous pressures, the energy dissipated by these flow structures might be important in the context of the work that the heart is required to do to provide adequate perfusion of the circulatory system. Figure 9.7 illustrates typical haemodynamic structures in the two different scenarios of the Stage 2 operation [36]. The increase in SVC pressure after the surgical operation is visible in the right panel; negligible differences are detectable from the two variants [30].

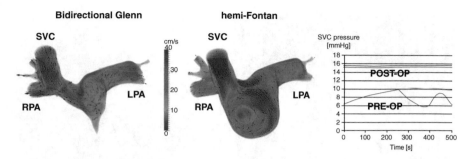

Fig. 9.7 Comparison of the haemodynamics of two different models of Stage 2 operation: (left) volume-rendered velocities at peak flow with velocity vectors; (right) pressure tracing in the pre- and post-operative scenarios. *SVC* superior vena cava, *RPA* right pulmonary artery, *LPA* left pulmonary artery

In one of the most sophisticated applications of simulation to the study of CHD, focusing on cardiac mechanics, patient-specific models of univentricular hearts following surgical treatment of hypoplastic left heart syndrome have been developed to investigate the interaction between myocardial mechanics and blood flow in diastole [15]. It was shown, see Fig. 9.8, that a more elliptical ventricular cavity shape can increase the intraventricular pressure gradients and filling capacity. In these personalised models the anatomy was determined from the segmentation of MR images at end diastole, and the models included representation of the fibre distribution in the myocardium.

9.4   Summary, Challenges and the Future of CFD in Cardiovascular Medicine

Computational fluid dynamics is a mature technology in the engineering industry and is used increasingly to provide insight into haemodynamic processes in cardiovascular application. Some of the most advanced applications, especially in the context of understanding of exercise pathophysiology, have been in congenital heart disease applications. Although there have been massive advances in anatomical personalisation of models based on exquisite modern imaging technology, it continues to be a challenge to personalise these models, especially the boundary conditions, to represent the range of physiological states (the physiological envelope) that an individual encounters as they lead their lives [5]. Huberts et al. [40] have presented a comprehensive review of the challenges that must be addressed to bring simulation into routine operation in the cardiovascular clinic. He asks a number of very pertinent questions, including:

- Are we calculating the information that the doctor needs?
- Where is the balance between model complexity and utility? It is possible to construct a very complex model, but it might be impossible to personalise such a

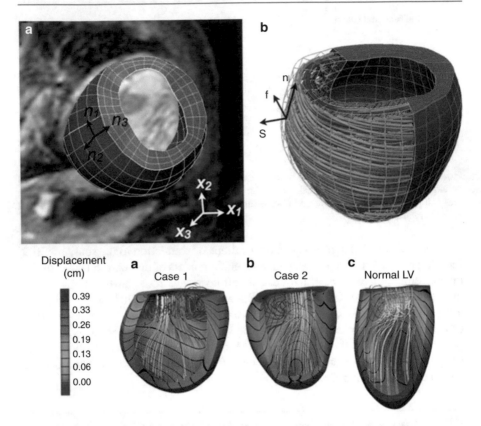

Fig. 9.8 (Top) Volume mesh from the manual segmentation of Dual Phase MRI contours. Anisotropic fibre model incorporated in the solid mesh; (bottom) instantaneous streamlines of blood flow and iso-contours of myocardial displacement at the peak E-wave of diastole in two baseline HLHS patients and a normal left ventricle: Vortex structures can be easily visualised and quantified. (Figure taken from [39] with permission, Springer)

model given the relatively sparse clinical information that is often available. Even if many clinical measurements, including comprehensive time series pressure or flow recordings, are available, the personalisation process might not be robust.
- What verification and validation of the model and the process is required for clinical confidence? … and how does the modelling process become embedded in a legal and regulatory framework? As indicated in the introduction there is recent significant progress, driven by the FDA, in these aspects.

In the same article, Huberts points out the absolute necessity to include recognition of model and parameter uncertainty in a clinically oriented pipeline. He proposes a new and carefully structured approach, termed the Medical Engineering modelling chain, and illustrates it with two clinical exemplars. An important series of articles covering the issues of verification, validation and uncertainty in biomedical simulation, edited by Steinman and Migliavacca [41], was published in a special issue of the *Journal of Cardiovascular Engineering and Technology* in 2018.

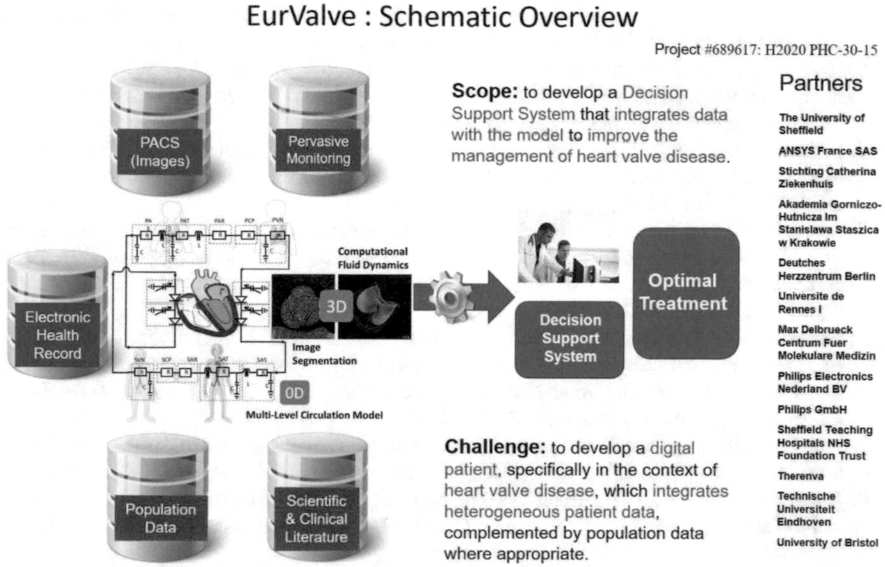
EurValve : Schematic Overview
Project #689617: H2020 PHC-30-15
PACS (Images)
Pervasive Monitoring
Scope: to develop a Decision Support System that integrates data with the model to improve the management of heart valve disease.
Partners
The University of Sheffield
ANSYS France SAS
Stichting Catherina Ziekenhuis
Akademia Gorniczo-Hutnicza Im Stanislawa Staszica w Krakowie
Deutches Herzzentrum Berlin
Universite de Rennes I
Max Delbrueck Centrum Fuer Molekulare Medizin
Philips Electronics Nederland BV
Philips GmbH
Sheffield Teaching Hospitals NHS Foundation Trust
Therenva
Technische Universiteit Eindhoven
University of Bristol
Electronic Health Record
Computational Fluid Dynamics
3D
Image Segmentation
0D
Multi-Level Circulation Model
Decision Support System
Optimal Treatment
Population Data
Scientific & Clinical Literature
Challenge: to develop a digital patient, specifically in the context of heart valve disease, which integrates heterogeneous patient data, complemented by population data where appropriate.

Fig. 9.9 Overview of model-based process, including a system model and a local three-dimensional computational fluid dynamics analysis, embedded in a data-rich environment and supporting a clinical decision support system: courtesy of the EurValve project (#689617: H2020 PHC-30-15)

We believe that the use of multi-scale, personalised computational models in clinical settings will accelerate over the next decade, and will become routine in the future. The first examples, such as the HeartFlow application for coronary FFR, have already secured regulatory approval and provide real clinical benefit. Figure 9.9 illustrates the embedding of a CFD analysis into a complete pipeline that ingests data from many sources to develop a personalised model that supports a clinical decision process. The framework now exists for development, evaluation and certification of appropriate computational pipelines. There remain real challenges in the personalisation of model parameters, going beyond anatomical fidelity, and in the assimilation of clinical data into the modelling process.

References

1. American Society of Mechanical Engineers. Codes and standards for verification and validation in computational modeling and simulation. n.d.. https://cstools.asme.org/csconnect/CommitteePages.cfm?Committee=100003367. Accessed 9 Jan 2020.
2. American Society of Mechanical Engineers. Verification, validation and uncertainty quantification (VVUQ). n.d.. https://www.asme.org/about-asme/standards/verification-validation-uncertainty. Accessed 9 Jan 2020.
3. van de Vosse FN, Stergiopulos N. Pulse wave propagation in the arterial tree. Annu Rev Fluid Mech. 2011;43:467–99. https://doi.org/10.1146/annurev-fluid-122109-160730.

4. Shi Y, Lawford P, Hose R. Review of Zero-D and 1-D models of blood flow in the cardiovascular system. Biomed Eng Online. 2011;10:33. https://doi.org/10.1186/1475-925X-10-33.
5. Hose DR, Lawford PV, Huberts W, Hellevik LR, Omholt SW, van de Vosse FN. Cardiovascular models for personalised medicine: where now and where next? Med Eng Phys. 2019;72:38–48. https://doi.org/10.1016/j.medengphy.2019.08.007.
6. Steinman DA, Pereira VM. How patient specific are patient-specific computational models of cerebral aneurysms? An overview of sources of error and variability. Neurosurg Focus. 2019;47:1–11. https://doi.org/10.3171/2019.4.FOCUS19123.
7. Stewart SFC, Paterson EG, Burgreen GW, Hariharan P, Giarra M, Reddy V, et al. Assessment of CFD performance in simulations of an idealized medical device: results of FDA's first computational interlaboratory study. Cardiovasc Eng Technol. 2012;3:139–60. https://doi.org/10.1007/s13239-012-0087-5.
8. Radaelli AG, Augsburger L, Cebral JR, Ohta M, Rüfenacht DA, Balossino R, et al. Reproducibility of haemodynamical simulations in a subject-specific stented aneurysm model - a report on the Virtual Intracranial Stenting Challenge 2007. J Biomech. 2008;41:2069–81. https://doi.org/10.1016/j.jbiomech.2008.04.035.
9. 2nd CFD challenge predicting patient-specific hemodynamics at rest and stress through an aortic coarctation. n.d.. http://www.vascularmodel.org/miccai2013/. Accessed 9 Jan 2020.
10. Doost SN, Zhong L, Su B, Morsi YS. The numerical analysis of non-Newtonian blood flow in human patient-specific left ventricle. Comput Methods Prog Biomed. 2016;127:232–47. https://doi.org/10.1016/j.cmpb.2015.12.020.
11. Singh PK, Marzo A, Howard B, Rufenacht DA, Bijlenga P, Frangi AF, et al. Effects of smoking and hypertension on wall shear stress and oscillatory shear index at the site of intracranial aneurysm formation. Clin Neurol Neurosurg. 2010;112:306–13. https://doi.org/10.1016/j.clineuro.2009.12.018.
12. Peskin CS, McQueen DM. A three-dimensional computational method for blood flow in the heart I. Immersed elastic fibers in a viscous incompressible fluid. J Comput Phys. 1989;81:239. https://doi.org/10.1016/0021-9991(89)90213-1.
13. De Hart J, Baaijens FPT, Peters GWM, Schreurs PJG. A computational fluid-structure interaction analysis of a fiber-reinforced stentless aortic valve. J Biomech. 2003;36:699. https://doi.org/10.1016/S0021-9290(02)00448-7.
14. Smith N, de Vecchi A, McCormick M, Nordsletten D, Camara O, Frangi AF, et al. euHeart: personalized and integrated cardiac care using patient-specific cardiovascular modelling. Interface Focus. 2011;1:349. https://doi.org/10.1098/rsfs.2010.0048.
15. De Vecchi A, Nordsletten DA, Remme EW, Bellsham-Revell H, Greil G, Simpson JM, et al. Inflow typology and ventricular geometry determine efficiency of filling in the hypoplastic left heart. Ann Thorac Surg. 2012;94:1562–9. https://doi.org/10.1016/j.athoracsur.2012.05.122.
16. Pant S, Corsini C, Baker C, Hsia TY, Pennati G, Vignon-Clementel IE. Data assimilation and modelling of patient-specific single-ventricle physiology with and without valve regurgitation. J Biomech. 2016;49:2162. https://doi.org/10.1016/j.jbiomech.2015.11.030.
17. Bertoglio C, Moireau P, Gerbeau JF. Sequential parameter estimation for fluid-structure problems: application to hemodynamics. Int J Numer Method Biomed Eng. 2012;28:434. https://doi.org/10.1002/cnm.1476.
18. Guyton AC, Coleman TG, Granger HJ. Circulation overall regulation. Annu Rev Physiol. 1972;34:13–44.
19. Lumens J, Delhaas T, Kirn B, Arts T. Three-wall segment (TriSeg) model describing mechanics and hemodynamics of ventricular interaction. Ann Biomed Eng. 2009;37:2234–55. https://doi.org/10.1007/s10439-009-9774-2.
20. Walmsley J, Arts T, Derval N, Bordachar P, Cochet H, Ploux S, et al. Fast simulation of mechanical heterogeneity in the electrically asynchronous heart using the Multipatch module. PLoS Comput Biol. 2015;11:1–23. https://doi.org/10.1371/journal.pcbi.1004284.
21. Arts T, Delhaas T, Bovendeerd P, Verbeek X, Prinzen FW. Adaptation to mechanical load determines shape and properties of heart and circulation: the CircAdapt model. Am J Physiol Heart Circ Physiol. 2005;288:1943–54. https://doi.org/10.1152/ajpheart.00444.2004.

22. Fox KAA. "Where everything comes together!" European Society of Cardiology Congress 2014. Eur Heart J. 2014;35:331–2. https://doi.org/10.1093/eurheartj/eht564.
23. Chopard B, Ouared R, Rüfenacht DA. A lattice Boltzmann simulation of clotting in stented aneurysms and comparison with velocity or shear rate reductions. Math Comput Simul. 2006;72:108–12. https://doi.org/10.1016/j.matcom.2006.05.025.
24. Halliday I, Atherton M, Care CM, Collins MW, Evans D, Evans PC, et al. Multi-scale interaction of particulate flow and the artery wall. Med Eng Phys. 2011;33:840–8. https://doi.org/10.1016/j.medengphy.2010.09.007.
25. Gijsen F, Katagiri Y, Barlis P, Bourantas C, Collet C, Coskun U, et al. Expert recommendations on the assessment of wall shear stress in human coronary arteries: existing methodologies, technical considerations, and clinical applications. Eur Heart J. 2019;40:3421–33. https://doi.org/10.1093/eurheartj/ehz551.
26. Transforming the diagnosis and management of coronary artery disease worldwide. n.d.. https://www.heartflow.com/. Accessed 9 Jan 2020.
27. Morris PD, Ryan D, Morton AC, Lycett R, Lawford PV, Hose DR, et al. Virtual fractional flow reserve from coronary angiography: modeling the significance of coronary lesions. Results from the VIRTU-1 (VIRTUal fractional flow reserve from coronary angiography) study. JACC Cardiovasc Interv. 2013;6:149–57. https://doi.org/10.1016/j.jcin.2012.08.024.
28. VirtuHeart. n.d.. http://virtuheart.com/. Accessed 9 Jan 2020.
29. Baretta A, Corsini C, Marsden AL, Vignon-Clementel IE, Hsia TY, Dubini G, et al. Respiratory effects on hemodynamics in patient-specific CFD models of the Fontan circulation under exercise conditions. Eur J Mech B/Fluids. 2012;35:61–9. https://doi.org/10.1016/j.euromechflu.2012.01.012.
30. Kung E, Corsini C, Marsden A, Vignon-Clementel I, Pennati G, Figliola R, et al. Multiscale modeling of superior cavopulmonary circulation: hemi-Fontan and bidirectional Glenn are equivalent. Semin Thorac Cardiovasc Surg. 2020;32:883–92. https://doi.org/10.1053/j.semtcvs.2019.09.007.
31. Kilner PJ, Balossino R, Dubini G, Babu-Narayan SV, Taylor AM, Pennati G, et al. Pulmonary regurgitation: the effects of varying pulmonary artery compliance, and of increased resistance proximal or distal to the compliance. Int J Cardiol. 2009;133:157–66. https://doi.org/10.1016/j.ijcard.2008.06.078.
32. de Leval MR, Kilner P, Gewillig M, Bull C. Total cavopulmonary connection: a logical alternative to atriopulmonary connection for complex Fontan operations. Experimental studies and early clinical experience. J Thorac Cardiovasc Surg. 1988;96:682–95.
33. de Leval MR, Dubini G, Migliavacca F, Jalali H, Camporini G, Redington A, et al. Use of computational fluid dynamics in the design of surgical procedures: application to the study of competitive flows in cavopulmonary connections. J Thorac Cardiovasc Surg. 1996;111:502–13. https://doi.org/10.1016/S0022-5223(96)70302-1.
34. Migliavacca F, Balossino R, Pennati G, Dubini G, Hsia TY, de Leval MR, et al. Multiscale modelling in biofluidynamics: application to reconstructive paediatric cardiac surgery. J Biomech. 2006;39:1010–20. https://doi.org/10.1016/j.jbiomech.2005.02.021.
35. Hsia TY, Cosentino D, Corsini C, Pennati G, Dubini G, Migliavacca F. Use of mathematical modeling to compare and predict hemodynamic effects between hybrid and surgical Norwood palliations for hypoplastic left heart syndrome. Circulation. 2011;124:204–10. https://doi.org/10.1161/CIRCULATIONAHA.110.010769.
36. Corsini C, Baker C, Kung E, Schievano S, Arbia G, Baretta A, et al. An integrated approach to patient-specific predictive modeling for single ventricle heart palliation. Comput Methods Biomech Biomed Eng. 2014;17:1572–89. https://doi.org/10.1080/10255842.2012.758254.
37. Louw JJ, Gewillig M. The fontan circulation: the known, the unknown and the plausible. Curr Pediatr Rep. 2013;1:69–74. https://doi.org/10.1007/s40124-013-0017-5.
38. Kung E, Perry JC, Davis C, Migliavacca F, Pennati G, Giardini A, et al. Computational modeling of pathophysiologic responses to exercise in fontan patients. Ann Biomed Eng. 2015;43:1335–47. https://doi.org/10.1007/s10439-014-1131-4.

39. De Vecchi A, Nordsletten DA, Razavi R, Greil G, Smith NP. Patient specific fluid-structure ventricular modelling for integrated cardiac care. Med Biol Eng Comput. 2013;51:1261–70. https://doi.org/10.1007/s11517-012-1030-5.
40. Huberts W, Heinen SGH, Zonnebeld N, van den Heuvel DAF, de Vries JPPM, Tordoir JHM, et al. What is needed to make cardiovascular models suitable for clinical decision support? A viewpoint paper. J Comput Sci. 2018;24:68. https://doi.org/10.1016/j.jocs.2017.07.006.
41. Steinman DA, Migliavacca F. Editorial: Special issue on verification, validation, and uncertainty quantification of cardiovascular models: towards effective VVUQ for translating cardiovascular modelling to clinical utility. Cardiovasc Eng Technol. 2018;9:539–43. https://doi.org/10.1007/s13239-018-00393-z.

3D Printing and Holography

10

Mari Nieves Velasco Forte, Ravi Vamsee,
and Tarique Hussain

10.1 Introduction

The increasing anatomical complexity of the patients undergoing congenital cardiac surgery over time has created the need for new techniques to assess cardiac morphology and structural defects, with multidetector computer tomography (CT) and cardiac magnetic resonance (CMR) being currently part of their routine evaluation. While 3D images could be generated using echocardiography, the absence of fixed imaging coordinates and operator dependency reduce the reliability. 3D images have therefore become more frequently available, with the limitation that although a 3D representation of the anatomy is provided, it is configured within the confines of a two-dimensional screen. The complexity of severe types of CHD precludes the understanding of the disease without the manipulation and direct visualization of the patient's heart features.

The first medical 3D printing techniques were aimed to plan cranial [1–4], maxillofacial [3–6], and orthopedic surgery [7, 8]. Since then, a wide variety of different materials and printing techniques have been developed, offering now the possibility of using them in different scenarios, including cardiovascular disease. In this chapter, we discuss how to create a patient-specific 3D model to be printed in different materials or presented as a hologram and their applications for patients with CHD.

M. N. Velasco Forte
School of Biomedical Engineering and Imaging Sciences, King's College London,
London, UK

Cardiovascular Pathology Unit, Institute of Biomedicine of Seville, IBIS, Virgen del Rocio
University Hospital, CSIC, University of Seville, Seville, Spain

R. Vamsee · T. Hussain (✉)
Department of Pediatrics, UT Southwestern Medical Center, Dallas, TX, USA
e-mail: Ravi.Vamsee@UTSouthwestern.edu; Mohammad.Hussain@UTSouthwestern.edu

© Springer Nature Switzerland AG 2021
P. Gallego, I. Valverde (eds.), *Multimodality Imaging Innovations In Adult
Congenital Heart Disease*, Congenital Heart Disease in Adolescents and Adults,
https://doi.org/10.1007/978-3-030-61927-5_10

10.2 How to Create a Patient-Specific 3D Representation of the Heart

10.2.1 Image Acquisition: What Type of Image Is Needed?

Most 3D models are created from CT or MRI whole-heart datasets. Some minimum requirements are necessary. Each slice must be contiguous to the preceding one, the image should be isotropic and any data element acquired must relate to every other image data point with a fixed relationship.

The preference between one imaging technique and another is based on the experience of the center, the main structure of interest and the age of the patient, with a tendency to use MRI in younger population to avoid radiation [9, 10]. Although being of significant relevance, the details for sequence acquisition are not always explained in clinical studies [11–13]. ECG-gated 3D balance steady-state free precession (SSFP) and contrast-enhanced MRI angiography are the most common reported techniques when MRI is the selected imaging method [9, 10, 14–18]. Image-based navigation for motion correction in 3D balance SSFP acquisition has been used for creation of models in complex interventional planning [10]. The sharpness of the borders of the cardiac contours and vessels and the small voxel size achieved with this technique help the operator perform a detailed segmentation of the patient's anatomy (Fig. 10.1).

Other studies using CT describe it as being one of the easiest modalities to segment anatomy for 3D printing [19]. Though a single procedure may not necessitate a high dose of radiation, an adult with congenital heart disease may be prone to repeated examinations over a lifetime with a high cumulative dose [20]. Newer generation CT machines and implementation of cardiac imaging protocols do however attenuate the effective radiation dose utilized [21–23]. Echocardiography has also been utilized when cardiac valves or atrial septal defects are the target of the

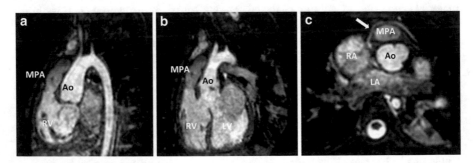

Fig. 10.1 Examples of multiplanar reformat of a 3D bSSFP acquisition using image-based navigation in a patient with double outlet right ventricle and malposition of the great arteries status post arterial switch operation. (**a**) Sagittal, (**b**) reformatted coronal, and (**c**) axial views. *Ao* aorta, *LA* left atrium, *LV* left atrium, *MPA* main pulmonary artery, *RA* right atrium, *RV* right ventricle, white arrow: coronary artery crossing around the MPA

segmentation, with more promising results when combining 3D echo with CT [24–27]. CT and 3D echocardiography have the advantage of usability in patients with intracardiac devices, or coils that preclude magnetic imaging.

As this field is still developing, new imaging modalities are emerging as possible options to reconstruct a 3D model. This is the case for rotational angiography, which allows tomographic slices to be routinely reconstructed with high spatial resolution. A short case series has been recently published, suggesting that this option may spread the opportunity to create 3D models to a larger number of centers [28].

10.2.2 Image Segmentation

Once the image is acquired, the data is imported into a segmentation software, where the anatomy of interest is delineated and separated from the surrounding tissues. There are several software packages available either commercially or as open-source access platforms [18, 29–33]. It is, however, quite common that the name of the software or program used is not mentioned in the study. A systematic review on image segmentation methodology showed that only 34% of journal publications provided sufficient detail for their methodology to be reproduced. A further 38% mentioned the methods that they had used, but did not explain how these had been applied and the remaining 29% of publications did not provide any description of their method whatsoever [18].

The segmentation process is carried out with the use of manual and semiautomatic methods. Brightness thresholding, region growing, and manual editing are the three most frequently used methods [18, 29, 34]. Depending on the complexity of anatomy, the quality of the images obtained, and the operator's experience, this process has the potential to be time intensive.

Once the segmentation is finished, the stereolithography file (.stl) created is exported to a computer-aided design (CAD) software, where refinement of the anatomy is performed. This process allows the creation of hollow models with smooth surfaces, as well as trimming the end of the vessels or cutting the model to show its inside. An example of the segmentation process using a free-access segmentation tool and computer-aided design methodology is provided in Fig. 10.2. Once the segmentation has concluded, the model can either be printed or exported into the virtual reality space to be represented as a hologram. An overview of this process is provided in Figs. 10.3 and 10.4.

10.2.3 3D Printing Technologies and Materials

Rapid prototyping is a method of fabricating 3D-printed specimens using 3D computer models, which involves using the computer-aided design files created from segmented images (as detailed above) to help a 3D printer build layer upon layer a

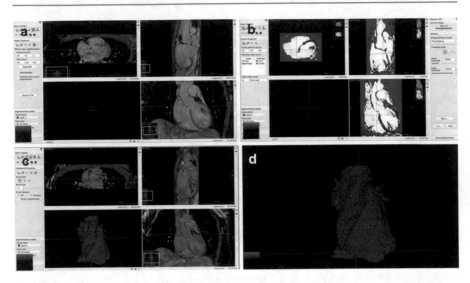

Fig. 10.2 Steps for the segmentation process using an open-access tool. (**a**) Image cropping. (**b**) Thresholding. (**c**) Manual editing of the anatomy. (**d**) Segmentation presented in 3D

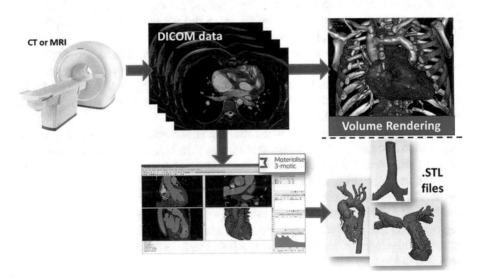

Fig. 10.3 The DICOM data from images acquired via cardiac CT or MRI scans may be loaded into a DICOM viewer to volume render the cardiac structure, which provides a quick and excellent representation of extracardiac anatomy. The raw DICOM data could also be imported into a segmentation software which is used to segment desired intra- or extracardiac anatomy and generate corresponding .STL files

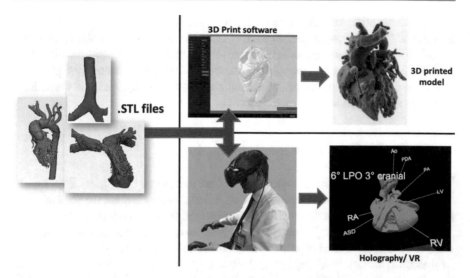

Fig. 10.4 The .STL files generated in the above step may be exported to 3D printer software which aids in developing 3D printer compatible files; and/or loaded into the virtual reality space using a VR headset attached to a computer

solid replica model [35]. Rapid prototyping technology can be subtractive or additive depending on the printing method used. Regarding subtractive techniques, only milling is applied in the medical field. Fused deposition modeling, polyjet printing, stereolithography, and selective laser sintering are the most common additive techniques utilized in medicine [33, 36, 37].

In fused deposition modeling, a thermoplastic filament is forced through a heated extrusion nozzle. The filament is melted while moving in vertical and horizontal directions. The layer of material hardens immediately after extrusion; the process is repeated layer by layer until the model is finished. A support material that is later dissolved is printed within the actual model.

Polyjet modeling works in a similar way to an ink-jet printer. During the process, layers of liquid photopolymers are jetted in the predefined shape using computer-aided files. Each layer hardens quickly under ultraviolet light. Multiple layers are incorporated until the model is complete.

Stereolithography builds the models through the polymerization of a photopolymeric resin. A digitally controlled ultraviolet beam hardens the surface of the resin layer by layer.

Selective laser sintering uses a high-power laser to fuse metal or ceramic powder. It offers highly accurate 3D models, used for functional prototypes or medical implants, but is also generally higher in cost when compared to other additive manufacturing techniques.

Several materials with different properties have been used to print cardiovascular structures. Initially, hard materials were utilized to show cardiac anatomy and great vessels [13, 38]. However, rubberlike models printed in a hollow fashion have become more common for the routine planning of interventions as they provide a more realistic representation of the patient's cardiac anatomy, which is essential to plan any surgical or interventional procedure [39].

10.2.4 Computer-Generated Holography

We define holography here as computer representation of 3D files. This can be done using *3-dimensional display* (3D TV), *Virtual reality* (where the viewer wears a visual headset and headphones and is immersed in a 3D environment such as a virtual room), *augmented reality* (where the viewer wears intelligent glasses that display additional virtual objects as an addition to the real environment), and *true projectional holographic displays* (which are not currently widely available). We will describe the process for rendering objects for virtual reality and the process is similar for any of these modalities, although simplification of the process via platform solutions is now becoming available. Once the DICOM data is imported into the segmentation software, and 3D files such as stereolithography files (.stl) are created, these could be imported into the software that runs virtual reality programs. The best experience with VR is usually achieved when using powerful hardware which is certified to be VR ready. Most computers designed to run PC games, video or graphics-intensive tasks have the necessary hardware to support VR connections. More powerful VR headsets like the Oculus Rift and HTC Vive were initially needed, but newer and lighter headsets with no attached wires can now be used independently of the computer. The VR headsets provide an immersive view of the 3D models that are generated. Using the handheld controls, viewers can easily, just to name a few functions, rotate, cut, zoom, hollow out, and perform a "walk through" the heart. Various scaled models of stents, devices, ventricular assist pumps, etc. can be pulled into the virtual space also and made to interact with the generated heart model. This provides not just an incredibly detailed view of the cardiac anatomy but makes it extremely intuitive for the planning of interventions as listed later on.

The quality of headsets available has been improving, with the technology getting cheaper with time, with the industry becoming more mainstream, and being increasingly adopted by the gaming community. Most of the software used to run the virtual reality headsets and load 3D models into the virtual space are available as freeware which reduces costs further. Once segmentation is performed, and 3D files are generated, there is little to no processing required to load the models into the VR space, thus saving time and material cost which are the major drawbacks with 3D printing. The ability to manipulate and mold the models in the virtual space based on need is also a feature that printed models lack.

10.3   Applications in Congenital Heart Disease

10.3.1 Clinical Practice

Recent reviews have extensively described the use of 3D printing and holography for procedural planning in a wide range of patients with congenital and structural heart disease [19, 29, 33, 34, 39].

While multiple centers around the world have used 3D models to help interventional planning, the use of virtual reality has been more limited in the field of congenital heart disease. More academic centers have started to use this technology on a case-by-case basis, and we have anecdotal reports, while randomized trials are pending [40, 41].

10.3.1.1   Surgical Planning

3D models have proven to be useful when complex anatomy precludes anatomical understanding using 2D images. A multicenter study involving ten hospitals from different countries showed high accuracy and fidelity of 3D-printed models segmented from CT and MRI images. Interestingly, during the planning phase, having access to the 3D model changed the management or surgical approach in 50% of patients [39]. Patients with double outlet right ventricle, tetralogy of Fallot, pulmonary atresia, and hypoplastic left heart syndrome seem to be the groups that have benefited the most from this emerging technique [17, 38, 42–46]. Another single-center study in patients with double outlet right ventricle and non-committed ventricular septal defect physiology using a 3D model over conventional imaging led to performing a successful bi-ventricular repair in three out of five patients [45]. A case report also illustrated the importance of 3D printing in a patient with double outlet right ventricle, dextrocardia, and supra-tricuspid ring [46].

Other studies continue to demonstrate the relevance of 3D printing hearts in patients with other complex cardiac disease, such as complex atrioventricular septal defect, congenitally corrected transposition of the great arteries, complex total anomalous pulmonary venous connection, multiple ventricular septal defects, criss-cross heart, or isomerism [39, 44].

In addition to CHD, rapid prototyping has been utilized for patients with different types of structural heart disease. Simulation of cardiac myomectomy has been performed in patients with severe forms of hypertrophic obstructive cardiomyopathy [47, 48]. In cases with cardiac tumors, 3D printing has been utilized to identify structures at risk and to determine appropriate therapeutic option and surgical approaches [30, 49–51].

A new procedure called PEARS (Personalized External Aortic Root Support) has emerged for the treatment of aortic root aneurysm in patients with Marfan syndrome, using 3D-printed models of the aortic root. These are made in thermoplastic by rapid prototyping, manufacturing a personalized support of a macroporous polymer mesh. The support is positioned around the aorta, closely applied from the aortoventricular junction to the proximal aortic arch, allowing sparing of the aortic valve and preserving the patient's coronary arteries [52–54].

10.3.1.2   Cardiac Catheterization: Interventional Planning and Performance

As the range of structural heart disorders treatable by percutaneous catheter interventions has increased, so has the complexity of these procedures. Visualization of patients' anatomy in three dimensions and the opportunity to manipulate it in our own hands or project it in a 3D hologram that can be navigated inside has allowed us to understand better the relationships between cardiac structures, opening new horizons in treatment for patients with CHD. High-risk patients in whom open heart surgery is not a therapeutic option can now benefit from palliative catheter-based interventional procedures. This is the case of patients receiving a MitraClip via cardiac catheterization. Although mimicking the properties of the tissue of the cardiac leaflets appears challenging when printing the heart, some groups have developed models with deformable leaflets. During simulations, patient-specific models helped to plan the best landing point and provided direct visualization of the morphological result [24, 55]. Various other catheter-based mitral valve interventions [56]; atrial septal, left atrial appendage, and Fontan fenestration device closure interventions are also now being planned and performed using advanced imaging modalities including 3D echocardiography [57, 58].

3D printing has also facilitated the implementation of transcatheter approach in the treatment of the aortic valve and the aortic arch [16, 59]. Aortic root 3D models have proven to accurately reproduce the anatomy of patients and aid prediction of paravalvular aortic regurgitation in transcatheter aortic valve replacement [60].

While interventional MRI procedures are seldom being performed on a non-research basis, holograms/virtual overlays of models generated for patients with congenital heart disease by CT or rapid sequence MRI to minimize radiation exposure have been used to supplement cardiac interventional catheterization procedures by providing live guidance of catheter position and three-dimensional orientation of vessels at the time of these interventions [61]. Segmented 3D models are loaded onto the lab fluoroscopy fusion software that has been developed by many leading healthcare companies and is currently available (Fig. 10.5).

A novel procedure to treat partial anomalous pulmonary venous drainage and sinus venous septal defect based on patient-specific models has recently been described. 3D models helped to demonstrate that stenting the superior vena cava towards the right atrium, occluding the sinus venous septal defect, and redirecting the pulmonary venous flow into the left atrium to correct this common defect diagnosed in adulthood are feasible via catheterization (Fig. 10.6). A retrospective analysis of anatomic variability of these defects was described in 28 patients to assess potential candidacy for transcatheter closure, and also look for anatomical reason that would preclude the same [62]. This new technique avoids cardiac bypass and allows the patient to be discharged home within 24 h [10].

Coronary fistulae tend to show tortuous course and unpredictable places of drainage. In patients with this condition, 3D models have an impact on decision-making within professionals in the medical field and on how to proceed with patients' management; they assist to plan the procedure and to explain to the patients and relatives the anatomy of their heart (Fig. 10.7) [9].

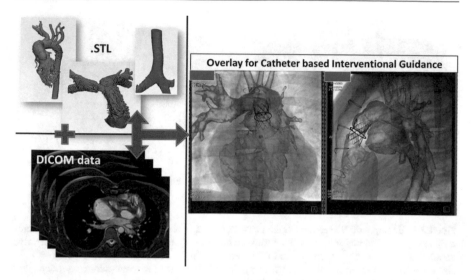

Fig. 10.5 STL models and DICOM data may be imported into compatible software, to generate 3D overlay maps to aid catheter-guided interventions

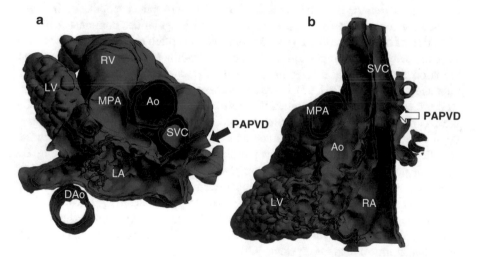

Fig. 10.6 3D segmentation of the heart of a patient with partial anomalous pulmonary venous drainage (PAPVD). (**a**) Axial reformat showing pathway of the right upper pulmonary vein (black arrow), draining into the SVC and continuing towards the left atrium. (**b**) Sagittal view of the heart showing right upper pulmonary vein (white arrow) draining into the SVC. *Ao* aorta, *DAo* descending aorta, *LA* left atrium, *LV* left atrium, *MPA* main pulmonary artery, *RA* right atrium, *RV* right ventricle, *SVC* superior vena cava

There are reports of use in individualized surgical planning for patients with complex anomalous coronary artery anatomy [63].

Patients with tetralogy of Fallot and other forms of right ventricular outflow tract abnormalities tend to need repeated surgical procedures through life to treat

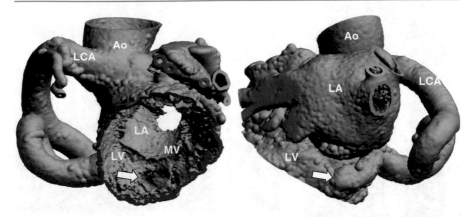

Fig. 10.7 Example of 3D segmentation in a patient with coronary fistula involving the left coronary artery and draining into the left ventricle (white arrow), in close relation to the mitral valve annulus. Anterior and posterior views of the anatomy (right and left images, respectively). *Ao* aorta, *LA* left atrium, *LCA* left coronary artery, *LV* left atrium, *MPA* main pulmonary artery, *MV* mitral valve, *RA* right atrium, *RV* right ventricle

pulmonary stenosis at different levels or pulmonary valve regurgitation. The use of transcatheter pulmonary valve replacement has slowly gained popularity in these cases. However, the density of trabeculations and irregularities combined with the dilatation of the right ventricle (RV) of these patients often makes it difficult to perform the percutaneous implantation of the valve, leading to prolonged procedure and radiation times. Several studies have aimed to plan the valve implantation using patient-specific models [64, 65], based on segmentations from MRI [66] and CT [67]. In these studies, 3D models helped the entire multidisciplinary team virtualize the intervention, attempt different strategies, and design individualized solutions for a population with widely differing cardiac anatomies [67], and also with more accurate selection of patients for percutaneous pulmonary valve implantation than using 2D MRI imaging alone [66], as well as better planning of the procedure in the context of complications like right ventricular outflow tract aneurysms [68]. Virtual 3D overlay imaging is slowly gaining popularity in this kind of procedures (Fig. 10.8).

3D printing and virtual reality have also found use during preprocedural planning of catheter ablation for treatment of arrhythmias in ACHD in conjunction with electro-anatomical mapping systems [69].

10.3.2 Education and Training

3D printing models have the potential to serve as unique educational tools for healthcare professionals. They have been used across a different range of medical personnel for training purposes.

Biglino et al. discussed the utility of using 3D models to teach nurses through a wide spectrum of CHD [70]. In their study, 100 pediatric and adult cardiac nurses

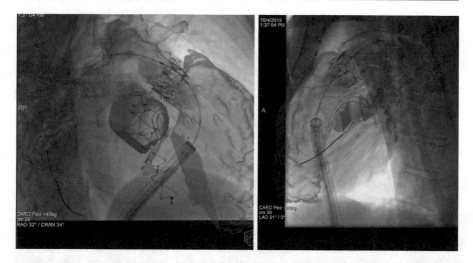

Fig. 10.8 Percutaneous Melody Valve positioned across the RVOT/Pulmonary valve (cyan) using advanced bi-plane overlay guidance, and then inflated. The aortic root and coronary relationship (blue) is helpful to predict or avoid coronary compression

were offered the possibility of handling 3D models of a healthy heart; repaired transposition of the great arteries (arterial switch operation); aortic coarctation; tetralogy of Fallot; pulmonary atresia with intact ventricular septum; and the three stages of palliated hypoplastic left heart syndrome. They concluded that 3D models helped in the appreciation of anatomy; however implementation of the models by using labels and colors to highlight the lesion of interest may help optimizing the 3D models for teaching and training purposes.

Other studies have offered expert input with a more orientated pattern of teaching on topics such as tetralogy of Fallot [71]. Surgical trainees have also benefitted from 3D printing on rubberlike materials. Fifty cardiac surgeons and trainees reported improvement of surgical skills with simulated surgeries using 3D-printed hearts [72]. Use of simulation techniques is being encouraged in the field of interventional procedures [73, 74], with studies showing benefits for procedures like vascular ring repair [75].

As illustrated by the above examples, the methodology of the teaching varies among studies. The lack of consistency makes the possibility of comparison between outcomes among studies challenging. Although results on improvements in knowledge acquisition when comparing 3D models against images alone remain controversial [70–72, 75, 76], there is a generally positive and enthusiastic feedback from participants and learners of different medical backgrounds, with a higher score in satisfaction when 3D-printed models are involved [71, 76].

The limited amount of original pathological specimens available for teaching purposes and the increasing number of clinical applications of these models as well as the current facility to share digital files make 3D models a desirable alternative to offer direct visualization of the anatomy to students and medical personnel in

training. Making 3D images available through online collections can provide hospitals and research centers with free access to a broad spectrum of heart conditions. A
wide range of anatomical variants for different spectrums of CHD has been gath-
ered with this purpose, including hypoplastic left heart syndrome and its surgical
stages, double outlet right ventricle, tetralogy of Fallot, and truncus arteriosus [77].

10.3.3 Communication with Patients and Relatives

Although the main areas of research in rapid prototyping have been focused on
presurgical planning and cardiac catheterization, there is an increasing awareness of
their importance in communication with patients. Biglino et al. [78] demonstrated
that parents find these models useful to understand their child's heart condition, and
were described in feedback as being more user friendly than medical images. The
employment of these aides did not significantly increase the duration of the consultation. Interestingly, the blind assessment performed to assess parent's knowledge
on the CHD did not improve significantly after the consultation regardless of the use
of the 3D model. However, their perceived understanding of the disease was rated
as higher. A study aiming to assess their impact on patients with hypertrophic
obstructive cardiomyopathy also showed high satisfaction rates [79].

Evaluation of their impact in transition-of-care clinics has also been carried out
[80], involving late adolescents with tetralogy of Fallot, transposition of the great
arteries, aortic coarctation, pulmonary atresia, aortic valve stenosis, double outlet
right ventricle, and Ebstein's anomaly. These teenagers reported to be impressed by
seeing their own heart and the level of detail in the models, and described the models as interesting, useful, and helpful in understanding their disease, with an increase
in their awareness of the impact of the disease on their lifestyle. Thirty percent of
the patients confessed that the models made them more anxious.

10.4   Limitations and Future Directions

Patient-specific 3D-printed models have extensively proven to have a significant
effect on clinical decision-making and procedure planning in open heart surgery or
cardiac catheterization, allowing for development of new techniques and approaches
in patients with CHD [9, 10, 16, 24, 38, 39, 42, 44–46, 48, 54, 55, 59, 60, 64, 66].
Special efforts are currently being made in order to improve on the materials the
models are built with in order to mimic the structural behavior of the myocardium,
the valve leaflets, and the great vessels' wall as closely as possible. Differences in
healthy and pathologic cardiac tissue are also to be considered. Holography at this
time has been limited by the price, availability, and lack of comfort with use of the
technology. The anatomic intricacies noted are somewhat limited by the resolution
of the displays in virtual reality headsets, which is not as good as a high definition

screen. There is loss of fidelity with smaller structures when zoomed in the virtual space. The segmentation process in rapid prototyping is based on their visual characteristics; therefore advances in imaging methods such as 3D echo are necessary before a more detailed characterization is achievable. This fact also brings on board another limitation: the segmentation process is time-consuming and requires familiarity with the software, the use of cross-sectional imaging, and a broad understanding on cardiac morphology. Manual editing of the segmentation process allows free creation and deletion of anatomical features; consequently expert's notion on the methodology is paramount to complete a reliable model.

The limited number of available pathological specimens makes 3D models an attractive option for teaching purposes. However, we believe that providing expert's input during the teaching session is essential, in the same way that imaging modalities in which MRI or echocardiography are explained during training. The involvement of the lecturer may improve the interaction of the students with the model and the understanding of the anatomy as reported in hands-on seminars [71, 72, 76]. Efforts are currently underway to create "virtual libraries" of 3D heart models from pathology museum specimens at multiple centers using CT and MRI [81–83] (Figs. 10.9 and 10.10). Virtual autopsies of the human heart have also been performed and may be a way of the future [84].

In future, automatic segmentation with minimal manual editing may reduce the amount of time invested in the process, therefore decreasing its costs and spreading its use across the world. Visualization of the anatomy in 3D will become routine practice before cardiac surgery, allowing for better planning of the procedure and selection of candidates for novel, less invasive techniques. The advent of augmented reality (AR) headsets has made interaction more realistic with a virtual overlay on top of the real world [85]. This means more intuitiveness in the use of this technology, with inlay into active use of this technology to assist the physician in real time during the performance of procedures.

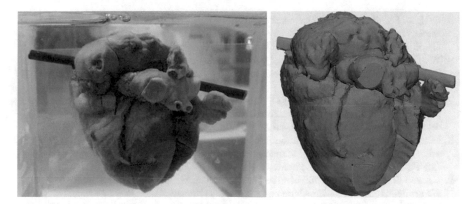

Fig. 10.9 3D virtual heart model using an MRI scan of an intact curated cardiac pathology specimens in a jar. (Specimen courtesy: Dr. K.M. Cherian, FARCS, Frontier Lifeline Hospital, India)

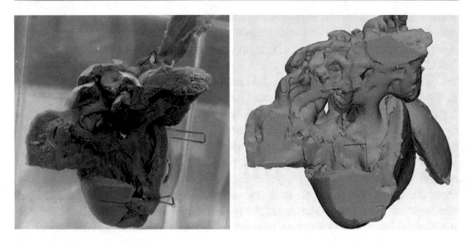

Fig. 10.10 A 3D model created from MRI images of a cut-open curated pathology specimen shows excellent intricate reproduction of internal anatomy including the valvar apparatus. (Specimen courtesy: Dr. K.M. Cherian, FARCS, Frontier Lifeline Hospital, India)

References

1. Heissler E, Fischer FS, Bolouri S, Lehmann T, Mathar W, Gebhardt A, et al. Custom-made cast titanium implants produced with CAD/CAM for the reconstruction of cranium defects. Int J Oral Maxillofac Surg. 1998;27(5):334–8. PubMed PMID: 9804194.
2. Sailer HF, Haers PE, Zollikofer CP, Warnke T, Carls FR, Stucki P. The value of stereolithographic models for preoperative diagnosis of craniofacial deformities and planning of surgical corrections. Int J Oral Maxillofac Surg. 1998;27(5):327–33. PubMed PMID: 9804193.
3. Park GC, Wiseman JB, Clark WD. Correction of congenital microtia using stereolithography for surgical planning. Plast Reconstr Surg. 2000;105(4):1444–7. PubMed PMID: 10744239.
4. Chang PS, Parker TH, Patrick CW Jr, Miller MJ. The accuracy of stereolithography in planning craniofacial bone replacement. J Craniofac Surg. 2003;14(2):164–70. PubMed PMID: 12621285.
5. D'Urso PS, Barker TM, Earwaker WJ, Bruce LJ, Atkinson RL, Lanigan MW, et al. Stereolithographic biomodelling in cranio-maxillofacial surgery: a prospective trial. J Craniomaxillofac Surg. 1999;27(1):30–7. PubMed PMID: 10188125.
6. Winder J, Bibb R. Medical rapid prototyping technologies: state of the art and current limitations for application in oral and maxillofacial surgery. J Oral Maxillofac Surg. 2005;63(7):1006–15. PubMed PMID: 16003630.
7. Munjal S, Leopold SS, Kornreich D, Shott S, Finn HA. CT-generated 3-dimensional models for complex acetabular reconstruction. J Arthroplast. 2000;15(5):644–53. https://doi.org/10.1054/arth.2000.6629. PubMed PMID: 10960004.
8. Minns RJ, Bibb R, Banks R, Sutton RA. The use of a reconstructed three-dimensional solid model from CT to aid the surgical management of a total knee arthroplasty: a case study. Med Eng Phys. 2003;25(6):523–6. PubMed PMID: 12787991.
9. Velasco Forte MN, Byrne N, Valverde Perez I, Bell A, Gomez-Ciriza G, Krasemann T, et al. 3D printed models in patients with coronary artery fistulae: anatomical assessment and interventional planning. EuroIntervention. 2017;13(9):e1080–e3. https://doi.org/10.4244/EIJ-D-16-00897. PubMed PMID: 28555593.
10. Velasco Forte MN, Byrne N, Valverde I, Gomez Ciriza G, Hermuzi A, Prachasilchai P, et al. Interventional correction of sinus venosus atrial septal defect and partial anomalous pul-

monary venous drainage: procedural planning using 3D printed models. JACC Cardiovasc Imaging. 2018;11(2 Pt 1):275–8. https://doi.org/10.1016/j.jcmg.2017.07.010. PubMed PMID: 28917677.

11. Sodian R, Weber S, Markert M, Rassoulian D, Kaczmarek I, Lueth TC, et al. Stereolithographic models for surgical planning in congenital heart surgery. Ann Thorac Surg. 2007;83(5):1854–7. https://doi.org/10.1016/j.athoracsur.2006.12.004. PubMed PMID: 17462413.

12. Sodian R, Schmauss D, Schmitz C, Bigdeli A, Haeberle S, Schmoeckel M, et al. 3-dimensional printing of models to create custom-made devices for coil embolization of an anastomotic leak after aortic arch replacement. Ann Thorac Surg. 2009;88(3):974–8. https://doi.org/10.1016/j.athoracsur.2009.03.014. PubMed PMID: 19699931.

13. Schmauss D, Haeberle S, Hagl C, Sodian R. Three-dimensional printing in cardiac surgery and interventional cardiology: a single-centre experience. Eur J Cardiothorac Surg. 2015;47(6):1044–52. https://doi.org/10.1093/ejcts/ezu310. PubMed PMID: 25161184.

14. Greil GF, Wolf I, Kuettner A, Fenchel M, Miller S, Martirosian P, et al. Stereolithographic reproduction of complex cardiac morphology based on high spatial resolution imaging. Clin Res Cardiol. 2007;96(3):176–85. https://doi.org/10.1007/s00392-007-0482-3. PubMed PMID: 17225916.

15. Mottl-Link S, Hubler M, Kuhne T, Rietdorf U, Krueger JJ, Schnackenburg B, et al. Physical models aiding in complex congenital heart surgery. Ann Thorac Surg. 2008;86(1):273–7. https://doi.org/10.1016/j.athoracsur.2007.06.001. PubMed PMID: 18573436.

16. Valverde I, Gomez G, Coserria JF, Suarez-Mejias C, Uribe S, Sotelo J, et al. 3D printed models for planning endovascular stenting in transverse aortic arch hypoplasia. Catheter Cardiovasc Interv. 2015;85(6):1006–12. https://doi.org/10.1002/ccd.25810. PubMed PMID: 25557983.

17. Valverde I, Gomez G, Gonzalez A, Suarez-Mejias C, Adsuar A, Coserria JF, et al. Three-dimensional patient-specific cardiac model for surgical planning in Nikaidoh procedure. Cardiol Young. 2015;25(4):698–704. https://doi.org/10.1017/S1047951114000742. PubMed PMID: 24809416.

18. Byrne N, Velasco Forte M, Tandon A, Valverde I, Hussain T. A systematic review of image segmentation methodology, used in the additive manufacture of patient-specific 3D printed models of the cardiovascular system. JRSM Cardiovasc Dis. 2016;5:2048004016645467. https://doi.org/10.1177/2048004016645467. PubMed PMID: 27170842, PubMed Central PMCID: PMCPMC4853939.

19. Otton JM, Birbara NS, Hussain T, Greil G, Foley TA, Pather N. 3D printing from cardiovascular CT: a practical guide and review. Cardiovasc Diagn Ther. 2017;7(5):507–26. https://doi.org/10.21037/cdt.2017.01.12. PubMed PMID: 29255693, PubMed Central PMCID: PMCPMC5716949.

20. Glatz AC, Purrington KS, Klinger A, King AR, Hellinger J, Zhu X, et al. Cumulative exposure to medical radiation for children requiring surgery for congenital heart disease. J Pediatr. 2014;164(4):789–94.e10. https://doi.org/10.1016/j.jpeds.2013.10.074. PubMed PMID: 24321535.

21. LaBounty TM, Earls JP, Leipsic J, Heilbron B, Mancini GB, Lin FY, et al. Effect of a standardized quality-improvement protocol on radiation dose in coronary computed tomographic angiography. Am J Cardiol. 2010;106(11):1663–7. https://doi.org/10.1016/j.amjcard.2010.07.023. PubMed PMID: 21094371.

22. Raff GL, Chinnaiyan KM, Share DA, Goraya TY, Kazerooni EA, Moscucci M, et al. Radiation dose from cardiac computed tomography before and after implementation of radiation dose-reduction techniques. JAMA. 2009;301(22):2340–8. https://doi.org/10.1001/jama.2009.814. PubMed PMID: 19509381.

23. Tanabe Y, Kido T, Kimura F, Kobayashi Y, Matsunaga N, Yoshioka K, et al. Japanese survey of radiation dose associated with coronary computed tomography angiography - 2013 data from a multicenter registry in daily practice. Circ J. 2020;84:601. https://doi.org/10.1253/circj.CJ-19-0843. PubMed PMID: 32074543.

24. Vukicevic M, Puperi DS, Jane Grande-Allen K, Little SH. 3D printed modeling of the mitral valve for catheter-based structural interventions. Ann Biomed Eng. 2017;45(2):508–19. https://doi.org/10.1007/s10439-016-1676-5. PubMed PMID: 27324801.
25. Scanlan AB, Nguyen AV, Ilina A, Lasso A, Cripe L, Jegatheeswaran A, et al. Comparison of 3D echocardiogram-derived 3D printed valve models to molded models for simulated repair of pediatric atrioventricular valves. Pediatr Cardiol. 2018;39(3):538–47. https://doi.org/10.1007/s00246-017-1785-4. PubMed PMID: 29181795.
26. Gosnell J, Pietila T, Samuel BP, Kurup HK, Haw MP, Vettukattil JJ. Integration of computed tomography and three-dimensional echocardiography for hybrid three-dimensional printing in congenital heart disease. J Digit Imaging. 2016;29(6):665–9. https://doi.org/10.1007/s10278-016-9879-8. PubMed PMID: 27072399, PubMed Central PMCID: PMCPMC5114226.
27. Yang HS. Three-dimensional echocardiography in adult congenital heart disease. Korean J Intern Med. 2017;32(4):577–88. https://doi.org/10.3904/kjim.2016.251. PubMed PMID: 28704916, PubMed Central PMCID: PMCPMC5511944.
28. Parimi M, Buelter J, Thangundla V, Condoor S, Parkar N, Danon S, et al. Feasibility and validity of printing 3D heart models from rotational angiography. Pediatr Cardiol. 2018;39:653. https://doi.org/10.1007/s00246-017-1799-y. PubMed PMID: 29305642.
29. Cantinotti M, Valverde I, Kutty S. Three-dimensional printed models in congenital heart disease. Int J Card Imaging. 2017;33(1):137–44. https://doi.org/10.1007/s10554-016-0981-2. PubMed PMID: 27677762.
30. Giannopoulos AA, Mitsouras D, Yoo SJ, Liu PP, Chatzizisis YS, Rybicki FJ. Applications of 3D printing in cardiovascular diseases. Nat Rev Cardiol. 2016;13(12):701–18. https://doi.org/10.1038/nrcardio.2016.170. PubMed PMID: 27786234.
31. Giannopoulos AA, Steigner ML, George E, Barile M, Hunsaker AR, Rybicki FJ, et al. Cardiothoracic applications of 3-dimensional printing. J Thorac Imaging. 2016;31(5):253–72. https://doi.org/10.1097/RTI.0000000000000217. PubMed PMID: 27149367, PubMed Central PMCID: PMCPMC4993676.
32. Suarez-Mejias C, Gomez-Ciriza G, Valverde I, Parra Calderon C, Gomez-Cia T. New technologies applied to surgical processes: virtual reality and rapid prototyping. Stud Health Technol Inform. 2015;210:669–71. PubMed PMID: 25991234.
33. Vukicevic M, Mosadegh B, Min JK, Little SH. Cardiac 3D printing and its future directions. JACC Cardiovasc Imaging. 2017;10(2):171–84. https://doi.org/10.1016/j.jcmg.2016.12.001. PubMed PMID: 28183437, PubMed Central PMCID: PMCPMC5664227.
34. Valverde I. Three-dimensional printed cardiac models: applications in the field of medical education, cardiovascular surgery, and structural heart interventions. Rev Esp Cardiol (Engl Ed). 2017;70(4):282–91. https://doi.org/10.1016/j.rec.2017.01.012. PubMed PMID: 28189544.
35. Webb PA. A review of rapid prototyping (RP) techniques in the medical and biomedical sector. J Med Eng Technol. 2000;24(4):149–53. https://doi.org/10.1080/03091900050163427. PubMed PMID: 11105287.
36. Kim MS, Hansgen AR, Carroll JD. Use of rapid prototyping in the care of patients with structural heart disease. Trends Cardiovasc Med. 2008;18(6):210–6. https://doi.org/10.1016/j.tcm.2008.11.001. PubMed PMID: 19185811.
37. Kim MS, Hansgen AR, Wink O, Quaife RA, Carroll JD. Rapid prototyping: a new tool in understanding and treating structural heart disease. Circulation. 2008;117(18):2388–94. https://doi.org/10.1161/CIRCULATIONAHA.107.740977. PubMed PMID: 18458180.
38. Ngan EM, Rebeyka IM, Ross DB, Hirji M, Wolfaardt JF, Seelaus R, et al. The rapid prototyping of anatomic models in pulmonary atresia. J Thorac Cardiovasc Surg. 2006;132(2):264–9. https://doi.org/10.1016/j.jtcvs.2006.02.047. PubMed PMID: 16872948.
39. Valverde I, Gomez-Ciriza G, Hussain T, Suarez-Mejias C, Velasco-Forte MN, Byrne N, et al. Three-dimensional printed models for surgical planning of complex congenital heart defects: an international multicentre study. Eur J Cardiothorac Surg. 2017;52(6):1139–48. https://doi.org/10.1093/ejcts/ezx208. PubMed PMID: 28977423.

40. Ong CS, Krishnan A, Huang CY, Spevak P, Vricella L, Hibino N, et al. Role of virtual reality in congenital heart disease. Congenit Heart Dis. 2018;13(3):357–61. https://doi.org/10.1111/chd.12587. PubMed PMID: 29399969.

41. Goo HW, Park SJ, Yoo SJ. Advanced medical use of three-dimensional imaging in congenital heart disease: augmented reality, mixed reality, virtual reality, and three-dimensional printing. Korean J Radiol. 2020;21(2):133–45. https://doi.org/10.3348/kjr.2019.0625. PubMed PMID: 31997589.

42. Kiraly L, Tofeig M, Jha NK, Talo H. Three-dimensional printed prototypes refine the anatomy of post-modified Norwood-1 complex aortic arch obstruction and allow presurgical simulation of the repair. Interact Cardiovasc Thorac Surg. 2016;22(2):238–40. https://doi.org/10.1093/icvts/ivv320. PubMed PMID: 26590304.

43. Shiraishi I, Yamagishi M, Hamaoka K, Fukuzawa M, Yagihara T. Simulative operation on congenital heart disease using rubber-like urethane stereolithographic biomodels based on 3D datasets of multislice computed tomography. Eur J Cardiothorac Surg. 2010;37(2):302–6. https://doi.org/10.1016/j.ejcts.2009.07.046. PubMed PMID: 19758813.

44. Riesenkampff E, Rietdorf U, Wolf I, Schnackenburg B, Ewert P, Huebler M, et al. The practical clinical value of three-dimensional models of complex congenitally malformed hearts. J Thorac Cardiovasc Surg. 2009;138(3):571–80. https://doi.org/10.1016/j.jtcvs.2009.03.011. PubMed PMID: 19698837.

45. Garekar S, Bharati A, Chokhandre M, Mali S, Trivedi B, Changela VP, et al. Clinical Application and Multidisciplinary Assessment of Three Dimensional Printing in Double Outlet Right Ventricle With Remote Ventricular Septal Defect. World J Pediatr Congenit Heart Surg. 2016;7(3):344–50. https://doi.org/10.1177/2150135116645604. PubMed PMID: 27142402.

46. Farooqi KM, Nielsen JC, Uppu SC, Srivastava S, Parness IA, Sanz J, et al. Use of 3-dimensional printing to demonstrate complex intracardiac relationships in double-outlet right ventricle for surgical planning. Circ Cardiovasc Imaging. 2015;8(5):e003043. https://doi.org/10.1161/CIRCIMAGING.114.003043. PubMed PMID: 25904574.

47. Hermsen JL, Burke TM, Seslar SP, Owens DS, Ripley BA, Mokadam NA, et al. Scan, plan, print, practice, perform: development and use of a patient-specific 3-dimensional printed model in adult cardiac surgery. J Thorac Cardiovasc Surg. 2017;153(1):132–40. https://doi.org/10.1016/j.jtcvs.2016.08.007. PubMed PMID: 27650000.

48. Yang DH, Kang JW, Kim N, Song JK, Lee JW, Lim TH. Myocardial 3-dimensional printing for septal myectomy guidance in a patient with obstructive hypertrophic cardiomyopathy. Circulation. 2015;132(4):300–1. https://doi.org/10.1161/CIRCULATIONAHA.115.015842. PubMed PMID: 26216088.

49. Son KH, Kim KW, Ahn CB, Choi CH, Park KY, Park CH, et al. Surgical planning by 3D printing for primary cardiac schwannoma resection. Yonsei Med J. 2015;56(6):1735–7. https://doi.org/10.3349/ymj.2015.56.6.1735. PubMed PMID: 26446661, PubMed Central PMCID: PMCPMC4630067.

50. Schmauss D, Gerber N, Sodian R. Three-dimensional printing of models for surgical planning in patients with primary cardiac tumors. J Thorac Cardiovasc Surg. 2013;145(5):1407–8. https://doi.org/10.1016/j.jtcvs.2012.12.030. PubMed PMID: 23312105.

51. Jacobs S, Grunert R, Mohr FW, Falk V. 3D-imaging of cardiac structures using 3D heart models for planning in heart surgery: a preliminary study. Interact Cardiovasc Thorac Surg. 2008;7(1):6–9. https://doi.org/10.1510/icvts.2007.156588. PubMed PMID: 17925319.

52. Golesworthy T, Lamperth M, Mohiaddin R, Pepper J, Thornton W, Treasure T. The Tailor of Gloucester: a jacket for the Marfan's aorta. Lancet. 2004;364(9445):1582. https://doi.org/10.1016/S0140-6736(04)17308-X. PubMed PMID: 15519627.

53. Pepper J, Golesworthy T, Utley M, Chan J, Ganeshalingam S, Lamperth M, et al. Manufacturing and placing a bespoke support for the Marfan aortic root: description of the method and technical results and status at one year for the first ten patients. Interact Cardiovasc Thorac Surg. 2010;10(3):360–5. https://doi.org/10.1510/icvts.2009.220319. PubMed PMID: 20007995.

54. Treasure T, Takkenberg JJ, Golesworthy T, Rega F, Petrou M, Rosendahl U, et al. Personalised external aortic root support (PEARS) in Marfan syndrome: analysis of 1-9 year outcomes by intention-to-treat in a cohort of the first 30 consecutive patients to receive a novel tissue and valve-conserving procedure, compared with the published results of aortic root replacement. Heart. 2014;100(12):969–75. https://doi.org/10.1136/heartjnl-2013-304913. PubMed PMID: 24395977, PubMed Central PMCID: PMCPMC4033204.

55. Little SH, Vukicevic M, Avenatti E, Ramchandani M, Barker CM. 3D printed modeling for patient-specific mitral valve intervention: repair with a clip and a plug. JACC Cardiovasc Interv. 2016;9(9):973–5. https://doi.org/10.1016/j.jcin.2016.02.027. PubMed PMID: 27151611.

56. Azran MS, Romig CB, Locke A, Whitley WS. Echo rounds: application of real-time 3-dimensional transesophageal echocardiography in the percutaneous closure of a mitral paravalvular leak. Anesth Analg. 2010;110(6):1581–3. https://doi.org/10.1213/ANE.0b013e3181da82aa. PubMed PMID: 20375301.

57. Obasare E, Mainigi SK, Morris DL, Slipczuk L, Goykhman I, Friend E, et al. CT based 3D printing is superior to transesophageal echocardiography for pre-procedure planning in left atrial appendage device closure. Int J Cardiovasc Imaging. 2018;34:821. https://doi.org/10.1007/s10554-017-1289-6.

58. Clegg SD, Chen SJ, Nijhof N, Kim MS, Salcedo EE, Quaife RA, et al. Integrated 3D echo-x ray to optimize image guidance for structural heart intervention. JACC Cardiovasc Imaging. 2015;8(3):371–4. https://doi.org/10.1016/j.jcmg.2014.06.024. PubMed PMID: 25772840.

59. Figulla HR, Webb JG, Lauten A, Feldman T. The transcatheter valve technology pipeline for treatment of adult valvular heart disease. Eur Heart J. 2016;37(28):2226–39. https://doi.org/10.1093/eurheartj/ehw153. PubMed PMID: 27161617.

60. Ripley B, Kelil T, Cheezum MK, Goncalves A, Di Carli MF, Rybicki FJ, et al. 3D printing based on cardiac CT assists anatomic visualization prior to transcatheter aortic valve replacement. J Cardiovasc Comput Tomogr. 2016;10(1):28–36. https://doi.org/10.1016/j.jcct.2015.12.004. PubMed PMID: 26732862, PubMed Central PMCID: PMCPMC5573584.

61. Goreczny S, Dryzek P, Morgan GJ, Lukaszewski M, Moll JA, Moszura T. Novel three-dimensional image fusion software to facilitate guidance of complex cardiac catheterization: 3D image fusion for interventions in CHD. Pediatr Cardiol. 2017;38(6):1133–42. https://doi.org/10.1007/s00246-017-1627-4. PubMed PMID: 28551818.

62. Tandon A, Burkhardt BEU, Batsis M, Zellers TM, Velasco Forte MN, Valverde I, et al. Sinus venosus defects: anatomic variants and transcatheter closure feasibility using virtual reality planning. JACC Cardiovasc Imaging. 2019;12(5):921–4. https://doi.org/10.1016/j.jcmg.2018.10.013. PubMed PMID: 30553676.

63. Shinbane JS, Baker C, Saremi F, Starnes V. Cardiovascular computed tomographic angiography as a virtual patient avatar for individualized surgical planning of complex anomalous coronary artery anatomy. World J Pediatr Congenit Heart Surg. 2019;10(4):502–3. https://doi.org/10.1177/2150135119854742. PubMed PMID: 31307300.

64. Valverde I, Sarnago F, Prieto R, Zunzunegui JL. Three-dimensional printing in vitro simulation of percutaneous pulmonary valve implantation in large right ventricular outflow tract. Eur Heart J. 2017;38(16):1262–3. https://doi.org/10.1093/eurheartj/ehw546. PubMed PMID: 28025232.

65. Pluchinotta FR, Sturla F, Caimi A, Giugno L, Chessa M, Giamberti A, et al. 3-Dimensional personalized planning for transcatheter pulmonary valve implantation in a dysfunctional right ventricular outflow tract. Int J Cardiol. 2020;309:33. https://doi.org/10.1016/j.ijcard.2019.12.006. PubMed PMID: 31839428.

66. Schievano S, Migliavacca F, Coats L, Khambadkone S, Carminati M, Wilson N, et al. Percutaneous pulmonary valve implantation based on rapid prototyping of right ventricular outflow tract and pulmonary trunk from MR data. Radiology. 2007;242(2):490–7. https://doi.org/10.1148/radiol.2422051994. PubMed PMID: 17255420.

67. Phillips AB, Nevin P, Shah A, Olshove V, Garg R, Zahn EM. Development of a novel hybrid strategy for transcatheter pulmonary valve placement in patients following transannular

patch repair of tetralogy of fallot. Catheter Cardiovasc Interv. 2016;87(3):403–10. https://doi.org/10.1002/ccd.26315. PubMed PMID: 26527499.

68. Jivanji S, Velasco Forte M, Byrne N, Valverde Perez I, Qureshi S, Rosenthal E. Complex percutaneous pulmonary venus P valve implantation with simultaneous device closure of RVOT aneurysm. The use of 3D modelling to perform mock intervention to aid in planning. Frankfurt: CSI; 2018.

69. Knecht S, Brantner P, Cattin P, Tobler D, Kuhne M, Sticherling C. State-of-the-art multimodality approach to assist ablations in complex anatomies-from 3D printing to virtual reality. Pacing Clin Electrophysiol. 2019;42(1):101–3. https://doi.org/10.1111/pace.13479. PubMed PMID: 30133862.

70. Biglino G, Capelli C, Koniordou D, Robertshaw D, Leaver LK, Schievano S, et al. Use of 3D models of congenital heart disease as an education tool for cardiac nurses. Congenit Heart Dis. 2017;12(1):113–8. https://doi.org/10.1111/chd.12414. PubMed PMID: 27666734.

71. Loke YH, Harahsheh AS, Krieger A, Olivieri LJ. Usage of 3D models of tetralogy of Fallot for medical education: impact on learning congenital heart disease. BMC Med Educ. 2017;17(1):54. https://doi.org/10.1186/s12909-017-0889-0. PubMed PMID: 28284205, PubMed Central PMCID: PMCPMC5346255.

72. Yoo SJ, Spray T, Austin EH III, Yun TJ, van Arsdell GS. Hands-on surgical training of congenital heart surgery using 3-dimensional print models. J Thorac Cardiovasc Surg. 2017;153(6):1530–40. https://doi.org/10.1016/j.jtcvs.2016.12.054. PubMed PMID: 28268011.

73. Green SM, Klein AJ, Pancholy S, Rao SV, Steinberg D, Lipner R, et al. The current state of medical simulation in interventional cardiology: a clinical document from the Society for Cardiovascular Angiography and Intervention's (SCAI) Simulation Committee. Catheter Cardiovasc Interv. 2014;83(1):37–46. https://doi.org/10.1002/ccd.25048. PubMed PMID: 23737458.

74. Gould DA, Reekers JA, Kessel DO, Chalmers NC, Sapoval M, Patel AA, et al. Simulation devices in interventional radiology: validation pending. J Vasc Interv Radiol. 2006;17(2 Pt 1):215–6. https://doi.org/10.1097/01.RVI.0000197480.16245.1A. PubMed PMID: 16517766.

75. Jones TW, Seckeler MD. Use of 3D models of vascular rings and slings to improve resident education. Congenit Heart Dis. 2017;12(5):578–82. https://doi.org/10.1111/chd.12486. PubMed PMID: 28608434.

76. Costello JP, Olivieri LJ, Su L, Krieger A, Alfares F, Thabit O, et al. Incorporating three-dimensional printing into a simulation-based congenital heart disease and critical care training curriculum for resident physicians. Congenit Heart Dis. 2015;10(2):185–90. https://doi.org/10.1111/chd.12238. PubMed PMID: 25385353.

77. Velasco Forte M. 3D printing for teaching clinicians; summary AEPC junior Grant 2015. In: 51st Annual Meeting of the Association for European Paediatric and Congenital Cardiology (AEPC). Lyon: Cardiology in the Young; 2017.

78. Biglino G, Capelli C, Wray J, Schievano S, Leaver LK, Khambadkone S, et al. 3D-manufactured patient-specific models of congenital heart defects for communication in clinical practice: feasibility and acceptability. BMJ Open. 2015;5(4):e007165. https://doi.org/10.1136/bmjopen-2014-007165. PubMed PMID: 25933810, PubMed Central PMCID: PMCPMC4420970.

79. Guo HC, Wang Y, Dai J, Ren CW, Li JH, Lai YQ. Application of 3D printing in the surgical planning of hypertrophic obstructive cardiomyopathy and physician-patient communication: a preliminary study. J Thorac Dis. 2018;10(2):867–73. https://doi.org/10.21037/jtd.2018.01.55. PubMed PMID: 29607159, PubMed Central PMCID: PMCPMC5864607.

80. Biglino G, Koniordou D, Gasparini M, Capelli C, Leaver LK, Khambadkone S, et al. Piloting the use of patient-specific cardiac models as a novel tool to facilitate communication during clinical consultations. Pediatr Cardiol. 2017;38(4):813–8. https://doi.org/10.1007/s00246-017-1586-9. PubMed PMID: 28214968, PubMed Central PMCID: PMCPMC5388703.

81. Jutras LC. Magnetic resonance of hearts in a jar: breathing new life into old pathological specimens. Cardiol Young. 2010;20(3):275–83. https://doi.org/10.1017/S1047951109991521. PubMed PMID: 20346199.

82. Kiraly L, Kiraly B, Szigeti K, Tamas CZ, Daranyi S. Virtual museum of congenital heart defects: digitization and establishment of a database for cardiac specimens. Quant Imaging Med Surg. 2019;9(1):115–26. https://doi.org/10.21037/qims.2018.12.05. PubMed PMID: 30788253, PubMed Central PMCID: PMCPMC6351808.
83. Shinohara G, Morita K, Hoshino M, Ko Y, Tsukube T, Kaneko Y, et al. Three dimensional visualization of human cardiac conduction tissue in whole heart specimens by high-resolution phase-contrast CT imaging using synchrotron radiation. World J Pediatr Congenit Heart Surg. 2016;7(6):700–5. https://doi.org/10.1177/2150135116675844. PubMed PMID: 27834761.
84. Jackowski C, Schweitzer W, Thali M, Yen K, Aghayev E, Sonnenschein M, et al. Virtopsy: postmortem imaging of the human heart in situ using MSCT and MRI. Forensic Sci Int. 2005;149(1):11–23. https://doi.org/10.1016/j.forsciint.2004.05.019. PubMed PMID: 15734105.
85. Philips and Microsoft Showcase augmented reality for image-guided minimally invasive therapies. 2019. https://www.dicardiology.com/content/philips-and-microsoft-showcase-augmented-reality-image-guided-minimally-invasive-therapies.

Part II

Novel Applications to ACHD

Cardiac Shunts

11

Lars Grosse-Wortmann and Cesar Gonzalez de Alba

Abbreviations

ASD	Atrial septal defect
CMR	Cardiac magnetic resonance
CTA	Computed tomography angiography
CW	Continuous wave
LV	Left ventricle/left ventricular
PAPVC	Partial anomalous pulmonary venous connection
PC	Phase contrast flow velocity mapping
PDA	Patent ductus arteriosus
PVR	Pulmonary vascular resistance
PW	Pulsed wave
Qp	Pulmonary blood flow
Qs	Systemic blood flow
RV	Right ventricle/right ventricular
VSD	Ventricular septal defect

11.1 Overview

The evaluation of shunt lesions requires a keen understanding of their anatomy and associated anomalies, as well as of the physical principles of volume and pressure changes throughout the circulation that accompany them. Echocardiography and cardiac catheterization have traditionally been the mainstay of their evaluation and

L. Grosse-Wortmann (✉) · C. G. de Alba
Oregon Health and Science University, Portland, OR, USA
e-mail: grossewo@ohsu.edu; Cesar.GonzalezdeAlba@childrenscolorado.org

© Springer Nature Switzerland AG 2021
P. Gallego, I. Valverde (eds.), *Multimodality Imaging Innovations In Adult Congenital Heart Disease*, Congenital Heart Disease in Adolescents and Adults, https://doi.org/10.1007/978-3-030-61927-5_11

continue to play important roles. Advances in the so-called "advanced" imaging techniques, foremost cardiac magnetic resonance (CMR), over the last quarter of a century have expanded the physicians' toolbox for the assessment of shunts. This chapter reviews the basic anatomical and pathophysiological concepts that apply to the evaluation of all shunt defects and across modalities, followed by a description of the individual modalities used in the contemporary care of patients with congenital heart disease.

11.1.1 Shunt Anatomy

Shunt defects are commonly categorized by two approaches: (1) intracardiac vs. extracardiac or (2) pre-tricuspid vs. post-tricuspid valve shunt defects. The first approach refers primarily to the anatomical location, while the second clusters lesions of comparable hemodynamic significance. For example, the pathophysiology of a ventricular septal defect (VSD) is relatively similar to that of a patent ductus arteriosus (PDA), although one is intra- and the other extracardiac, while the hemodynamics of a VSD and an atrial septal defect (ASD) are quite different, although both are intracardiac. Approaching the subject from a hemodynamic angle rather than purely anatomical, the authors prefer the categorization into "pre-tricuspid" vs. "post-tricuspid" and apply it to this chapter.

11.1.1.1 Pre-tricuspid Shunt Defects
In "pre-tricuspid" lesions, shunting occurs between vessels or chambers localized upstream from the tricuspid valve (or single atrioventricular valve in single-ventricle cases). These include deficiencies of the interatrial septum, unroofed coronary sinus, and partial anomalous pulmonary venous connection (PAPVC).

11.1.1.2 Post-tricuspid Shunt Defects
These are communications between vessels or chambers where shunting occurs downstream from the tricuspid valve. They include VSD, PDA, aorto-pulmonary window, major aortopulmonary collateral arteries, and coronary-cameral fistulae.

In addition to congenital shunt lesions, surgically created communications are frequently used to palliate congenital heart disease, typically to augment and/or control pulmonary blood flow. Shunts may also be created as "pop-offs" when pulmonary vascular resistance (PVR) is too high for the circulation "to work." An example is the fenestration placed between the Fontan conduit and the pulmonary venous atrium [1].

11.1.1.3 Shunt Direction
The blood flow direction across a shunt is typically described as left-to-right or right-to-left. Commonly, left-to-right shunting refers to oxygenated blood traveling to a chamber or a vessel carrying deoxygenated blood (systemic venous blood). Right-to-left shunting is the opposite: deoxygenated blood moves to an area of oxygenated blood. As such, left-to-right shunts lead to volume overload in the lungs, while right-to-left shunts lead to hypoxemia [2, 3].

There are situations, however, in which this rule is broken, for instance in unrepaired transposition of the great arteries in which blood flow across a VSD reaches the lungs, although it travels from the right to the left ventricle (RV and LV respectively). In these scenarios it is preferable to describe the path of the blood and to explain whether there is more or less pulmonary blood flow than systemic blood flow, rather than relying on an abbreviated description.

11.1.1.4 Shunt Magnitude

The magnitude of the shunt is expressed by the ratio of pulmonary blood flow to systemic blood flow, or Qp:Qs. In a normal heart the two circulations are balanced and the ratio is approximately 1:1. A Qp:Qs > 1 denotes a net left-to-right shunt while a Qp:Qs < 1 indicates a right-to-left shunt. Patients with Qp:Qs <1.5 are typically asymptomatic, while most with a Qp:Qs > 2 will display signs and symptoms of volume overload (e.g., shortness of breath, dyspnea on exertion), although the association of symptoms and Qp:Qs severity is loose. It is important to note that several shunts can co-exist within the same patient, sometimes with opposing directions, such as systemic to pulmonary venous collaterals and aorto-pulmonary collaterals in patients with single-ventricle physiology.

11.1.1.5 Intrapulmonary Shunts

Systemic veins may connect to pulmonary veins as in the case of veno-venous collaterals. These are common in single-ventricle patients after Glenn and Fontan surgeries with associated high pulmonary arterial pressures. Connections between pulmonary arteries and pulmonary veins, also known as pulmonary arteriovenous malformations, can be primary/congenital or secondary, for example in palliated single-ventricle physiology. Both veno-venous collaterals and pulmonary arteriovenous malformations bypass lung capillaries and therefore are right-to-left shunts.

11.1.2 Volume Overload

Right heart enlargement, including the right atrium and RV, usually occurs with pre-tricuspid shunt defects. Rarely, RV enlargement will occur with VSDs, especially when the shunt volume is large. High-volume post-tricuspid shunts result in left heart enlargement (left atrium and ventricle). The main and branch pulmonary arteries are prone to enlargement with any left-to-right shunt, regardless of whether it is located before or after the tricuspid valve. The degree of right or left heart enlargement is reflective, to some degree, of Qp:Qs.

11.1.3 Pressure Overload

Pressure overload on the receiving chamber or vessels (typically the RV or pulmonary arteries) is dependent on the defect size and any associated restrictions to blood flow through it. Large defects transmit pressure directly to the receiving chamber or vessel, thus yielding a small pressure gradient across the communication. The pressure gradient may be diminished by an outflow obstruction of the receiving chamber, which serves to elevate its intracavitary pressure, e.g., pulmonary valve stenosis or pulmonary hypertension in a patient with a VSD.

The pressure gradient determinates the flow direction across a defect. In ASDs, for example, the direction of flow depends on the right and left atrial pressures which are, in turn, reflective of the compliance of their respective ventricles. Some patients with long-standing unrestrictive post-tricuspid shunts develop irreversible pulmonary vascular changes which lead to pulmonary hypertension. Once the pulmonary supersedes the systemic blood pressure, the shunt direction across the VSD becomes right-to-left, also known as Eisenmenger physiology [4–6].

11.1.4 Associated Lesions

When evaluating a shunt defect it is important to investigate associated lesions that can affect the shunt physiology, as exemplified in the previous paragraph. Conversely, the shunt can either mask or exaggerate the effects from concomitant defects: For example, the augmented Qp from an ASD may increase the gradient across the pulmonary valve and make it appear more stenotic than it intrinsically is. On the other hand, an ASD in the presence of left-sided obstructive lesions may mask the true degree of stenosis into or out of the LV by shunting some of the blood flow away from the stenotic LV inflow or outflow tract.

Volume loading can lead to mitral or tricuspid valve annular dilation. When this results in mitral and tricuspid valve leakage, the resultant volume overload can further worsen the chamber dilation which, in turn, aggravates the valvar regurgitation.

11.1.5 Confounders in Shunt Assessment

Certain systemic conditions can alter hemodynamics and, consequently, shunt volumes. High-output states as seen in thyroid disorders, fever, or anemia can interfere with laminar blood flow [7, 8]. Thus, hyperdynamic states that increase blood flow velocity or decrease its viscosity result in turbulent blood flow, which in turn may erroneously increase gradients across vessels and other shunts.

11.2 Modalities Used in Shunt Evaluation

The comprehensive evaluation of a shunt lesion includes the anatomical and physiological description of the shunt. Table 11.1 includes the aspects in both categories that need to be examined. No single imaging modality is capable of delivering optimally on all of these and, frequently, an approach using more than one technique is warranted.

Table 11.1 Anatomical and physiological characteristics of shunt defects

Anatomical description, location, size, and number of defect(s)
Flow direction and velocity across the shunt
Atrial and ventricular volume/enlargement
Right and left ventricular function
Ventricular and arterial pressure
Pulmonary to systemic arterial flow ratio
Associated lesions, particularly limitations to blood flow and lesions affected by the shunt
Pulmonary vascular health, pulmonary vascular resistance

11.3 Echocardiography

Echocardiography has been in use since the early 1950s when Edler and Hertz first described M-mode ultrasound of the heart [9]. Today, Doppler color flow, 2D, 3D, and 4D technologies are at our disposal for assessing shunt lesions [7, 8, 10].

11.3.1 Delineation of Shunt Anatomy and Flow Direction

11.3.1.1 2D and 3D Echocardiography
Echocardiography allows the study of the anatomy of the shunt, including number of defects, location, sizes as well as associated lesions. Three-dimensional echocardiography is particularly useful for the evaluation of heart valves, but also awards comprehensive views of ASDs and VSDs as illustrated in Fig. 11.1 [11–13].

11.3.1.2 Color Doppler
Color Doppler imaging encodes blood flow direction into a color scale and is useful in the assessment of the presence and direction of shunts (Fig. 11.2) [14, 15]. When interrogating shunt lesions with color flow, setting an appropriate Nyquist limit, i.e., the highest detectable velocity, is instrumental. High velocity shunts (i.e., pressure restrictive defects) require a high Nyquist limit (Fig. 11.3), while low-velocity shunt defects should be evaluated with a lower Nyquist setting (Fig. 11.4), as using a higher limit may falsely "hide" a defect. This is especially useful when evaluating interatrial communications, veno-venous collaterals, and PAPVCs, which have low-velocity venous flow, but also large major aorto-pulmonary connections or PDAs in the setting of high PVR, all marked by relatively low velocities across the shunt. Of note, a color signal may be attenuated or even absent when evaluating defects whose shunting direction is perpendicular to the ultrasound beam.

11.3.1.3 Contrast Studies
Contrast echocardiograms use microbubble injections (agitated saline solution or a mix of saline and blood) via a peripheral intravenous line, when there is suspicion of or it is important to rule out with certainty shunting lesions not readily seen by

Fig. 11.1 Three-dimensional transthoracic echocardiography: The reconstruction shows a large muscular ventricular septal defect (white asterisk) seen *en face* from the right ventricular aspect. (Image courtesy of Christopher Marcella RDCS FASE, Oregon Health and Science University)

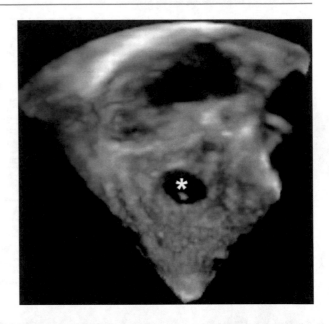

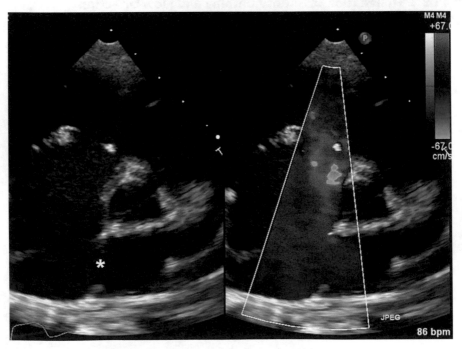

Fig. 11.2 Transthoracic echocardiogram of an atrial septal defect: Parasternal short axis view with color Doppler comparison demonstrates left-to-right shunting across a large atrial septal defect (asterisk)

Fig. 11.3 Transthoracic echocardiogram in patent ductus arteriosus: The parasternal long axis view with color Doppler demonstrates continuous high velocity left-to-right shunting across a moderate-sized duct (red flow), suggesting a high-pressure gradient between the aorta and main pulmonary artery

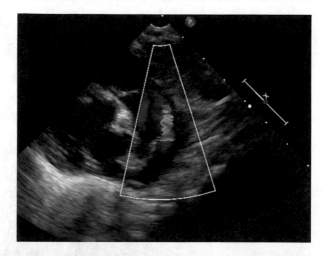

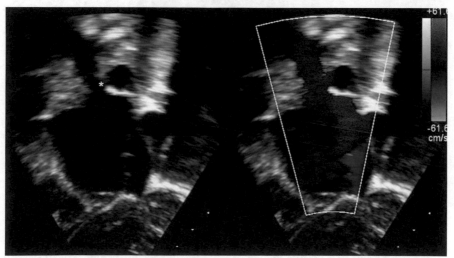

Fig. 11.4 Subcostal echocardiogram with color Doppler comparison in a patient with partial anomalous pulmonary venous connection. A lower Nyquist limit is used to demonstrate a right pulmonary vein connecting anomalously to the right atrium—superior vena cava junction (white asterisk)

2D or color Doppler [16]. In a heart with no shunt defects, microbubbles should appear in the right atrium and RV following a venous injection, to be then removed in the pulmonary capillaries. In patients with right-to-left shunt defects, microbubbles will appear in the left atrium and ventricle. Intracardiac defects such as ASDs and VSDs will typically show microbubbles in the left atrium within the first three beats of right atrial/ventricular opacification, while they take 3–5 beats or longer to appear in the left atrium in the case of pulmonary arteriovenous malformations or veno-venous collaterals (Fig. 11.5) [16–18].

Fig. 11.5 Echocardiographic bubble study in a patient with bidirectional cavo-pulmonary connection and pulmonary arteriovenous malformations: The apical four-chamber view shows contrast bubbles entering the common atrium via the pulmonary veins 1–2 beats after injection into the left pulmonary artery (during cardiac catheterization), consistent with an arteriovenous connection in the lungs that bypasses the pulmonary capillary bed

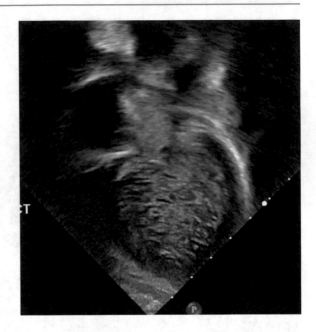

11.3.2 Flow Assessment

11.3.2.1 Simplified Bernoulli's Equation

This formula uses velocity measurements on both sides of a pressure drop—across a shunt or other narrowing to estimate pressure gradients across that lesion:

$$\Delta P = 4V^2$$

where ΔP (in mmHg) denotes the pressure gradient and V is the velocity (in m/s) distal to the shunt or narrowing, respectively. If the proximal velocity is <1.5 m/s, this value should be added to the equation as follows ($\Delta P = 4V_2^2 - 4V_1^2$).

It is important to note that this equation estimates peak *instantaneous* pressure gradients, which are almost always greater than the *peak-to-peak* gradients obtained by cardiac catheterization.

11.3.2.2 Doppler Modalities

Continuous wave (CW) and pulsed-wave (PW) Doppler ultrasound both measure flow velocities which, using the modified Bernoulli equation, provide an estimate of the pressure drop across a shunt lesion. While CW Doppler is able to measure higher maximum flow velocities, but without the ability to identify the location of the fastest flow along the insonation beam, PW offers the benefit of measuring flow speeds at user-defined depths. These properties make CW Doppler the technique of choice in shunt lesions where fast flows are expected, including VSDs, PDAs, and aorto-pulmonary windows, whereas PW Doppler is commonly employed to measure velocities/gradients across ASDs, with PAPVCs, or veno-venous collaterals.

11.3.3 Quantification of Shunt Magnitude

11.3.3.1 Atrial and Ventricular Volumes and Function

Right or left heart enlargement can be assessed qualitatively or quantitatively by echocardiography. The preferred methods of quantification of ventricular volume and function are beyond the scope of this chapter. In brief, the size and function of the atria and of the RV are commonly evaluated qualitatively, while the LV, for which greater standardization and more widely accepted normative values exist, is commonly measured quantitatively.

11.3.3.2 Ventricular and Arterial Pressure Load

Depending on the type of shunt defect, pressure load can be assessed by qualitative and quantitative methods. In VSDs for example, the velocity across the defect is used to estimate the systolic pressure gradient between the LV and RV. Provided that the LV systolic pressure, which usually is similar to the systolic blood pressure, is known, the RV pressure can be calculated:

$$\text{Right ventricular systolic pressure} (\text{RV}p) = \text{systolic blood pressure} - \left(4 \times \text{VSD}v^2\right)$$

where $\text{VSD}v$ = velocity across the VSD. As mentioned above, RV or branch pulmonary artery obstructive lesions as well as elevated pulmonary vascular resistance can yield a lower pressure gradient, even though the defect itself may be restrictive.

Right ventricular systolic pressure can also be estimated by using the tricuspid valve regurgitation velocity (TRv) in the simplified Bernoulli equation and adding the assumed right atrial pressure (RAp):

$$\text{Right ventricular pressure} (\text{RV}p) = \left(4 \times \text{TR}v^2\right) + \text{RA}p$$

The qualitative assessment of RV pressure overload includes presence of RV hypertrophy, as well as interventricular septal flattening during systole, assessed in the parasternal short axis view.

11.3.3.3 Qp:Qs Assessment

In principle, volumetric flow assessments are feasible by echocardiography and follow the same principle as phase contrast (PC) magnetic resonance imaging (below), using the following equation:

$$Q = V \times \text{CSA}$$

where Q = flow volume, V = mean velocity, and CSA = cross-sectional area of flow [15]. Mean velocities are calculated as velocity time integrals (VTI) divided by the flow period of the traced beat. The shortcoming of flow measurements based on ultrasound is that the true mean velocity across the entire cross-sectional area of the vessel is difficult to ascertain and the value obtained by VTI is only an approximation.

Fig. 11.6 Transesophageal echocardiogram in the same patient as in Fig. 11.2: The color Doppler acquisition at the mid-esophageal level reveals left-to-right shunting across the atrial septal defect

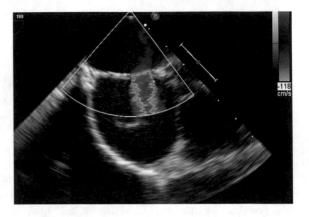

11.3.4 Strengths and Limitations

The greatest advantages of echocardiography are its widespread availability, low cost, and noninvasive nature, along with excellent temporal resolution and a wealth of real-time functional information. Its limitations reside in its operator and acoustic window dependency. The estimation of RV and pulmonary arterial pressures by echocardiography is imperfect and the quantification of the shunt magnitude relies on indirect markers. The use of contrast studies with microbubbles improves the blood-tissue contrast, but requires placement of an intravenous line.

11.4   Transesophageal Echocardiography

Traditionally, transesophageal echocardiography has been widely used to characterize intracardiac shunts, especially with addition of bubble study [19–22]. However, with the arrival of harmonics, image resolution of transthoracic echo has greatly improved [23, 24]. Today, its use in shunt lesions is largely limited to intraoperative evaluations and assistance to percutaneous procedures in the catheterization laboratory (Fig. 11.6) [25–27].

11.5   Cardiac Catheterization

11.5.1 Basic Principles

Assessment of blood flow by cardiac catheterization is based on measuring oxygen content in the blood and oxygen consumption, using the Fick principle: Knowledge of the concentration of a tracer (oxygen) in the blood before and after a known amount of it was added allows computing the volume of blood [28]. Quantifying the added oxygen per time interval (typically "minute") allows the calculation of blood flow volume during the same period.

Applying the Fick equation to both the pulmonary and the systemic circulation yields the pulmonary to systemic flow ratio, or Qp:Qs. If only the ratio and not the absolute flow amounts for each circulation are needed, this can be derived from the following formula:

$$Qp : Qs = \frac{Aorta\,sat - MV\,sat}{PV\,sat - PA\,sat}$$

where sat = oxygen saturation, MV = mixed venous, PV = pulmonary venous, and PA = pulmonary arterial. In cases where Qp:Qs ratio is >3, the difference between the pulmonary vein and pulmonary artery oxygen saturation is small; in this scenario, it is suggested to report Qp:Qs as "greater than 3:1" rather than providing a particular ratio.

11.5.2 Shunt Evaluation

It is important to understand the concept of effective pulmonary blood flow (Q_{EP}) and effective systemic blood flow (Q_{ES}). Effective pulmonary blood flow represents the total amount of deoxygenated (or "blue") blood returning from the systemic venous circulation, represented by the mixed venous oxygen saturation that passes through the lungs to be re-oxygenated (pulmonary venous oxygen saturation). In the absence of a shunt defect, Q_{EP} equals Q_P [29–31].

Similarly, Q_{ES} represents the total flow of blood oxygenated in the lungs ("red" blood) returned via the pulmonary veins to the left atrium that eventually reaches the systemic capillary circulation. Once again, in a person without a significant shunt, Q_{ES} roughly equals Q_S (and $Q_{EP} = Q_{ES}$).

In a patient with a left-to-right shunt, the total amount of blood flow arriving via the pulmonary arteries (Q_p) will comprise both "blue" and "red" blood. The additional "shunted" blood flow into the lungs ("red" portion of Q_p) can be calculated as:

$$Q_{L-R} \left(\text{left to right shunt volume}\right) = Q_p - Q_{EP}$$

Conversely, in a right-to-left shunt (R − L), "blue" is added to the "red" blood. Therefore, the R − L shunt volume is:

$$Q_{R-L} \left(\text{right to left shunt volume}\right) = Q_s - Q_{ES}$$

11.5.3 Pulmonary and Systemic Vascular Resistance

Pulmonary vascular resistance (PVR) informs on the health of the pulmonary vascular bed: The lower the PVR, the more permissive the lung vessels are towards an increased blood flow volume via a shunt. In patients with a shunt defect a high PVR may indicate that the arteries and capillaries have been irreversibly damaged. Resistance is calculated using Ohm's law, which incorporates the change in pressure drop and the blood flow volume across the vasculature (Q_p):

$$PVR = \Delta P / Q_p$$

The change in pressure across the pulmonary vascular bed is obtained by subtracting the mean left atrial (or pulmonary arterial wedge) pressure from the mean pulmonary artery or pulmonary venous wedge pressure.

11.5.4 Strengths

Cardiac catheterization allows for calculation of blood flows and shunt volumes. Importantly, invasive manometry is the only modality that directly measures pulmonary blood pressures and, as such, is instrumental in assessing PVR. "Step-ups" or "step-downs" of oxygen saturations between chambers can indicate the location of a shunt.

Fluoroscopic angiography delivers exquisite blood-tissue contrast and depicts the location and size of a shunt, as illustrated in Figs. 11.7 and 11.8. In contrast to cardiac magnetic resonance and, to a lesser degree, computed tomography, metallic objects do not produce artifacts on fluoroscopic images.

Fig. 11.7 Cardiac catheterization in a patient with veno-venous collateral: The fluoroscopic angiography with injection of contrast into the proximal left innominate vein in a patient with single-ventricle physiology and Glenn anastomosis shows a large decompressing vein

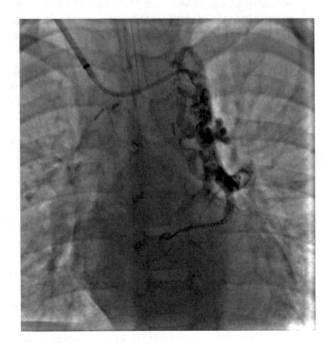

Fig. 11.8 Cardiac catheterization angiography in a patient with patent ductus arteriosus: The straight lateral view with contrast injection in the proximal descending aorta reveals a moderate-sized duct (white asterisk). *DA* descending aorta, *MPA* main pulmonary artery

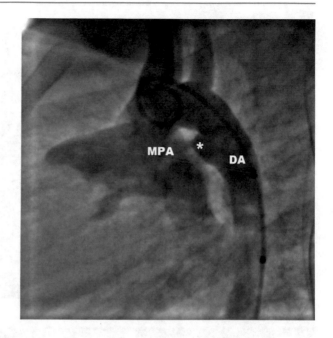

11.5.5 Limitations

The greatest limitation of cardiac catheterization is its invasive nature and use of ionizing radiation. Further, the collection sites of blood samples for invasive oxygen measurements impact and may skew the resultant flow measurements. For example, streaming of oxygenated blood from a PDA may lead to the collection of a blood sample that is not representative of the saturation in the distal pulmonary arteries. The quantification of oxygen consumption is complex and constitutes another Achilles' heel of hemodynamic evaluation by cardiac catheterization. Lastly, apart from rotational angiography, cardiac catheterization is a two-dimensional modality, offering limited representation of septal defects as illustrated in Fig. 11.9 and complex three-dimensional structures [32, 33].

11.6   Cardiac Magnetic Resonance Imaging

Cardiac magnetic resonance plays out many of its strengths in the evaluation of intra- and extracardiac shunt lesions: It is a three-dimensional modality with superb blood-tissue contrast and affords an accurate quantification of blood flow.

11.6.1 Basic Principles

A variety of techniques are applied in CMR to assess the anatomy and hemodynamics of shunt lesions. Phase contrast flow velocity mapping (PC) is the gold standard of flow quantification and highly accurate as long as flow is laminar [34–36]. In

Fig. 11.9 Cardiac catheterization in a patient with a secundum-type atrial septal defect: The fluoroscopic angiogram with contrast injection into the left atrium via a catheter crossing the atrial septum shows contrast shunting from left-to-right atrium consistent with an atrial septal defect (asterisk). Septal defect anatomy delineation is limited compared to other imaging modalities

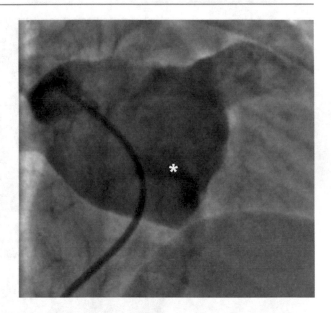

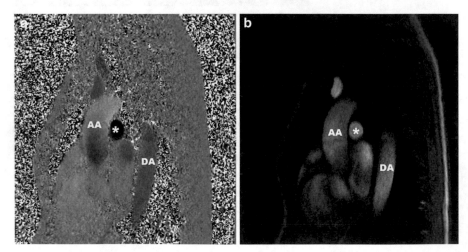

Fig. 11.10 Magnetic resonance phase contrast acquisition: The magnitude image (**a**) and velocity maps (**b**) show the right pulmonary artery *en face* (asterisk). *AA* ascending aorta, *DA* descending aorta

contrast to cardiac catheterization, blood flow volumes are measured directly (Figs. 11.10 and 11.11), instead of being calculated using the Fick principle. When comparing blood flows derived in the catheterization laboratory to those from CMR, it is essential for the clinician to be aware that most CMR centers quantify Qp as the total pulmonary venous flow [37, 38]. In the absence of aorto-pulmonary collateral arteries, pulmonary venous flow is identical to pulmonary arterial flow and, in principle, similar to Qp by invasive oximetry and Fick. However, in the presence of

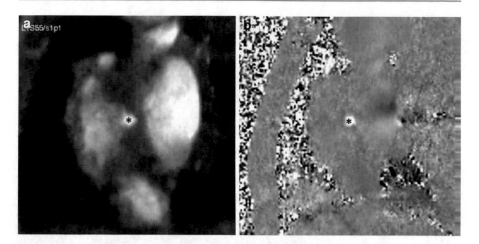

Fig. 11.11 Magnetic resonance phase contrast flow velocity mapping in a patient with hypoplastic left heart syndrome and fenestrated Fontan conduit: The magnitude image (**a**) and phase contrast flow velocity map (**b**) are *en face* with the shunt across the Fontan fenestration seen directly (asterisk)

collaterals, Qp by catheterization is affected by the location of blood sampling for oxygen saturation measurements and, typically, lower than Qp by CMR PC. In fact, the latter technique can be used to quantify the left-to-right shunt via aorto-pulmonary collateral arteries as the difference between Qp and pulmonary arterial flow, which has been shown to be a prognostic factor after the Fontan completion.

Another way to measure Qp:Qs by CMR is as the ratio of RV-to-LV stroke volumes. Given the simplicity and superior accuracy of PC, however, as well as the confounders of shunt assessment via stroke volumes, the latter method is rarely used, and only applicable in the absence of significant valvar regurgitation.

11.6.2 Shunt Evaluation

By convention, as illustrated above, Qp is defined as the volume of blood that passes through the lungs, irrespective of the source, and that is returned via the pulmonary veins. Qs is the blood that passes through the systemic capillary bed and is returned via the caval veins. Within the systemic or the pulmonary circulation and, in fact, between them as long as no shunt is present, the flow volume is preserved. As a consequence, in many clinical scenarios, Qp:Qs by PC CMR can be obtained by more than one equation: For example, in PAPVC, it is the ratio of main pulmonary artery to aortic flows, but also the ratio of the sum of branch pulmonary artery flows to the sum of descending aortic and superior caval vein flows. The authors recommend applying more than one method for Qp/Qs quantification as a means of internal validation of the measurements.

In addition to the shunt amount, PC provides the net direction of the shunt (either left-to-right or right-to-left) as illustrated in Fig. 11.12. Furthermore, it offers the

Fig. 11.12 Cardiac magnetic resonance image in the same patient as Fig. 11.11: The fenestration jet (white asterisk) into the common atrium causes a dephasing artifact on the steady-state-free precession images. *F* Fontan, *RV* right ventricle

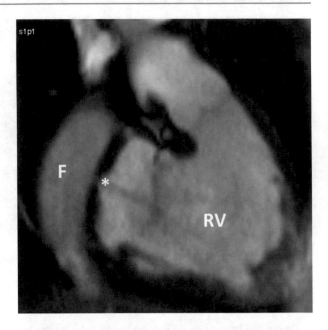

Fig. 11.13 Cardiac magnetic resonance examination in a patient with superior sinus venosus atrial septal defect: The still frame from a steady-state-free precession acquisition in the axial plane shows the deficient wall (asterisk) between the superior vena cava and the right upper pulmonary vein, causing anomalous drainage of the pulmonary vein flow into the right atrium

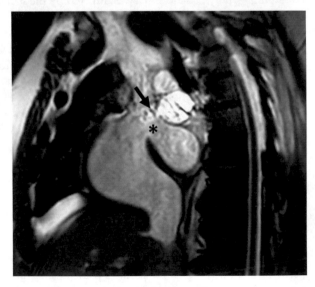

unique ability to quantify the contribution of each of several co-existing left-to-right shunt lesions, such as a VSD and PDA or PAPVC with an atrial septal defect (Fig. 11.13) [39, 40]. This knowledge can be relevant to determine the appropriate treatment strategy (e.g., percutaneous, operative, or a combination of both).

11.6.3 Anatomy

As mentioned in Table 11.1, there are key anatomical features that need to be evaluated for each defect. An exhaustive description of CMR techniques is beyond the scope of this chapter. In synopsis, the most common CMR tools for the delineation of anatomy include ECG-gated non-contrast-enhanced white blood techniques, using steady-state-free precession (Figs. 11.14 and 11.15) or spoiled gradient-echo

Fig. 11.14 Cardiac magnetic resonance in a patient with an atrial septal defect: The four-chamber view, acquired using a white blood steady-state-free precession approach, shows severe right heart enlargement due to a secundum atrial septal defect (asterisk). This patient had an indexed right ventricular end-diastolic volume of 268 mL/m²

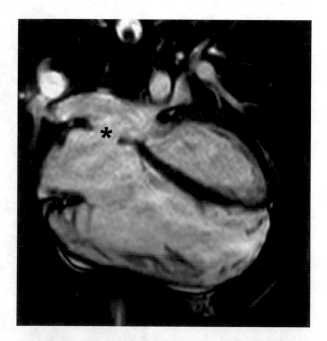

Fig. 11.15 Cardiac magnetic resonance image in a patient with superior sinus venosus atrial septal defect and anomalous pulmonary venous connection: The sagittal cut demonstrates the interatrial connection (asterisk) and the anomalous pulmonary venous connection (arrow)

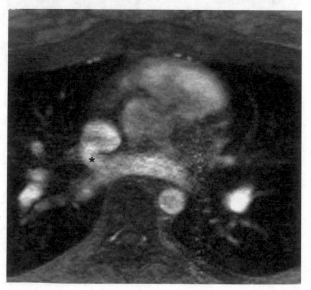

approaches. Contrast-enhanced magnetic resonance angiography yields high-resolution three-dimensional images (Fig. 11.16) and volume-rendered reconstructions (Fig. 11.17). In contrast, turbo-spin-echo-based black blood sequences have largely fallen out of favor, although they retain a role in the delineation of airways,

Fig. 11.16 Cardiac magnetic resonance angiogram in a patient with scimitar syndrome: The multiplanar reformat reveals stenosis of the supra-hepatic inferior vena cava at the entrance of the hepatic veins, resulting in congestion of the latter. *HV* hepatic vein, *SV* scimitar vein

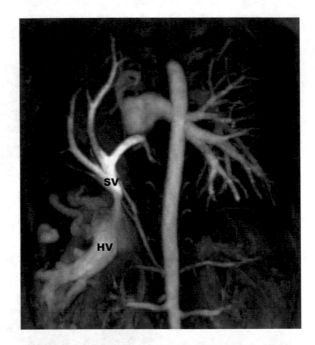

Fig. 11.17 Volume-rendered reconstruction of a three-dimensional contrast-enhanced magnetic resonance angiogram. The right upper and middle pulmonary (asterisks) connect to the superior vena cava (SVC)

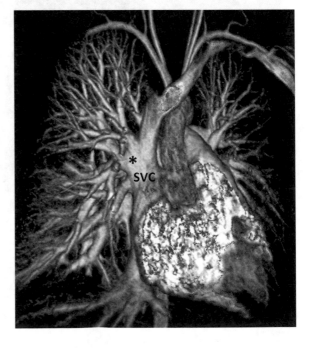

in order to overcome image artifacts from metallic implants, and in patient populations in whom high spatial resolution without the use of gadolinium contrast is desired, such as neonates and young infants.

11.6.4 Strengths

One of the major strengths of CMR is that it allows for cross-sectional imaging while avoiding ionizing radiation. It is noninvasive except for the administration of intravenous gadolinium. In contrast to cardiac catheterization, CMR has the ability to quantify blood flows in parts of the pulmonary or of the systemic circulation: For example, in patients with tetralogy of Fallot, pulmonary atresia, and major aorto-pulmonary collateral arteries, CMR is capable of quantifying the importance of each collateral for the pulmonary circulation [41].

11.6.5 Limitations

The most important limitation of CMR in the evaluation of shunt lesions is its inability to measure pressures directly. This is particularly important in cases where PVR is suspected to be elevated enough to be a barrier towards surgical repair, such as in some VSDs, PDAs, as well as in single-ventricle palliative repairs (Glenn and Fontan). However, in "simple" left-to-right shunt lesions, a Qp:Qs >2.5 has been shown to predict an acceptably low PVR of 3.5 Woods units*m^2 or less with a sensitivity of 83% and specificity of 100% [42]. Given the turbulence of flow across most shunt lesions, CMR is unable to quantify intracardiac shunts directly, although an approximation is often feasible with reasonable accuracy (Fig. 11.11) [43]. Other limitations include a comparatively long study duration and limited availability of CMR as compared to echocardiography. Electromagnetic implants are a common source of image artifacts and, in some cases, contraindications towards performing CMR [44, 45].

11.7 Computed Tomography Angiography

Contrast-enhanced computed tomography angiography (CTA) is an excellent cross-sectional imaging technique for the evaluation of cardiovascular anatomy, including vascular shunts [46]. Ventricular functional evaluation and volume quantification by CTA are possible as well; however, this comes at the expense of additional ionizing radiation [47, 48].

11.7.1 Strengths

Computed tomography is more widely available than CMR, requires less patient compliance, and offers superior anatomical delineation [49, 50].

11.7.2 Limitations

The most important limitations of CTA are the use of ionizing radiation and the scarce functional information that it yields. The administration of contrast is routinely necessary and may be contraindicated in patients with decreased renal function or a history of allergic reactions to contrast.

11.8 Nuclear Medicine Imaging

Given the increasing availability of noninvasive and nonradiating alternatives such as echocardiography and CMR, along with the limited fidelity of nuclear medicine modalities, the role of the latter for the evaluation of shunt lesions has diminished. Quantification of shunts by this modality requires administration of radiopharmaceutical agents, most commonly technetium 99-m in macro-aggregated albumin.

Radiopharmaceutical activity is tracked across the heart, lungs, and other extrathoracic organs (i.e., kidneys and brains) [51, 52]. Higher levels of activity measured in the LV or extra-thoracic organs compared to the lungs indicate a right-to-left shunt, while the presence of a second spike of radiopharmaceutical activity in the lungs is indicative of a left-to-right shunt.

11.9 Multimodality Imaging in Evaluating Shunt Defects

While transthoracic echocardiography is typically the first-line modality in the evaluation of shunt lesions, the results from ultrasound sometimes need to be supplemented with information from one of the other imaging modalities discussed in this chapter.

The choice of additional imaging modality to evaluate a shunt defect depends on the information that is missing and whether this information is required for clinical decision-making. Examples include a VSD where cardiac catheterization may be indicated in order to measure PVR prior to repair or major aorto-pulmonary collateral arteries, which often necessitate CMR, CTA, or cardiac catheterization in order to complete the anatomic evaluation. Table 11.2 summarizes the advantages and limitations of each modality, along with examples for lesions where each modality excels.

Other considerations that play into the choice of imaging modality include (a) whether there are concomitant lesions that need evaluation, (b) whether the patient is able to comply with the examination or requires sedation or anesthesia, (c) patient body habitus, presence of concomitant cardiac lesions, as well as (d) any contraindications to the desired study.

In some cases, imaging modalities can be combined to increase their sensitivity and specificity or guide interventions when needed [53]. For instance, atrial septal defects can be closed in the cardiac catheterization lab with simultaneous use of echocardiography, thereby significantly decreasing and in some institutions altogether avoiding the need for angiography [54–56]. Magnetic resonance and computed tomography angiographies can be co-registered during an interventional procedure in the catheter laboratory during complex vascular interventions, adding three-dimensional information and reducing the need for fluoroscopic angiographies [57–59]. Further, rapid prototyping based on CMR or CTA data yields 3D printed models of the anatomy, which can be used to practice interventions or even custom-design implants.

Table 11.2 Strengths and limitations of imaging modalities in the evaluation of shunt defects

Imaging modality	Strengths	Limitations	Particularly useful for the following lesions
Transthoracic echocardiography	Noninvasive, no radiation or intravenous contrast (except for bubble study) Excellent blood-soft tissue contrast for anatomical delineation of defect location, size, concomitant lesions, especially valvar Functional information on shunt direction, pressure gradients (Indirect) quantification of shunt magnitude via ventricular volumes and estimates of ventricular and arterial pressure No image degradation from implants or indwelling catheters	Degraded image quality in patients with poor acoustic windows Often limited visualization of vasculature, particularly in the lungs No absolute quantification of shunt amount	Baseline modality in virtually all shunt lesions, particularly useful in: Atrial septal defect Partial anomalous pulmonary venous connection Ventricular septal defect Coronary-cameral fistula Aorto-pulmonary window Patent ductus arteriosus Pulmonary arteriovenous malformations and veno-venous collaterals via bubble study
Transesophageal echocardiography	Largely the same as transthoracic echocardiography plus: Better echo image resolution in patients with poor acoustic windows through the chest Superior imaging of heart valves, vegetations, and clots	Invasive Requires sedation (degree varies on patient population and center) Risk of patient extubation, dental trauma, laceration or perforation of oropharynx, esophagus, and stomach	Same as transthoracic echocardiography, but rarely used as a first-line modality Commonly used for guidance of interventional procedures (e.g., closure of septal defects) and in the operating room

(continued)

Table 11.2 (continued)

Imaging modality	Strengths	Limitations	Particularly useful for the following lesions
Cardiac catheterization and angiography	Very good visualization of shunt lesions, particularly outside of the heart Direct measurement of pressures Absolute quantification of blood flow volumes and shunt amounts Opportunity for percutaneous closure of certain lesions	Invasive Requires ionizing radiation and typically administration of contrast Flow quantification is subject to errors, especially in patients with complex shunt lesions	Many lesions; frequently used in: Coronary-cameral fistula Aorto-pulmonary collateral arteries Patent ductus arteriosus Surgically placed shunt Veno-venous collaterals
Cardiac magnetic resonance	Anatomical evaluation of defects Gold standard for flow measurements, including selective blood flow quantification in subcomponents of the circulation Gold standard of ventricular volume and function assessment Evaluation of vascular anatomy	Unable to measure pressures Precise size of atrial septal defects may be difficult to visualize Artifacts and possible contraindications due to metallic implants Intravenous contrast may be required	Essentially all shunt lesions in which an exact quantification of Qp/Qs is warranted
Computed tomography	Excellent anatomical delineation and spatial resolution, particularly useful for small vessels Lower requirements for patient compliance as compared to CMR Gold standard for evaluation of pulmonary parenchymal pathology	Use of intravenous contrast and ionizing radiation Only indirect information on shunt magnitude and limited information on cardiac size and function (unless study is multiphasic)	Often reserved for extracardiac shunts Coronary-cameral fistula Aorto-pulmonary collateral arteries Patent ductus arteriosus Surgically placed shunt Veno-venous collaterals
Nuclear medicine imaging	Quantification of Qp:Qs and of right vs. left lung perfusion	Use of ionizing intravenous contrast Limited spatial resolution and functional information	Used primarily when CMR is contraindicated and invasive cardiac catheterization is to be avoided

CMR cardiac magnetic resonance, *Qp* pulmonary blood flow, *Qs* systemic blood flow

References

1. Li D, Li M, Zhou X, An Q. Comparison of the fenestrated and non-fenestrated Fontan procedures: a meta-analysis. Medicine (Baltimore). 2019;98(29):e16554. https://doi.org/10.1097/MD.0000000000016554.
2. Rudolph A. Congenital diseases of the heart. 3rd ed. Oxford: Wiley; 2009.
3. Joffe DC, Shi MR, Welker CC. Understanding cardiac shunts. Paediatr Anaesth. 2018;28(4):316–25. https://doi.org/10.1111/pan.13347.
4. Eisenmenger V. Die angeborenen Defecte der Kammerscheidewand des Herzens. Z Klin Med. 1897;32(suppl):1–28.
5. Wood P. The Eisenmenger syndrome or pulmonary hypertension with reversed central shunt: I. Br Med J. 1958;2:701–9.
6. Wood P. The Eisenmenger syndrome or pulmonary hypertension with reversed central shunt. Br Med J. 1958;2:755–62.
7. Awasthy N, Radhakrishnan S. Stepwise evaluation of left to right shunts by echocardiography. Indian Heart J. 2013;65(2):201–18. https://doi.org/10.1016/j.ihj.2013.03.003.
8. Yoganathan AP, Cape EG, Sung HW, Williams FP, Jimoh A. Review of hydrodynamic principles for the cardiologist: applications to the study of blood flow and jets by imaging techniques. J Am Coll Cardiol. 1988;12(5):1344–53.
9. Singh S, Goyal A. The origin of echocardiography: a tribute to Inge Edler. Tex Heart Inst J. 2007;34(4):431–8.
10. Deri A, English K. Educational series in congenital heart disease: echocardiographic assessment of left to right shunts: atrial septal defect, ventricular septal defect, atrioventricular septal defect, patent arterial duct. Echo Res Pract. 2018;5(1):R1–R16. https://doi.org/10.1530/ERP-17-0062.
11. Simpson JM, van den Bosch A. Educational series in congenital heart disease: three-dimensional echocardiography in congenital heart disease. Echo Res Pract. 2019;6(2):R75–86. https://doi.org/10.1530/ERP-18-0074.
12. Simpson J, Lopez L, Acar P, Friedberg MK, Khoo NS, Ko HH, et al. Three-dimensional echocardiography in congenital heart disease: an expert consensus document from the European Association of Cardiovascular Imaging and the American Society of Echocardiography. J Am Soc Echocardiogr. 2017;30(1):1–27. Epub 2016 Nov 9. https://doi.org/10.1016/j.echo.2016.08.022.
13. McGhie JS, van den Bosch AE, Haarman MG, Ren B, Roos-Hesselink JW, Witsenburg M, Geleijnse ML. Characterization of atrial septal defect by simultaneous multiplane two-dimensional echocardiography. Eur Heart J Cardiovasc Imaging. 2014;15:1145–51. https://doi.org/10.1093/ehjci/jeu098.
14. Hedrick WR, Hykes DL, Starchman DE. Ultrasound physics and instrumentation: practice examinations. St. Louis, MO: Mosby-Year Book; 1995. p. 1–90.
15. Friedberg MK. Hemodynamic measurements. In: Lai WW, Mertens LL, Cogehn MS, Geva T, editors. Echocardiography in pediatric and congenital heart disease: from fetus to adult. 2nd ed. Chichester, West Sussex; Hoboken, NJ: Wiley-Blackwell; 2009. p. 73–95.
16. Porter TR, Abdelmoneim S, Belcik JT, McCulloch ML, Mulvagh SL, Olson JJ, Porcelli C, Tsutsui JM, Wei K. Guidelines for the cardiac sonographer in the performance of contrast echocardiography: a focused update from the American Society of Echocardiography. J Am Soc Echocardiogr. 2014 Aug;27(8):797–810. https://doi.org/10.1016/j.echo.2014.05.011.
17. Gupta SK, Shetkar SS, Ramakrishnan S, Kothari SS. Saline contrast echocardiography in the era of multimodality imaging—importance of "bubbling it right". Echocardiography. 2015;32(11):1707–19 . Epub 2015 Aug 7. https://doi.org/10.1111/echo.13035.
18. Chang RK, Alejos JC, Atkinson D, et al. Bubble contrast echocardiography in detecting pulmonary arteriovenous shunting in children with univentricular heart after cavopulmonary anastomosis. J Am Coll Cardiol. 1999;33(7):2052–8.

19. Frazin L, Talano JV, Stephanides L, et al. Esophageal echocardiography. Circulation. 1976;54:102–8. PMid:1277411. https://doi.org/10.1161/01.CIR.54.1.102.
20. Kerut EK, Norfleet WT, Plotnick GD, Giles TD. Patent foramen ovale: a review of associated conditions and the impact of physiological size. J Am Coll Cardiol. 2001;38:613–23.
21. Belkin RN, Pollack BD, Ruggiero ML, Alas LL, Tatini U. Comparison of transesophageal and transthoracic echocardiography with contrast and color flow Doppler in the detection of patent foramen ovale. Am Heart J. 1994;128(3):520–5.
22. Thanigaraj S, Valika A, Zajarias A, Lasala JM, Perez JE. Comparison of transthoracic versus transesophageal echocardiography for detection of right-to-left atrial shunting using agitated saline contrast. Am J Cardiol. 2005;96(7):1007–10.
23. Caidahal K, Kazzam E, Lindberg J, Neumann-Andersen G, Nordanstig J, Dahlqvist SR, Waldenstrom A, Wikh R. New concept in echocardiography: harmonic imaging of tissue without contrast agent. Lancet. 1998;352:1264–70.
24. Kornbluth M, Liang DH, Paloma A, Schnittger I. Native tissue harmonic imaging improves endocardial border definition and visualization of cardiac structures. J Am Soc Echocardiogr. 1998;11:693–701.
25. Eltzschig HK, Rosenberger P, Löffler M, Fox JA, Aranki SF, Shernan SK. Impact of intraoperative transesophageal echocardiography on surgical decisions in 12,566 patients undergoing cardiac surgery. Ann Thorac Surg. 2008;85:845–52.
26. Click RL, Abel MD, Schaff HV. Intraoperative transesophageal echocardiography: 5-year prospective review of impact on surgical management. Mayo Clin Proc. 2000;75:241–7.
27. Kihara C, Murata K, Wada Y, Hadano Y, Ohyama R, Okuda S, Tanaka T, Nose Y, Fukagawa Y, Yoshino H, Susa T, Mikamo A, Furutani A, Kobayashi T, Hamano K, Matsuzaki M. Impact of intraoperative transesophageal echocardiography in cardiac and thoracic aortic surgery: experience in 1011 cases. J Cardiol. 2009;54:282–8.
28. Vargo TA. Cardiac catheterization: hemodynamic measurements. In: Garson Jr A, Bricker JT, Fisher DJ, Neish SR, editors. The science and practice of pediatric cardiology. 2nd ed. Baltimore, MD: Williams & Wilkins; 1998. p. 961–93.
29. Lock JE, Keane JF, Fellows KE. Diagnostic and interventional catheterization in congenital heart disease. Boston, MA: Martinus Nijhoff; 1987.
30. Yang SS, Bentivoglio LG, Maranhao V, Goldberg H. From cardiac catheterization data to hemodynamic parameters. 2nd ed. Philadelphia, PA: FA Davis Co.; 1978.
31. Taggart NW, Cabalka AK. Cardiac catheterization and angiography. In: Allen HD, Shaddy RE, Penny DJ, Cetta F, Feltes TF, editors. Moss and Adams' heart disease in infants, children, and adolescents: including the fetus and young adult. 9th ed. Philadelphia: Wolters Kluwer; 2016. p. 436–65.
32. Hirshfeld JW Jr, Balter S, Brinker JA, et al. ACCF/AHA/HRS/SCAI clinical competence statement on physician knowledge to optimize patient safety and image quality in fluoroscopically guided invasive cardiovascular procedures: a report of the American College of Cardiology Foundation/American Heart Association/American College of Physicians Task Force on clinical competence and training. J Am Coll Cardiol. 2004;44:2259–82.
33. Bergersen L, Marshall A, Gauvreau K, et al. Adverse event rates in congenital cardiac catheterization—a multi-center experience. Catheter Cardiovasc Interv. 2010;75:389–400.
34. Goo HW, Al-Otay A, Grosse-Wortmann L, Wu S, Macgowan CK, Yoo SJ. Phase-contrast magnetic resonance quantification of normal pulmonary venous return. J Magn Reson Imaging. 2009;29:588–94.
35. Beerbaum P, Korperich H, Barth P, Esdorn H, Gieseke J, Meyer H. Noninvasive quantification of left-to-right shunt in pediatric patients: phase-contrast cine magnetic resonance imaging compared with invasive oximetry. Circulation. 2001;103:2476–82.
36. Nayak KS, Nielsen JF, Bernstein MA, Markl M, Gatehouse PD, Botnar RM, Saloner D, Lorenz C, Wen H, Hu BS, Epstein FH, Oshinski JN, Raman SV. Cardiovascular magnetic resonance phase contrast imaging. J Cardiovasc Magn Reson. 2015;17:71. https://doi.org/10.1186/s12968-015-0172-7.

37. Grosse-Wortmann L, Al-Otay A, Yoo SJ. Aortopulmonary collaterals after bidirectional cavopulmonary connection or Fontan completion: quantification with MRI. Circ Cardiovasc Imaging. 2009;2(3):219–25 . Epub 2009 Mar 25. https://doi.org/10.1161/CIRCIMAGING.108.834192.
38. Whitehead KK, Harris MA, Glatz AC, et al. Status of systemic to pulmonary arterial collateral flow after the fontan procedure. Am J Cardiol. 2015;115(12):1739–45. https://doi.org/10.1016/j.amjcard.2015.03.022.
39. Holmvang G, Palacios IF, Vlahakes GJ, et al. Imaging and sizing of atrial septal defects by magnetic resonance. Circulation. 1995;92:3473–80.
40. Festa P, Ait-Ali L, Cerillo AG, De Marchi D, Murzi B. Magnetic resonance imaging is the diagnostic tool of choice in the preoperative evaluation of patients with partial anomalous pulmonary venous return. Int J Cardiovasc Imaging. 2006;22:685–93.
41. Kilner PJ, Geva T, Kaemmerer H, Trindade PT, Schwitter J, Webb GD. Recommendations for cardiovascular magnetic resonance in adults with congenital heart disease from the respective working groups of the European Society of Cardiology. Eur Heart J. 2010;31(7):794–805. Epub 2010 Jan 11. https://doi.org/10.1093/eurheartj/ehp586.
42. Bell A, Beerbaum P, Greil G, Hegde S, Toschke AM, Schaeffter T, Razavi R. Noninvasive assessment of pulmonary artery flow and resistance by cardiac magnetic resonance in congenital heart diseases with unrestricted left-to-right shunt. JACC Cardiovasc Imaging. 2009;2(11):1285–91. https://doi.org/10.1016/j.jcmg.2009.07.009.
43. Grosse-Wortmann L. Assessing shunts. In: Lombardi M, editor. The EACVI textbook of cardiovascular magnetic resonance. 1st ed. Oxford: Oxford University Press; 2018. p. 509–15.
44. Ibrahim E, Horwood L, Stojanovska J, et al. Safety of CMR in patients with cardiac implanted electronic devices. J Cardiovasc Magn Reson. 2016;18(Suppl 1):O123. Published online 2016 Jan 27. https://doi.org/10.1186/1532-429X-18-S1-O123.
45. Schwitter J, Gold MR, Al Fagih A, et al. Image quality of cardiac magnetic resonance imaging in patients with an implantable cardioverter defibrillator system designed for the magnetic resonance imaging environment. Circ Cardiovasc Imaging. 2016;9(5):e004025. https://doi.org/10.1161/CIRCIMAGING.115.004025.
46. Ellis AR, Mulvihill D, Bradley SM, Hlavacek AM. Utility of computed tomographic angiography in the pre-operative planning for initial and repeat congenital cardiovascular surgery. Cardiol Young. 2010;20(3):262–8.
47. Rizvi A, Deaño RC, Bachman DP, Xiong G, Min JK, Truong QA. Analysis of ventricular function by CT. J Cardiovasc Comput Tomogr. 2015;9(1):1–12. https://doi.org/10.1016/j.jcct.2014.11.007.
48. Nicolay S, Salgado RA, Shivalkar B, Van Herck PL, Vrints C, Parizel PM. CT imaging features of atrioventricular shunts: what the radiologist must know. Insights Imaging. 2016;7(1):119–29. https://doi.org/10.1007/s13244-015-0452-7.
49. Taylor AJ, Cerqueira M, Hodgson JM, Mark D, Min J, O'Gara P, Rubin GD, Kramer CM, Berman D, Brown A, Chaudhry FA, Cury RC, Desai MY, Einstein AJ, Gomes AS, Harrington R, Hoffmann U, Khare R, Lesser J, McGann C, Rosenberg A, Schwartz R, Shelton M, Smetana GW, Smith SC Jr, American College of Cardiology Foundation Appropriate Use Criteria Task F, Society of Cardiovascular Computed T, American College of R, American Heart A, American Society of E, American Society of Nuclear C, North American Society for Cardiovascular I, Society for Cardiovascular A, Interventions, Society for Cardiovascular Magnetic R. ACCF/SCCT/ACR/AHA/ASE/ASNC/NASCI/SCAI/SCMR 2010 appropriate use criteria for cardiac computed tomography. A report of the American College of Cardiology Foundation Appropriate Use Criteria Task Force, the Society of Cardiovascular Computed Tomography, the American College of Radiology, the American Heart Association, the American Society of Echocardiography, the American Society of Nuclear Cardiology, the North American Society for Cardiovascular Imaging, the Society for Cardiovascular Angiography and Interventions, and the Society for Cardiovascular Magnetic Resonance. J Am Coll Cardiol. 2010;56:1864–94.
50. Broberg C, Meadows AK. Advances in imaging: the impact on the care of the adult with congenital heart disease. Prog Cardiovasc Dis. 2011;53(4):293–304.

51. MacDonald A, Burrell S. Infrequently performed studies in nuclear medicine: part 1. J Nucl Med Technol. 2008;36(3):132–43; quiz 145. Epub 2008 Aug 14. https://doi.org/10.2967/jnmt.108.051383.

52. Treves S. Detection and quantitation of cardiovascular shunts with commonly available radiopharmaceuticals. Semin Nucl Med. 1980;10:16–26.

53. Silvestry FE, Cohen MS, Armsby LB, Burkule NJ, Fleishman CE, Hijazi ZM, Lang RM, Rome JJ, Wang Y. American Society of Echocardiography; Society for Cardiac Angiography and Interventions. Guidelines for the echocardiographic assessment of atrial septal defect and patent foramen ovale: from the American Society of Echocardiography and Society for Cardiac Angiography and Interventions. J Am Soc Echocardiogr. 2015;28:910–58. https://doi.org/10.1016/j.echo.2015.05.015.

54. Rana BS. Echocardiography guidance of atrial septal defect closure. J Thorac Dis. 2018;10(Suppl 24):S2899–908. https://doi.org/10.21037/jtd.2018.07.126.

55. Balzer J, van Hall S, Rassaf T, et al. Feasibility, safety, and efficacy of real-time three-dimensional transoesophageal echocardiography for guiding device closure of interatrial communications: initial clinical experience and impact on radiation exposure. Eur J Echocardiogr. 2010;11(1):1–8.

56. Van der Velde ME, Sanders SP, Keane JF, Perry SB, Lock JE. Transesophageal echocardiographic guidance of transcatheter ventricular septal defect closure. J Am Coll Cardiol. 1994;23(7):1660–5.

57. Ciske BR, Speidel MA, Raval AN. Improving the cardiac cath-lab interventional imaging ecosystem. Transl Pediatr. 2018;7(1):1–4. https://doi.org/10.21037/tp.2017.09.03.

58. Fagan TE, Truong UT, Jone PN, et al. Multimodality 3-dimensional image integration for congenital cardiac catheterization. Methodist Debakey Cardiovasc J. 2014;10(2):68–76. https://doi.org/10.14797/mdcj-10-2-68.

59. Glöckler M, Halbfaβ J, Koch A, Achenbach S, Dittrich S. Multimodality 3D-roadmap for cardiovascular interventions in congenital heart disease—a single-center, retrospective analysis of 78 cases. Catheter Cardiovasc Interv. 2013;82(3):436–42. Epub 2013 Mar 18. https://doi.org/10.1002/ccd.24646.

Repaired Tetralogy of Fallot

12

Magalie Ladouceur, Tal Geva, and Francesca Raimondi

M. Ladouceur
Université de Paris, PARCC, INSERM, Paris, France

Medico-Surgical Unit of Adult Congenital Heart Disease, Assistance Publique Hôpitaux de Paris, Hôpital Européen Georges Pompidou-AP-HP, Paris University, Paris, France

Adult Congenital Heart Disease Unit, Centre de référence des Malformations Cardiaques Congénitales Complexes, M3C, Paris, France
e-mail: magalie.ladouceur@aphp.fr

T. Geva
Université de Paris, Paris, France

Department of Pediatrics, Harvard Medical School, Boston, MA, USA
e-mail: Tal.Geva@cardio.chboston.org

F. Raimondi (✉)
Université de Paris, Paris, France

Pediatric Cardiology, Centre de référence des Malformations Cardiaques Congénitales Complexes, M3C, Hôpital Universitaire Necker Enfants-Malades, Paris, France

Pediatric Radiology Unit, Hôpital Universitaire Necker Enfants-Malades, Paris, France

School of Biomedical Engineering and Imaging Sciences, King's College London, Lambeth Wing St. Thomas' Hospital, London, UK

Decision and Bayesian Computation, Computation Biology Department, CNRS, URS 3756, Neuroscience Department, CNRS UMR 3571, Institut Pasteur, Paris, France
e-mail: francesca.raimondi@aphp.fr

© Springer Nature Switzerland AG 2021
P. Gallego, I. Valverde (eds.), *Multimodality Imaging Innovations In Adult Congenital Heart Disease*, Congenital Heart Disease in Adolescents and Adults, https://doi.org/10.1007/978-3-030-61927-5_12

221

12.1 Introduction: Role of Imaging in the Assessment of Pathophysiology and Risk Stratification in Repaired Tetralogy of Fallot

Tetralogy of Fallot (TOF) is the most common cyanotic heart defect (CHD), accounting for 3–5% of all infants born with CHD [1]. The advent of cardiac surgery has led to improved survival to adulthood with about 17 per 100,000 adults currently living with repaired TOF (rTOF) [2, 3]. Adult survivors are, however, not cured, and many are left with residual hemodynamic lesions. Structural and functional abnormalities encountered in rTOF are summarized in Table 12.1. In the majority of patients with rTOF repair, relief of the RV outflow tract (RVOT) obstruction with the use of a transannular patch or pulmonary valvuloplasty results in moderate or severe pulmonary valve regurgitation (PR) [5].

Chronic PR results in volume overload leading to RV dilatation and dysfunction. In addition, scar tissue and noncontracting RVOT free wall, which can progress to become an aneurysm, further contribute to RV functional impairment [6, 7]. Conduction abnormalities with right bundle branch block are near universal after

Table 12.1 Structural and functional abnormalities encountered in patients with repaired TOF (adapted from Valente et al. [4])

Structural abnormalities	Functional abnormalities
Inherent to TOF repair	RV volume overload
Partial or complete removal of pulmonary valve leaflets	Pulmonary regurgitation
Infundibulotomy scar/patch	Tricuspid regurgitation
Resection of RV/infundibular muscle bundles	Left-to-right shunt
Right atriotomy scar	Ventricular septal defect
VSD patch	Atrial septal defect
Residual or recurrent lesions	Systemic-to-pulmonary collaterals
RV outflow tract obstruction	RV pressure overload
Main or branch pulmonary artery stenosis	RVOT obstruction or pulmonary artery stenosis
Ventricular septal defect	Pulmonary vascular disease
Atrial septal defect	Pulmonary venous hypertension secondary to LV diastolic dysfunction
Acquired lesions	RV systolic or diastolic dysfunction
Tricuspid valve abnormalities	LV systolic or diastolic dysfunction
RV outflow tract aneurysm	Aortic regurgitation
RV fibrosis	

Associated anomalies
  Dilated aorta
  Additional congenital cardiovascular anomalies
  Noncardiac anomalies
Genetic anomalies
	Ventricular conduction delay and dyssynchrony
	Arrhythmias
	  Atrial flutter
	  Atrial fibrillation
	  Ventricular tachycardia
	Comorbidities
	  Renal, pulmonary, musculoskeletal, neurodevelopmental abnormalities

TOF repair and contribute to RV dyssynchrony and dysfunction [8, 9]. Although the pathologic remodeling process first affects the RV, it also impacts left ventricular mechanics through ventricular-ventricular interaction [10]. Moreover, additional residual lesions such as RVOT obstruction, atrial septal defect, ventricular septal defect, tricuspid regurgitation, and aortic regurgitation can worsen ventricular dysfunction. Finally, most patients with rTOF live long enough to develop acquired cardiovascular disease such as coronary artery disease (CAD) or hypertension that could contribute to cardiac complications onset. Consequently, late survival is significantly lower in rTOF patients compared with the general population, and sudden cardiac death and heart failure are major contributors to late mortality [11, 12]. The incidences of arrhythmias, exercise intolerance, heart failure, and death increase coincides with progressive dilation and dysfunction of both the left and right ventricles [5] and there is growing evidence of a link between RV dysfunction and poor outcomes, such as death or sustained ventricular tachycardia [12, 13]. Pathophysiology pathways leading to RV dysfunction and impaired clinical status after TOF repair are illustrated in Fig. 12.1.

Management strategy mainly consists of preventing RV and LV dysfunction. For this reason, cardiac imaging is a mainstay of surveillance in patients with rTOF by assessing the severity of residual cardiac lesions, aiding in risk stratification, and helping in management decision such as when to recommend pulmonary valve replacement (PVR) and other transcatheter or surgical procedures. Summary of the main elements for reporting is provided in Table 12.2.

PVR has been advocated to reduce RV volume overload and, thereby, improve RV performance and reduce morbidity and mortality. However, the indications and optimal timing of intervention have yet to be established. The current indications for PVR in rTOF with hemodynamically significant PR according to the most recent

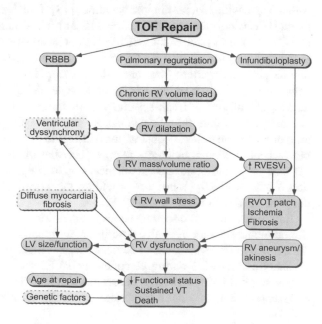

Fig. 12.1 Pathophysiology of right ventricular (RV) dysfunction and clinical status impairment (adapted from Geva T. Journal of Cardiovascular Magnetic Resonance 2011, 13:9). *LV* left ventricle, *RBBB* right bundle branch block, *RVOT* right ventricle outflow tract, *RVESVi* RV end-systolic volume indexed, *VT* ventricular tachycardia

Table 12.2 Essential imaging data elements in patients with repaired TOF (adapted from Valente et al. [4])

• RV volumes, function, and mass	• LV volumes, function, and mass
• RV systolic pressure	• Size of the aortic root and ascending aorta
• Regional RV wall motion abnormalities	• Degree and mechanism of aortic regurgitation
• Presence, degree, and location of RVOT obstruction	• Aortic arch sidedness and branching pattern
• Presence and extent of RVOT aneurysm	• Origin and proximal course of the left and right coronary arteries—assess risk of compression by an implanted valve
• Assessment of the main and branch pulmonary arteries for stenosis	• Myocardial viability—extent and location of gross scar tissue
• Differential pulmonary artery flow	• Diffuse myocardial fibrosis
• Degree of pulmonary regurgitation	• Residual intracardiac and extracardiac shunts
• Tricuspid regurgitation (degree and mechanism)	• Extent and location of systemic-to-pulmonary collaterals
• Right atrial size	• Associated anomalies (e.g., anomalies of the systemic or pulmonary veins)

guidelines are based on the presence of symptoms (Class I) [15, 16]. In asymptomatic patients, several data indicate that PVR performed prior to specific ventricular size is associated with normalization of RV volumes [17], even if it is not yet evident that criteria based on RV diastolic volume are associated with any clinical benefit such as improved morbidity or mortality. A recent study from Boston Children's Hospital found no evidence that mild or even moderate RV dilatation after PVR—the target of intervention based on end-diastolic volume criteria alone—is associated with adverse clinical outcomes [18]. Imaging parameters are essential to guide decision-making in this setting [15, 16]. They include measurements of RV and LV volumes, systolic function, mass, right atrial size, flow measurements (e.g., pulmonary regurgitation fraction, tricuspid regurgitation fraction, differential branch pulmonary artery flow, and other). Examples of imaging-based threshold values often used in deciding when to intervene include RV end-diastolic volume index ≥ 160 mL/m^2, RV end-systolic volume index ≥ 80 mL/m^2, RV end-diastolic volume $\geq 2 \times$ LV end-diastolic volume, RV mass-to-volume ratio > 0.3, and RV systolic pressure due to RVOT obstruction $\geq 2/3$ systemic pressure [16]. Other imaging biomarkers of clinical outcomes (e.g., myocardial fibrosis, myocardial strain, and 4D flow-based indices of flow dynamics such as shear stress) are under investigation. CMR is ideally suited for providing the relevant data elements to inform decision-making in rTOF (Table 12.3).

Before any surgical or percutaneous intervention in patients with rTOF, workup should include a comprehensive description of the origins and proximal courses of the coronary arteries. Abnormal coronary artery anatomy has a substantial risk for coronary compression during percutaneous PVR or direct injury to the coronary during surgical PVR. Similarly, the relationship between cardiovascular structures and sternum should be carefully studied before any new sternotomy.

Table 12.3 Role of CMR in informing the decision for pulmonary valve replacement in patients with repaired tetralogy of Fallot (Adapted from Geva T [14]). Criteria based on CMR are marked with (*)

Indications for pulmonary valve replacement in patients with repaired TOF or similar physiology with moderate or severe pulmonary regurgitation (regurgitation fraction ≥25%)

I.   Asymptomatic patient with 2 or more of the following criteria:
  (a)   *RV end-diastolic volume index >160 mL/m^2 or Z-score >6. In patients whose body surface area falls outside published normal data: RV/LV end-diastolic volume ratio >2
  (b)   *RV end-systolic volume index >80 mL/m^2
  (c)   *RV ejection fraction <48%
  (d)   *LV ejection fraction <55%
  (e)   *Large RVOT aneurysm
  (f)   RV mass-to-volume ratio >0.3 g/mL
  (g)   Sustained tachyarrhythmia related to right heart volume load
  (h)   Other hemodynamically significant abnormalities:
    (i)   RVOT obstruction with RV systolic pressure ≥2/3 systemic
    (ii)   Severe branch pulmonary artery stenosis (<30% flow to affected lung) not amenable to transcatheter therapy
    (iii)   ≥Moderate tricuspid regurgitation
    (iv)   Left-to-right shunt from residual atrial or ventricular septal defects with pulmonary-to-systemic flow ratio ≥1.5
    (v)   Severe aortic regurgitation
    (vi)   Severe aortic dilatation (diameter >5 cm or progressive dilatation >0.5 cm/year)

II.   Symptoms and signs attributable to severe RV volume load documented by CMR or alternative imaging modality, fulfilling ≥1 of the quantitative criteria detailed above. Examples of symptoms and signs include:
  (a)   Exercise intolerance not explained by extracardiac causes (e.g., lung disease, musculoskeletal anomalies, genetic anomalies, obesity), with documentation by exercise testing with metabolic cart (≤70% predicted peak VO$_2$ for age and gender not explained by chronotropic incompetence)
  (b)   Signs and symptoms of heart failure (e.g., dyspnea with mild effort or at rest not explained by extracardiac causes, peripheral edema)
  (c)   Syncope attributable to arrhythmia

III.   Special considerations:
  (a)   Due to higher risk of adverse clinical outcomes in patients who underwent TOF repair at age ≥ 3 years, [5] PVR may be considered if fulfilling ≥1 of the quantitative criteria in section I
  (b)   Women with severe PR and RV dilatation and/or dysfunction may be at risk for pregnancy-related complications [19]. Although no evidence is available to support benefit from pre-pregnancy PVR, the procedure may be considered if fulfilling ≥1 of the quantitative criteria in section I

In case of advanced heart failure, accurate evaluation of LV and RV function and anatomy of distal pulmonary arteries are essential to decide appropriate course of action, particularly in deciding if a patient may be appropriate for mechanical circulatory support or heart transplant. Despite numerous studies that identified factors associated with malignant ventricular arrhythmias and sudden cardiac death, risk stratification remains imperfect. Implantable cardioverter defibrillator (ICD) for primary prevention should be considered in patients who meet standard qualifying criteria (i.e., LV ejection fraction ≤35% with NYHA class II or III symptoms), but additional imaging parameters such as CMR-derived RV ejection fraction [20], focal [21] and diffuse fibrosis [22], diastolic LV dysfunction [23], or ventricular dyssynchrony [8, 9] may improve selection of candidates for ICD implantation in rTOF. A prospective large study including these imaging parameters would improve risk stratification of sudden cardiac death in this population.

12.2   Imaging Methods

12.2.1 Echocardiography

Echocardiography is the first-line technique for assessing intracardiac anatomy, residual shunts, left and right ventricular dimensions and function, RV fractional area change (FAC), tricuspid annular plane systolic excursion (TAPSE), RV and LV tissue Doppler systolic velocity, RV and LV longitudinal strain, valve function (regurgitation or stenosis), and right ventricular pressure. Principal recommended measures of right heart structures by echocardiography are listed in Table 12.2.

Recent advances by echocardiography in patients with rTOF include analysis of myocardial deformation and dyssynchrony [24–26], demonstrating associations between adverse clinical outcomes and myocardial deformation echocardiographic parameters. Regarding evaluation of RV anatomy, the complex geometry and retrosternal location of the chamber hamper echocardiographic assessment of volumes and function, leaving cardiac MRI as the gold standard method for functional assessment in patients with rTOF.

12.2.2 Cardiac MRI

Cardiac MRI has emerged as a reference standard for anatomic and functional evaluation of rTOF patients. Principal recommended measures of right heart structures by cardiac MRI are listed in Table 12.3.

The strength of cardiac MRI is its versatility, reproducibility of measurements, and ability to comprehensively evaluate of all anatomic, functional, and tissue parameters in patients with rTOF regardless of body habitus (Figs. 12.2, 12.3, 12.4, 12.5, 12.6 and 12.7).

Recently emerging technology as 4D Flow CMR improved markedly CMR capacity to perform comprehensive non-invasive hemodynamic analysis. As detailed in Chapter 8, 4D flow MRI is an emerging tool to evaluate anatomy and hemodynamics in a new noninvasive way. 4D flow acquisition data set includes a full dynamic volume of the thorax with kinetic and vectorial data, allowing reconstruction and analysis of ventricular function, cardiac, and vessel anatomy, and flow physiology (stroke volume, valve regurgitation and stenosis, vessel stenosis) [27] (Figs. 12.8, 12.9, 12.10, 12.11, 12.12, 12.13, and 12.14). Pulmonary perfusion

Fig. 12.2 3D angiography after contrast injection, coronal view showing PA trunk and right pulmonary artery with visualization of peripheral pulmonary vessel

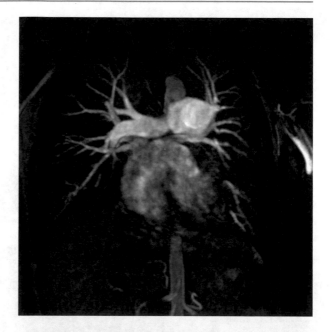

Fig. 12.3 3D angiography after contrast injection, coronal view showing left pulmonary artery with. visualization of peripheral pulmonary vessel

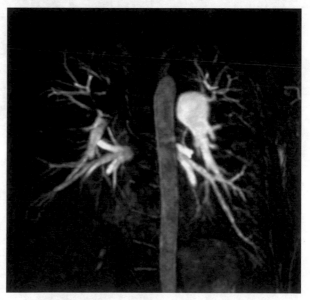

analysis could also be reliably explored by 4D flow MRI, even in presence of stent material, detecting anomalies not suspected by echocardiography.

CMR also allows assessment of cardiac mechanics, including measurements of myocardial deformation and strain and ventricular dyssynchrony. A growing body of literature has been published about this topic but the actual contribution of mechanical analysis to risk stratification is still debated. Moon et al. [28] demonstrated in 2014 that patients with TOF who experienced adverse outcomes had

Fig. 12.4 3D respiratory-navigated balanced steady-state free precession sequence, axial view, showing visualization of right coronary ostium

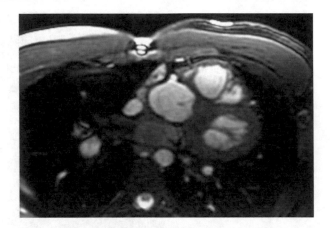

Fig. 12.5 3D respiratory-navigated balanced steady-state free precession sequence, axial view, showing visualization of left coronary artery

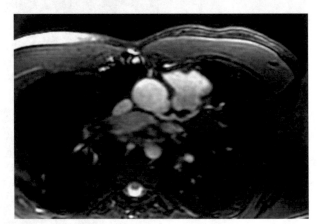

Fig. 12.6 Image derived from 4-chamber cine sequence showing dilated right ventricle

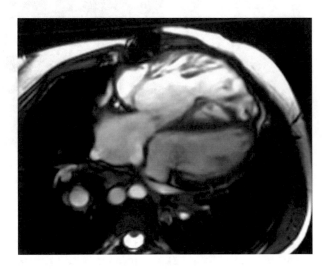

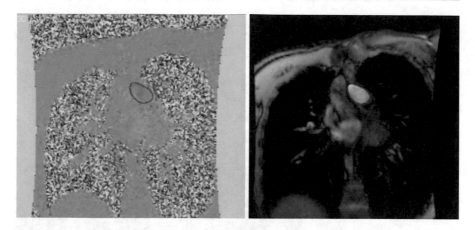

Fig. 12.7 Example of right ventricular outflow tract stroke volume calculation from 2D phase contrast sequence

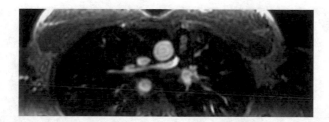

Fig. 12.8 3D respiratory-navigated balanced steady-state free precession sequence, axial view, showing visualization of stented right ventricular outflow tract and pulmonary arteries

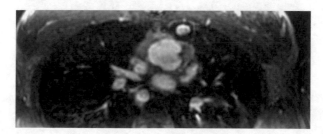

Fig. 12.9 3D respiratory-navigated balanced steady-state free precession sequence, axial view, showing visualization of stented right ventricular outflow tract

Fig. 12.10 4D flow sequence, oblique view showing stent at the origin of left pulmonary artery

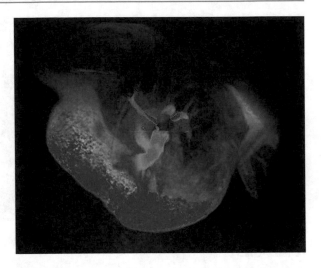

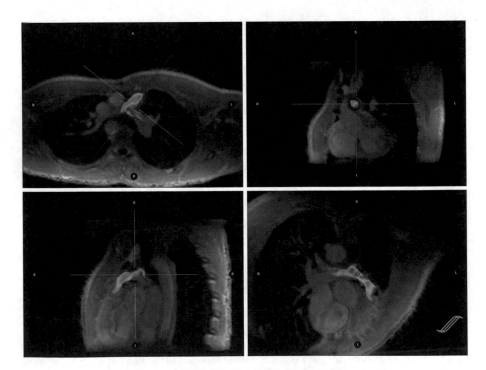

Fig. 12.11 4D flow sequence including all thoracic volume and multiplanar visualization showing right ventricular outflow tract (Contegra conduit n°20)

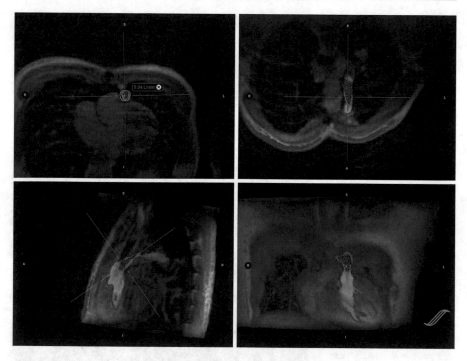

Fig. 12.12 4D flow sequence including all thoracic volume and multiplanar visualization showing stenosis (red) of right ventricular outflow tract (V_{max} 4.9 m/s)

Fig. 12.13 4D flow sequence in axial view with only anatomic data, showing a spatial resolution for anatomical details of right ventricular outflow tract (Contegra conduit n°20) and pulmonary arteries

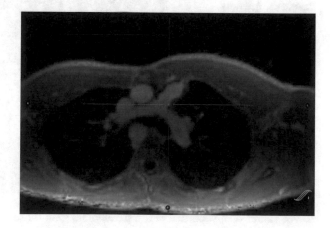

Fig. 12.14 4D flow sequence in oblique view with only anatomic data, showing a spatial resolution for anatomical details of right ventricular outflow tract

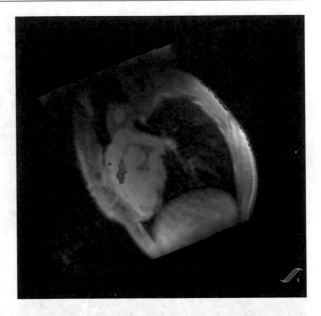

Fig. 12.15 Late gadolinium enhancement sequence in short axis view showing fibrosis in RV-LV junction, in right ventricular outflow tract (patch, RVOT) and right ventricular free wall (RVFW)

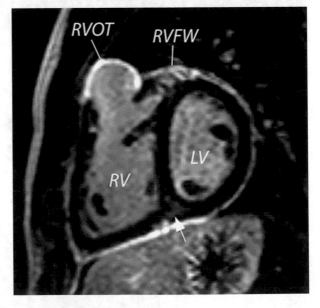

lower values of myocardial strain parameters than those who did not and impaired longitudinal strain was strongly associated with adverse clinical outcomes. In the meantime Jing et al. [29] in 2016 showed that the ability to predict deterioration in ventricular function by CMR-derived strain parameters was limited.

Adverse myocardial remodeling in rTOF is also characterized by expansion of extracellular volume fraction (ECV), involving development of myocardial fibrosis (Fig. 12.15). Myocardial fibrosis and increased ECV are associated with RV volume overload and arrhythmia.

Cardiac MRI is the only imaging tool capable of identifying this kind of myocardial abnormalities, improving risk stratification, and tailoring therapeutic strategies [30, 31].

12.2.3 Cardiac CT

Cardiac CT is used for anatomic evaluation of cardiac anatomy and pulmonary vasculature in patients who have contraindications to cardiac MRI such as incompatible implantable pacemakers and defibrillators. It also provides detailed imaging of the coronary arteries, presence of calcification, and lung parenchymal features.

Low-dose protocols and advanced technology (e.g., dual source CT) allow to sensibly reduce radiation dose delivery without impairing image quality [32, 33] (Fig. 12.16).

Using cardiac CT, a novel 3D strategy was recently developed to plan percutaneous PVR. In Pluchinotta et al. [34] the authors proposed a combination of imaging and bioengineering methods to improve patient selection and assess feasibility of percutaneous PVR in an aneurysmal RVOT-patched anatomy. The paper reported a successful percutaneous PVR procedure in a young boy with a dilated RVOT, borderline for conventional intervention. In this case, the patient was studied with ECG-gated CT angiography and acquired every 10% of the cardiac cycle. The innovation lies in the postprocessing of the 3D CT dataset through bioengineering algorithms able to capture local shape changes of specific cross-sections, which are usually reference points for interventionists, such as the ventricular side outflow tract, the proximal and distal main pulmonary trunk, and the pulmonary arteries (Fig. 12.17). The dynamic CT assessment showed that the RVOT anatomy was at the upper limit of the percutaneous PVR acceptable range but provided interventional cardiologists with insights into the RVOT/PA function, and finally a nonconventional pulmonary jailing intervention was successfully performed.

Fig. 12.16 3D rendering of a dual source CT scan showing relationship between right coronary artery and right ventricular outflow tract conduit

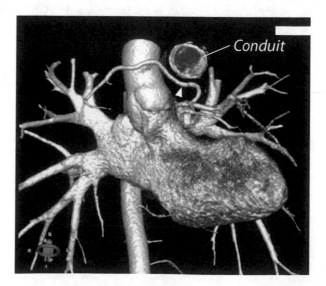

Conduit

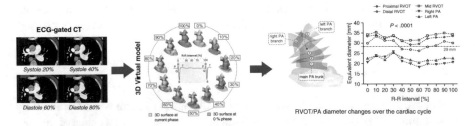

Fig. 12.17 Left side image: ECG-gated CT angiography; middle image: RVOT/PA reconstruction from 0% to 100% of the cardiac cycle with CT-derived 3D dataset; right side image: RVOT/PA dynamic changes computed over the cardiac cycle in five anatomical regions of interests (i.e., proximal RVOT, mid-RVOT, distal RVOT, left PA and right PA). (Figure courtesy of Dr. Francesca Pluchinotta, IRCCS Policlinico San Donato)

12.3 Advanced Imaging

12.3.1 Deep Learning Imaging Analysis

Machine learning algorithms may be applied to patients affected by CHD to estimate prognosis [35]. Several studies are ongoing, based on clinical and imaging data. Diller et al. [36], using data from the German Competence Network for Congenital Heart Disease, identified a subgroup of repaired TOF patients at risk of adverse outcome (HR 2.1) by a composite score of enlarged atrial area and depressed right ventricular longitudinal function. The score was generated by deep learning-based image analysis of 372 cardiac MRI study over a period of 10 years of follow-up. They demonstrated the utility of machine learning-based deep learning algorithms to predict prognosis directly and to serve as surrogate of labor intensive manually obtained parameters in repaired TOF, with reduced interobserver variability.

12.3.2 Virtual Surgery for RVOT and Conduit Reconstruction

MRI-derived anatomic and functional data may also help in preoperative modeling of RVOT reconstruction. Virtual surgery can be useful to simulate implantation and to tailor devices to individual patients characteristics. Chin Siang Ong et al. utilized preoperative MRI data to build a 3D model to simulate surgical implantation of 3 different sizes of RV-PA conduit [37] (Figs. 12.18 and 12.19). Yang et al. performed mechanical analysis of human right ventricle with MRI-based RV/LV combination model with fluid structure with promising results towards clinical application and patient-specific surgical planning [38].

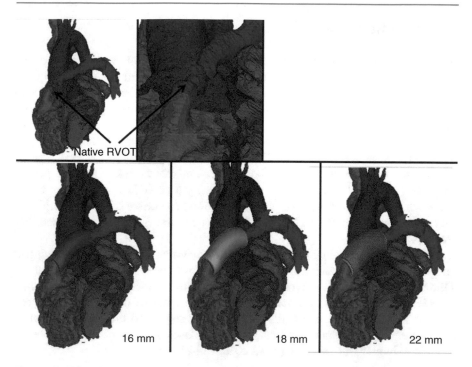

Fig. 12.18 Virtual right ventricle outflow tract (RVOT) conduit reconstruction surgery with 3 different sizes of conduits, 18, 20, and 22 mm. (Figure courtesy of Dr. Laura Olivieri and Dr. Yue-Hin Loke, Children's National Hospital, Washington, DC)

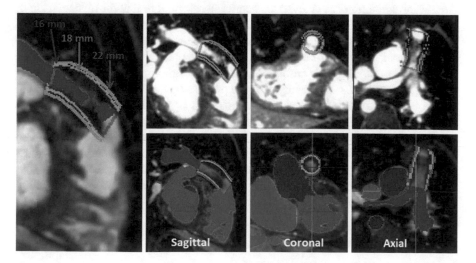

Fig. 12.19 Virtual simulated right ventricle outflow tract conduit superimposed on MRI images of the patient with 3 different sizes of conduits, 18, 20, and 22 mm. (Figure courtesy of Dr. Laura Olivieri and Dr. Yue-Hin Loke, Children's National Hospital, Washington, DC)

12.3.3 3D Modeling

3D CT reconstruction of the right heart in systole and diastole is used to calculate RVOT dimensions including lengths, diameters, and circumference along the length of the potential deployment zone. Then virtual "implants" of the device in systole and diastole is possible with evaluation of the extent of device contact with vessel wall. The complexity of the RVOT anatomy often makes implantation of percutaneous devices challenging. Schievano et al. demonstrated a large variety of outflow types, dividing them into different mathematical groups [39, 40]. Several efforts are underway to customize balloon expandable valves to specific patient anatomy [41–44]. The importance of developing a sophisticated imaging-based approach to customization of device implantation in a variety of RVOT morphologies is highlighted by the high screen failure rate in the Harmony early feasibility study [45].

Advanced 3D modeling from cardiac MRI or cardiac CT scan data is helping to go forward an individualized approach to tailor procedures on a specific patient. As Jolley et al. [46] demonstrated in reproducing a virtual device implant in 4 bovine models, assumption of a rigid vessel may limit the accuracy of current approaches to valve selection for native outflow tracts. They suggested that incorporation of vessel elasticity and other empiric dynamic feedback may be needed to improve virtual pre-implant modeling (Figs. 12.20 and 12.21).

12.4 Challenges and Outlook

Noninvasive imaging has evolved to become an essential tool in the management of the growing population of adults with rTOF. The future of surveillance, risk stratification, and image-guidance of therapeutic interventions lies in integration of information from existing and future modalities and techniques, including ultrasound-based, magnetic resonance, computed tomography, nuclear, and other evolving technologies. Increasingly, image processing and the analytical tools used to process the resulting data involve methods such as deep learning and other artificial intelligence methods. Finally, the concept of multiparametric imaging biomarkers is expected to evolve to generate more comprehensive insights incorporating information on tissue biomechanics, cellular and molecular characteristics, and the interaction between the ventricles and their respective vascular beds. Such advances will advance our ability to risk stratify adults with rTOF and inform the development of new therapies.

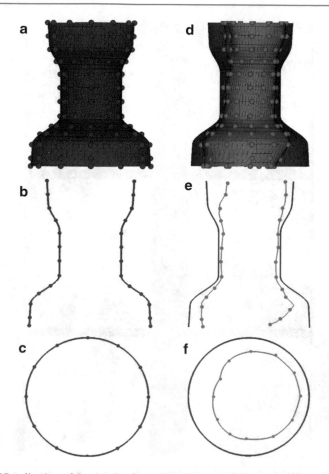

Fig. 12.20 Visualization of Device Conformation. (**a**) Front view of unconformed device (red) with handles (red spheres) which can be adjusted to conform the device. (**b**) Sagittal cutting plane of unconformed device. (**c**) Transverse cutting plane of unconformed device. (**d**) Front view of conformed device (blue) compared to unconformed device (red). (**e**) Sagittal cutting plane of conformed device (blue) compared to unconformed device (red). (**f**) Transverse cutting plane of conformed device (blue) compared to unconformed device (red). (Figure courtesy of Dr. Matthew A. Jolley and Hannah H. Nam from the Division of Cardiology and Department of Anesthesia at the Children's Hospital of Philadelphia, Philadelphia, PA, and Dr. Andras Lasso from the Laboratory for Percutaneous Surgery, Queen's University, Kingston, Ontario, Canada)

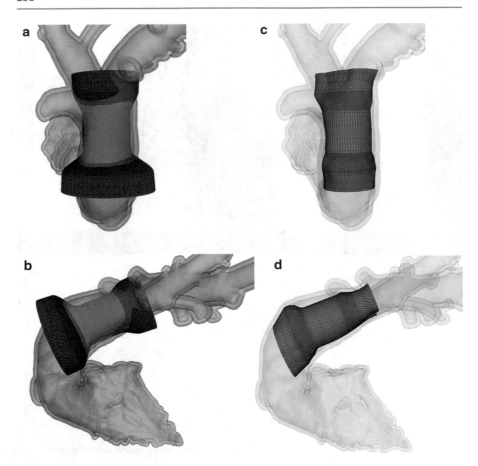

Fig. 12.21 Visualization of Virtual Device Placement in the RVOT from Pre-implant CT Scan. (**a**) Unconformed device viewed from the front. (**b**) Unconformed device viewed from the lateral side. (**c**) Conformed device viewed from the front. (**d**) Conformed device viewed from the lateral side. (Figure courtesy of Dr. Matthew A. Jolley and Hannah H. Nam from the Division of Cardiology and Department of Anesthesia at the Children's Hospital of Philadelphia, Philadelphia, PA, and Dr. Andras Lasso from the Laboratory for Percutaneous Surgery, Queen's University, Kingston, Ontario, Canada)

References

1. Apitz C, Webb GD, Redington AN. Tetralogy of Fallot. Lancet. 2009;374(9699):1462–71.
2. Hickey EJ, Veldtman G, Bradley TJ, Gengsakul A, Manlhiot C, Williams WG, Webb GD, McCrindle BW. Late risk of outcomes for adults with repaired tetralogy of Fallot from an inception cohort spanning four decades. Eur J Cardiothorac Surg. 2009;35(1):156–64.
3. Marelli AJ, Mackie AS, Ionescu-Ittu R, Rahme E, Pilote L. Congenital heart disease in the general population: changing prevalence and age distribution. Circulation. 2007;115(2):163–72.
4. Valente AM, Geva T. How to image repaired tetralogy of Fallot. Circ Cardiovasc Imaging. 2017;10(5):e004270.

5. Geva T, Sandweiss BM, Gauvreau K, Lock JE, Powell AJ. Factors associated with impaired clinical status in long-term survivors of tetralogy of Fallot repair evaluated by magnetic resonance imaging. J Am Coll Cardiol. 2004;43(6):1068–74.
6. Davlouros PA, Kilner PJ, Hornung TS, Li W, Francis JM, Moon JCC, et al. Right ventricular function in adults with repaired tetralogy of Fallot assessed with cardiovascular magnetic resonance imaging: detrimental role of right ventricular outflow aneurysms or akinesia and adverse right-to-left ventricular interaction. J Am Coll Cardiol. 2002;40(11):2044–52.
7. Wald RM, Idith H, Ron W, Marie VA, Powell Andrew J, Tal G. Effects of regional dysfunction and late gadolinium enhancement on global right ventricular function and exercise capacity in patients with repaired tetralogy of Fallot. Circulation. 2009;119(10):1370–7.
8. Jing L, Haggerty CM, Suever JD, Alhadad S, Prakash A, Cecchin F, et al. Patients with repaired tetralogy of Fallot suffer from intra- and inter-ventricular cardiac dyssynchrony: a cardiac magnetic resonance study. Eur Heart J Cardiovasc Imaging. 2014 Dec 1;15(12):1333–43.
9. Zakaria J, Frédéric S, Emmanuelle F, Hubert C, Nicolas D, Michel H, et al. Right ventricular electrical activation in patients with repaired tetralogy of Fallots. Circ Arrhythm Electrophysiol. 2019;12(6):e007141.
10. Dragulescu A, Friedberg MK, Grosse-Wortmann L, Redington A, Mertens L. Effect of chronic right ventricular volume overload on ventricular interaction in patients after tetralogy of Fallot repair. J Am Soc Echocardiogr. 2014;27(8):896–902.
11. Cuypers JAAE, Menting ME, Konings EEM, Opić P, Utens EMWJ, Helbing WA, et al. Unnatural history of tetralogy of Fallot: prospective follow-up of 40 years after surgical correction. Circulation. 2014;130(22):1944–53.
12. Valente AM, Gauvreau K, Assenza GE, Babu-Narayan SV, Schreier J, Gatzoulis MA, et al. Contemporary predictors of death and sustained ventricular tachycardia in patients with repaired tetralogy of Fallot enrolled in the INDICATOR cohort. Heart. 2014;100(3):247–53.
13. Knauth AL, Gauvreau K, Powell AJ, Landzberg MJ, Walsh EP, Lock JE, et al. Ventricular size and function assessed by cardiac MRI predict major adverse clinical outcomes late after tetralogy of Fallot repair. Heart. 2008;94(2):211–6.
14. Geva T. Is MRI the preferred method for evaluating right ventricular size and function in patients with congenital heart disease? Circ Cardiovasc Imaging. 2014;7:190–7.
15. Baumgartner H, Bonhoeffer P, De Groot NMS, de Haan F, Deanfield JE, Galie N, et al. ESC guidelines for the management of grown-up congenital heart disease (new version 2010). Eur Heart J. 2010;31(23):2915–57.
16. Stout KK, Daniels CJ, Aboulhosn JA, Bozkurt B, Broberg CS, Colman JM, et al. 2018 AHA/ACC guideline for the Management of Adults with Congenital Heart Disease: a report of the American College of Cardiology/American Heart Association task force on clinical practice guidelines. J Am Coll Cardiol. 2019;73(12):e81–192.
17. Oosterhof T, van Straten A, Vliegen HW, Meijboom FJ, van Dijk AP, Spijkerboer AM, Bouma BJ, Zwinderman AH, Hazekamp MG, de Roos A, Mulder BJ. Preoperative thresholds for pulmonary valve replacement in patients with corrected tetralogy of Fallot using cardiovascular magnetic resonance. Circulation. 2007;116(5):545–51.
18. Pastor TA, Geva T, Lu M, Duarte VE, Drakeley S, Sleeper LA, et al. Relation of right ventricular dilation after pulmonary valve replacement to outcomes in patients with repaired tetralogy of Fallot. Am J Cardiol. 2020;125(6):977–81.
19. Khairy P, Ouyang DW, Fernandes SM, Lee-Parritz A, Economy KE, Landzberg MJ. Pregnancy outcomes in women with congenital heart disease. Circulation. 2006;113(4):517–24.
20. Bokma JP, de Wilde KC, Vliegen HW, van Dijk AP, van Melle JP, Meijboom FJ, et al. Value of cardiovascular magnetic resonance imaging in noninvasive risk stratification in tetralogy of Fallot. JAMA Cardiol. 2017;2(6):678–83.
21. Babu-Narayan SV, Kilner PJ, Wei L, Moon James C, Omer G, Davlouros Periklis A, et al. Ventricular fibrosis suggested by cardiovascular magnetic resonance in adults with repaired tetralogy of Fallot and its relationship to adverse markers of clinical outcome. Circulation. 2006;113(3):405–13.

22. Cochet H, Iriart X, Allain-Nicolaï A, Camaioni C, Sridi S, Nivet H, et al. Focal scar and diffuse myocardial fibrosis are independent imaging markers in repaired tetralogy of Fallot. Eur Heart J Cardiovasc Imaging. 2019;20(9):990–1003.

23. Khairy P, Harris L, Landzberg MJ, Viswanathan S, Barlow A, Gatzoulis MA, et al. Implantable cardioverter-defibrillators in tetralogy of Fallot. Circulation. 2008;117(3):363–70.

24. Orwat S, Diller GP, Kempny A, Radke R, Pcters B, Kühne T, Boethig D, Gutberlet M, Dubowy KO, Beerbaum P, Sarikouch S, Baumgartner H, German Competence Network for Congenital Heart Defects Investigators. Myocardial deformation parameters predict outcome in patients with repaired tetralogy of Fallot. Heart. 2016;102:209–15.

25. Diller GP, Kempny A, Liodakis E, Alonso-Gonzalez R, Inuzuka R, Uebing A, Orwat S, Dimopoulos K, Swan L, Li W, Gatzoulis MA, Baumgartner H. Left ventricular longitudinal function predicts life-threatening ventricular arrhythmia and death in adults with repaired tetralogy of Fallot. Circulation. 2012;125:2440–6.

26. Menting ME, Eindhoven JA, van den Bosch AE, Cuypers JA, Ruys TP, van Dalen BM, McGhie JS, Witsenburg M, Helbing WA, Geleijnse ML, Roos-Hesselink JW. Abnormal left ventricular rotation and twist in adult patients with corrected tetralogy of Fallot. Eur Heart J Cardiovasc Imaging. 2014;15:566–74.

27. Isorni MA, Martins D, Ben Moussa N, Monnot S, Boddaert N, Bonnet D, Hascoet S, Raimondi F. 4D flow quantification of pulmonary flow: comparison to conventional MRI in patients after tetralogy of Fallot repair. Int J Cardiol. 2020;300:132–6.

28. Moon TJ, Choueiter N, GevaT VAM, Gauvreau K, Harrild DM. Relation in biventricular strain and dyssynchrony in repaired tetralogy of Fallot measured by cardiac magnetic resonance to death and sustained ventricular tachycardia. Am J Cardiol. 2015;115:676–80.

29. Jing L, Wehner GJ, Suever J, Charnigo RJ, Aldhad S, Stearns E, Mojsejenko D, Haagerty CM, Hickey K, Valente AM, Geva T, Powell AJ, Fornwalt BK. Left and right ventricular dyssynchrony and strains from cardiovascular magnetic resonance feature tracking do not predict deterioration of ventricular function in patients with repaired tetralogy of Fallot. J Cardiovasc Magn Reson. 2016;18(1):49.

30. Chen C, Dusenbery Susan M, Valente AM, Powell AJ, Geva T. Myocardial ECV fraction assessed by CMR is associated with type of hemodynamic load and arrhythmia in repaired tetralogy of Fallot. J Am Coll Cardiol Img. 2016;9:1–10.

31. Cochet H, Iriart X, Allain-Nicolaï A, Camaioni C, Sridi S, Nivet H, Fournier E, Dinet ML, Jalal Z, Laurent F, Montaudon M, Thambo JB. Focal scar and diffuse myocardial fibrosis are independent imaging markers in repaired tetralogy of Fallot. Eur Heart J Cardiovasc Imaging. 2019;20:990–1003.

32. Rashed M, Banka P, Barthur A, MacDougal RD, Rathod R, Powell AJ, Prakash A. Effect of dose reduction on diagnostic image quality of coronary computed tomography in children using a third generation dual source computed tomography scanner. Am J Cardiol. 2018;122:1260–4.

33. Schicchi N, Fogante M, Pirani PE, Agliata G, Basile MC, Oliva M, Agostini A, Giovagnoni A. Third generation dual source dual energy CT in pediatric congenital heart disease patients: state-of-the art. Radiol Med. 2019;124(12):1238–52.

34. Pluchinotta FR, Sturla F, Caimi A, et al. 3-dimensional personalized planning for transcatheter pulmonary valve implantation in a dysfunctional right ventricular outflow tract. Int J Cardiol. 2020;309:33–9.

35. Samad MD, Wehner GJ, Arbabshirani MR, Jing L, Geva T, Powell AJ, Haggerty CM, Fornwalt BK. Predicting deterioration of ventricular function in patients with repaired tetralogy of Fallot using machine learning. Eur Heart J Cardiovasc Imaging. 2018;19:730–8.

36. Diller GP, Orwat S, Vahle J, Bauer UMM, Urban A, Sarikouch S, Berger F, Beerbaum P, Baumgartner H. Prediction of prognosis in patients with tetralogy of Fallot based on deep learning imaging analysis. Heart. 2020;106:1007–14.

37. Ong CS, Loke YH, Opfermann J, Olivieri L, Vricella L, Krieger A, Hibino N. Virtual surgery for conduit reconstruction of the right ventricular outflow tract. World J Pediatr Congenit Heart Surg. 2017;8:391–3.

38. Yang C, Tang D, Haber I, Geva T, del Nido PJ. In vivo MRI-based 3D FSI RV/LV models for human right ventricle and patch design for potential computed aided surgery. Comput Struct. 2007;85:988–97.
39. Schievano S, Coats L, Migliavacca F, et al. Variations in right ventricular outflow tract morphology following repair of congenital heart disease: implications for percutaneous pulmonary valve implantation. J Cardiovasc Magn Reson. 2007;9(4):687–95.
40. Schievano S, Migliavacca F, Coats L, et al. Percutaneous pulmonary valve implantation based on rapid prototyping of right ventricular outflow tract and pulmonary trunk from MR data. Radiology. 2007;242(2):490–7.
41. Capelli C, Taylor AM, Migliavacca F, Bonhoeffer P, Schievano S. Patient-specific reconstructed anatomies and computer simulations are fundamental for selecting medical device treatment: application to a new percutaneous pulmonary valve. Philos Trans A Math Phys Eng Sci. 2010;368(1921):3027–38.
42. Lurz P, Bonhoeffer P. Percutaneous implantation of pulmonary valves for treatment of right ventricular outflow tract dysfunction. Cardiol Young. 2008;18(3):260–7.
43. Bergersen L, Benson LN, Gillespie MJ, et al. Harmony feasibility trial: acute and short-term outcomes with a self-expanding transcatheter pulmonary valve. JACC Cardiovasc Interv. 2017;10(17):1763–73.
44. Tang D, del Nido P, Yang C, Zuo H, Huang X, Rathod RH, Gooty V, Tang A, Wu Z, Billiar KL, Geva T. Patient-specific MRI-based right ventricle models using different zero-load diastole and systole geometries for better cardiac stress and strain calculations and pulmonary valve replacement surgical outcome predictions. PLoS One. 2016;11:e0162986.
45. Gillespie MJ, Benson LN, Bergersen L, et al. Patient selection process for the harmony Transcatheter pulmonary valve early feasibility study. Am J Cardiol. 2017;120(8):1387–92.
46. Jolley M, Lasso A, Nam JH, Dihn PV, et al. Toward predictive modeling of catheter-based pulmonary valve replacement into native right ventricular outflow tracts. Catheter Cardiovasc Interv. 2018;93:E143–52.

Aortic Disease: Bicuspid Aortic Valve, Aortic Coarctation, Marfan Syndrome

13

Alessandra Frigiola, Froso Sophocleous, and Giovanni Biglino

Abbreviations

3D PC	Three-dimensional phase-contrast
AAo	Ascending aorta
AS	Aortic stenosis
AVR	Aortic valve replacement
BAV	Bicuspid aortic valve
CFD	Computational fluid dynamics
CHD	Congenital heart disease
CoA	Coarctation
CT	Computed tomography
LV	Left ventricle
MRI	Magnetic resonance imaging

Supplementary Information The online version of this chapter (https://doi.org/10.1007/978-3-030-61927-5_13) contains supplementary material, which is available to authorized users.

A. Frigiola (✉)
Cardiovascular Department, Guy's and St Thomas's Hospital, London, UK

Imaging Science Division, King's College London, London, UK
e-mail: alessandra.frigiola@gstt.nhs.uk

F. Sophocleous
Bristol Medical School, University of Bristol, Bristol, UK
e-mail: fs16815@bristol.ac.uk

G. Biglino
Bristol Medical School, University of Bristol, Bristol, UK

National Heart and Lung Institute, Imperial College London, London, UK
e-mail: g.biglino@bristol.ac.uk

© Springer Nature Switzerland AG 2021
P. Gallego, I. Valverde (eds.), *Multimodality Imaging Innovations In Adult Congenital Heart Disease*, Congenital Heart Disease in Adolescents and Adults, https://doi.org/10.1007/978-3-030-61927-5_13

OSI   Oscillatory shear index
PEARS   Personalised external aortic root support
SSM   Statistical shape modelling
WSS   Wall shear stress

13.1   Introduction

In this chapter we explore the role of multimodality imaging for three important aortic lesions: bicuspid aortic valve, coarctation of the aorta and Marfan syndrome.

Routine transthoracic echocardiogram (TTE), cardiovascular magnetic resonance imaging (CMR) and computed tomography (CT) are the key imaging modalities guiding clinical decision-making alongside the clinical picture (examination, medical history, exercise capacity, etc.) in any of the above-mentioned lesions. 4D flow, computational fluid dynamics and statistical shape modelling represent innovative imaging developments which have the potential to offer a further insight in predicting disease progression, mechanics and results following catheter or surgical interventions. We will also explore the role of virtual stenting and 3D printing in the clinical practice including their current and future applications.

13.2   Background

13.2.1 Bicuspid Aortic Valve

Bicuspid aortic valve (BAV) is the most common congenital heart disease (CHD) accounting for up to 2% of all CHD lesions [1] and is characterised by a very heterogeneous clinical presentation. BAV can be found in isolation or in association with congenital left-sided obstructive lesions (i.e. coarctation of the aorta, Shone complex) [2], ventricular septal defect, and syndromic conditions (i.e. Turner, Loeys-Dietz), and familial TAA and dissection disease due to smooth muscle α-actin (ACTA2) gene mutations, as well [3–6].

Whether truly bicuspid or functionally bicuspid, the aortic valve is subject to early degeneration with a high intervention rate in patients younger than 50 years of age. Aneurysm formation of the aortic root and ascending aorta is also common and may lead to surgical indication for aortic root-ascending aorta replacement or personalised external arterial support (PEARS) surgery even in the absence of significant aortic valve dysfunction [7, 8]. Current guidelines recommend surgery when the aortic size exceeds >55 mm, or ≥45 mm if concomitant AVR is being performed [9, 10]. The aneurysm formation may involve predominantly the root (sinuses of Valsalva) or the tubular-ascending portion of the aorta, with the latter being the most common phenotype (60%–70% of dilated aortas) with the fastest growing rate in adults (≈0.4–0.6 mm/year), irrespective of BAV morphology and function [11, 12]. In addition, these patients are more prone to develop infective endocarditis due to the turbulent flow patterns in the proximal ascending aorta and finally they are at

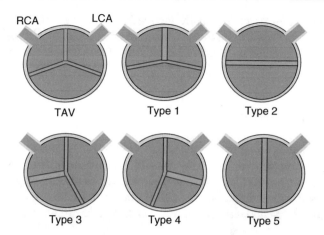

Fig. 13.1 BAV phenotypes including the fusion of the left and right coronary cusps or A-P orientation of the free edge if truly bicuspid (top middle and figures) and examples of fusion of either right or left with the non-coronary cusps or L-R orientation of the free edge if truly bicuspid (bottom figures). *RCA* right coronary artery; *LCA* left coronary artery; *TAV* trileaflet aortic valve for reference of normal anatomy

risk of aortic dissection although this remains relatively low and very difficult to predict based on aortic size [5, 13, 14].

Various BAV phenotypes (Fig. 13.1) have been identified and the most common forms are represented by the fusion of the left and right coronary cusps or A-P orientation of the free edge if truly bicuspid (BAV-AP 56% ca) followed by the fusion of either right or left coronary cusp with the non-coronary cusp or L-R orientation of the free edge if truly bicuspid (BAV R-L 44% combined). These phenotypes are associated with differences in valvar dysfunction pattern with regurgitation being the predominant mechanism of dysfunction in the BAV A-P phenotype and stenosis being the main mechanism of dysfunction in the BAV R-L phenotypes. Hierarchic cluster analysis showed 3 different types of bicuspid aortopathy according to the pattern of aortic dilation: type 1 (aortic enlargement confined to the sinuses of Valsalva), type 2 (aortic enlargement involving the ascending aorta), and type 3 (aortic enlargement extending to the transverse aortic arch). Kang et al.'s work showed that BAV A-P phenotype was mostly associated with type 1 aortic enlargement, whereas type 3 aortopathy was present in up to 40% of patients with BAV R-L [15].

Having said that, BAV remains a very heterogeneous lesion with mechanical and genetic factors involved in disease progression. Screening of first-degree family member is mandatory given the high penetrance of the condition [16] and patients with a diagnosis of BAV need to remain under routine surveillance with the interval between appointments dictated by the severity of valvar dysfunction, aortopathy and possible associated lesions. In patients with significant valvar dysfunction, serial echocardiogram and exercise testing are performed on a 6–12 months basis with 3D imaging generally being performed every 12 months (CMR for being the method of choice in order to acquire also volumetric and functional assessment unless specific contraindications are present). Imaging protocol will then be tailored to the surgical or percutaneous technique required, when indication for intervention is given.

13.2.2 Marfan Syndrome

Marfan syndrome is an autosomal dominant connective tissues disease caused by mutations in FBN1 gene on chromosome 15q21 encoding a large glycoprotein of the extracellular matrix, called fibrillin-1. Deficiency of fibrillin may lead to weakening of the supporting tissues. Over 1,000 mutations have been found in the FBN1 gene and in 10% of patients with clinical criteria of Marfan, a mutation cannot be found.

Marfan syndrome is characterised by a variable degree of cardiovascular, skeletal and ocular abnormalities and has a prevalence of 2–3/10,000 newborn (25–30% are new mutations). Prognosis is mainly related to the cardiovascular complications such as progressive dilatation of the aorta leading to dissection and death at young age [17]. Mean survival in untreated patients is 40 years but the variance is large. Dilatation of the sinuses of Valsalva is found in 60–80% of adult patients but the rate of progressive dilatation varies. The risk of dissection increases with the aortic diameter but can occur also in patients with non- or only mildly dilated aorta.

Diagnosis of Marfan syndrome is made on clinical ground following the Ghent criteria [18] and requires the occurrence of a major manifestation in two different organ systems and involvement of a third organ system.

Once diagnosis is made patients require strict surveillance with 3D imaging in order to monitor potential aortic dilatation and its rate of progression. CMR is the first-line investigation since radiation free whereas CT can be used if there are contraindications to CMR or for specific treatment planning such as PEARS procedure as explained later on in the chapter.

It is recommended to investigate first-degree relatives (siblings and parents) of a subject with Marfan syndrome to identify a familial form in which relatives all have a 50% chance of carrying the family mutation/disease. Once a familial form of the syndrome is highly suspected, it is recommended to refer the patient to a geneticist for family investigation and molecular testing [19].

When aortic dilatation is present medical therapy with beta-blocker or ARB antagonist is indicated to slow down the progression rate of dilatation. Recent studies suggest that statins may also play a role in limiting disease progression by reducing the formation of cholesterol precursors, therefore reducing the pro-inflammatory mediators known to be involved in aneurysm formation such as protein kinase-c (PKC) and TGF-β [20].

Prophylactic surgery on the dilated aorta is performed when the diameter exceeds 50 mm or 45 mm in the presence of a family history of dissection or if the rate of dilatation progression is greater than 3 mm/year [21]. Surgical procedures have evolved from classical aortic root replacement, including valve replacement with a

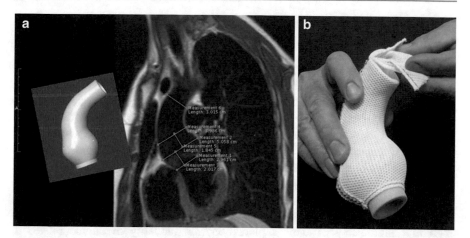

Fig. 13.2 (a) Aortic root and ascending aorta dilatation with diameters measured on 3D MR images and personalised aortic scaffold CAD model. (b) Textile mesh on 3D printing scaffold. (Reproduced with permission and courtesy of Tal Golesworthy)

mechanical or biological valve (Bentall procedure) to valve sparing techniques (David and Yacoub procedures) and even external procedures (personalised external aortic root support, PEARS procedure, Fig. 13.2) performed off pump, where the aortic root is left in place and reinforced by a sleeve from the outside [22]. For women with Marfan syndrome contemplating pregnancy, it is reasonable to prophylactically replace or "wrap" the aortic root and ascending aorta if the diameter exceeds 4.0 cm [21].

13.2.3 Coarctation of the Aorta

Coarctation of the aorta (CoA) was first described by Morgagni in 1760 [23] during an autopsy of a monk and refers to a complex cardiovascular disorder characterised by a generalised arteriopathy presenting with a discreet narrowing of the thoracic aorta generally opposite the arterial duct in adults or as a diffuse tubular hypoplasia involving the aortic arch or the aorta distal to the left subclavian artery. It accounts for 5–8% of all congenital heart lesions with a male predominance up to twice more frequent than in female. CoA can be found in isolation or associated with other congenital defects such as bicuspid aortic valve (up to 80%), ventricular septal defect, mitral valve abnormalities, intracranial aneurysm (most frequently Berry aneurysm of the circle of Willis) or genetic abnormalities such as Turner, Williams-Beuren, and Noonan syndromes. CoA can also be associated with more complex CHD such as double inlet left ventricle, tricuspid atresia, and hypoplastic left heart syndrome. Left untreated and based on its severity and associated anomalies, mortality can be as high as 90% in the first year of life. Aortic medial abnormalities may be present and account for an increased aortic stiffness and pulse wave velocity [24] which may persist after good anatomical repair. In those patients who survive the first 2 years of life, mortality has been described as high as 50% before the age of 30–31 years [25].

In infancy the diagnosis of coarctation of the aorta is generally made when patients present with congestive heart failure (CHF); however hypertension or CoA-related complications such as left ventricular failure (28%), intracranial haemorrhage (12%), infective endocarditis (18%), aortic rupture/dissection (21%), and premature coronary artery disease may be the first signs/symptoms in adults [26].

The first surgical repair of CoA was performed by Clarence Crafoord in 1944 using an end-to-end anastomosis technique in an 11 years old boy [27]. Several surgical techniques such as subclavian flap repair, patch aortoplasty, and interposition graft subsequently developed each with their potential complications. Nowadays, treatment of coarctation of the aorta can be surgical or percutaneous including angioplasty or stent implantation; the modality of choice relates to patient's age, anatomy and associated lesions. The general rule for intervention is the presence of a gradient greater than 20 mmHg across the CoA site. A percutaneous approach is mostly performed in adult patients, whereas surgery is generally the method of choice in infants. Despite satisfactory results patients may still suffer from chronic long-term complication, and long-term survival continues to be lower than that of the general population mainly due to cardiovascular complications; the presence of a bicuspid aortic valve is predictive for aortic valve procedures, and both, a brachial-ankle gradient difference greater than 20 mmHg and an impaired left ventricular function, are predictive for major cardiovascular events [28]. Cardiovascular complications include arterial hypertension, re-coarctation at the site of previous repair/stent, coronary artery disease, aneurysm formation, malfunction of the BAV when associated and infective endocarditis.

Patients require lifelong follow-up in order to screen for potential complications and to be treated medically or with an intervention as required. Follow-up includes regular clinical consultation with transthoracic echocardiogram performed on the day, 12 lead ECG, 24-h blood pressure monitoring, and 3D imaging such as cardiac MRI and CT. CMR is particularly useful as it provides 3D anatomical information of the CoA site, pre- and post-repair, and helps planning intervention especially in native CoA [29, 30]. In addition, CMR allows visualisation and assessment of collateral flows, provides haemodynamic information such as gradient across the CoA site, valvular and ventricular function as well as information on associated defects.

13.3 Multimodality Imaging Assessment

13.3.1 Echocardiography

Echocardiography with its wide range of approaches (transthoracic, transoesophageal, 3D, contrast, and stress) generally represents the first-line imaging modality in all congenital heart diseases including BAV, aortic coarctation and Marfan syndrome [31–33]. Protocols should be targeted to the lesions under investigation with a systematic approach in order to guarantee reproducibility, particularly important for patients under surveillance, where changes need careful monitoring.

Transthoracic echocardiogram (TTE) allows accurate assessment of valvar function with higher spatial and temporal resolution than CMR. Gradient across the aortic valve can be obtained using continuous wave Doppler interrogation from apical 5 chambers view and 3 chambers view. Parasternal long and short axis views alongside the apical 5 chambers view and 3 chambers views are used to assess valvar regurgitation. When significant aortic valve regurgitation is present, interrogation of the proximal descending aorta is performed to assess the presence of retrograde flow. Regurgitation is graded as mild, moderate or severe based on the width of the regurgitant jet, pressure half time and presence of retrograde flow in the proximal descending aorta [34]. Stenosis will be graded as mild if peak velocity is less than 3 m/s, moderate when >3 but <4 m/s and severe when >4 m/s. A mean aortic gradient higher than 40–50 mmHg and a valve area less than 1 cm^2 also indicate the presence of severe stenosis [35]. M-mode assessment of the left ventricle (LV) is used to provide measurements of the LV diameters, wall thickness and parameters of systolic function (shortening fraction and ejection fraction). LV volumes and function are however more accurately assessed using 2D Simpson volumetric assessment [36]. Using mitral valve inflow data combined with tissue Doppler echocardiographic velocity, information on LV diastolic function can be accurately obtained [37]. Left ventricular functional assessment can also be complemented by tissue Doppler indices of LV myocardial velocities such as strain and strain rate using speckle tracking which have been demonstrated to correlate with outcomes [38].

TTE also allows two-dimensional assessment of aortic root, proximal ascending aorta and transverse arch diameters; however, we must bear in mind that 2D dimensions may differ from 3D measures obtained with CMR or CT given the potential elliptical shape of the vessel and suboptimal angulation. Correlation with 3D imaging modality is therefore needed before using TTE for routine surveillance especially when diameters of the aortic root and ascending aorta are greater than 4 cm [13]. In patients with coarctation of the aorta, gradient across the coarctation site (before or after repair or stenting) can be obtained from supra-sternal view using continuous wave Doppler interrogation.

3D imaging adds value in assessing valvar morphology since it provides en face visualisation of the valve which can be easily interpreted by the surgeons guiding decision towards valve repair or replacement (Video 13.1). In addition, in the presence of multiple haemodynamic abnormalities, it allows sizing of valve stenosis and provides live dynamic geometric guidance during the interventional procedures, e.g. 3D transoesophageal echocardiography (TOE) [39]. 3D assessment of LV volumes and ejection fraction is preferred to 2D indices if acoustic window allows although 3D is still not routinely used in all echo laboratories.

If coronary artery disease is suspected, stress echocardiogram [pharmacological (DSE) or exercise induced] is a valuable technique in expert hands to assess the presence of inducible ischaemia and its regionality [40]. The addition of layer-specific strain by speckle tracking echocardiography may add value to DSE in detecting coronary artery disease [41].

13.3.2 Cardiovascular Magnetic Resonance Imaging

Cardiovascular magnetic resonance imaging (CMR) is a well-established, non-invasive and radiation-free imaging modality, essential in the management of patients with congenital heart diseases [31, 32]. CMR allows accurate assessment of ventricular parameters such as volumes, wall thickness, myocardial mass, myocardial scarring, systolic function, as well as valvar function with the possibility to measure the degree of stenosis and regurgitation. Importantly, CMR allows accurate and reproducible assessment of cardiac anatomy including 3D information of the aorta which is crucial for longitudinal monitoring of aneurysm formation in patients with BAV aortopathy or Marfan syndrome, to diagnose aortic coarctation and delineate its anatomy thus guiding surgical or catheter procedures and finally to unravel potential complications such as aneurysmal formation or dissection, and myocardial scarring using late gadolinium enhancement in patients with previous myocardial infarction as a result of coronary artery disease. Ventricular volumes are obtained from semi-automatic segmentation with manual correction of end-systolic and end-diastolic cine images, generally acquired from a short axis stack, whereas flows are acquired using through-plane or in-plane phase-contrast images. It is important to note that in patients with bicuspid aortic valve, flow turbulences in the aortic root may affect accuracy of the acquired data especially in the assessment of aortic valve regurgitation; comparison with ventricular stroke volumes and mitral valve inflow may help in estimating more accurately the degree of AR. Correlation with echocardiography is generally recommended. In patients with aortic coarctation, it is important to assess the velocity at the coarctation site but also the presence of continuous diastolic flow (Fig. 13.3), which informs about the haemodynamic significance of the narrowing. Flow needs to be accurately planned to avoid underestimation of the true velocity (Fig. 13.4). In-plane flow assessment can also be performed and is particularly useful in the presence of multiple sites of narrowing (Videos 13.2, 13.3 and 13.4).

In patients who underwent coarctation of the aorta stenting, choosing the right imaging sequence is key to delineate patency of the stent. Image quality is dependent on stent material, diameter and design [42, 43], so the right sequence needs to be used. Den Harder and colleague demonstrated that overall reliability of CMR was similar to that of CT using a 1.5T scanner and either a multi-slice T2-weighted turbo spin echo, an RF-spoiled three-dimensional T1-weighted Fast Field Echo or a balanced turbo field echo 3D sequence [44]. Theirs was an in vitro study and stents did not have stenosis or narrowing but it does highlight good resolution that can be obtained with CMR. In general, more T1-weighted sequences yield less stent artefacts and are the preferred choice with the least affected being black blood images.

13.3.3 Computed Tomography

Cardiac multidetector computed tomography (CT) is now in routine clinical use as an alternative to CMR. It is particularly useful in patients who have contraindications

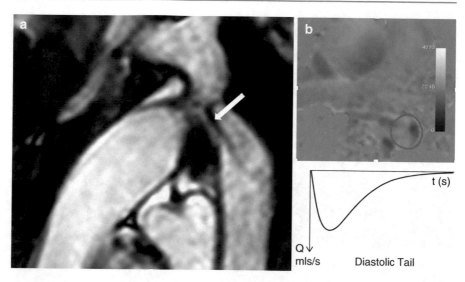

Fig. 13.3 (a) MR cine image of aortic coarctation showing continuous diastolic flow immediately distal to the narrow site; (b) Through-plane phase-contrast MR flow assessment confirming the continuous diastolic flow (diastolic tail) which suggests significant coarctation

Fig. 13.4 Through-plane flow assessment of aortic coarctation. Measured peak velocity is highly dependent on accurate planning

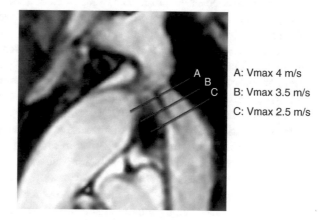

A: Vmax 4 m/s

B: Vmax 3.5 m/s

C: Vmax 2.5 m/s

to CMR due to metallic implants or in patients who cannot tolerate the MRI procedure due to claustrophobia or the inability to lie still for a long period of time. Although there is a recognised burden of ionising radiation and the need for intravenous iodinated contrast in MDCT, the newer generation of dual source CT technology, acquisition and postprocessing protocols have allowed for further reductions in radiation exposure while maintaining a high spatial resolution and short acquisition time [45]. The high-resolution imaging allows for the visualisation of coronary artery anatomy and potential coronary artery disease as well as providing good visualisation of peripheral vascular tree, stents and extracardiac structures such as the lungs and thoracic cage.

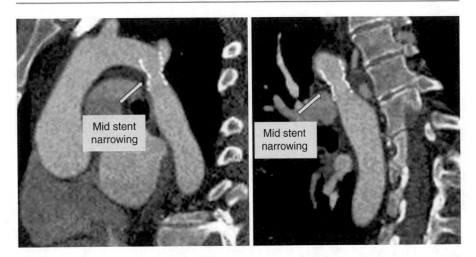

Fig. 13.5 Cross-sectional CT images of aortic coarctation stent. Arrows indicate area of stent narrowing

In the presence of vascular stents (such as coarctation of the aorta), image quality allows accurate assessment of stent patency or mechanism of failure in cases where re-coarctation is observed (Fig. 13.5, Videos 13.5, 13.6 and 13.7) [46, 47]. Stent material affects image quality with the worse obtained where covered stents made of platinum iridium were implanted [46].

In patients undergoing PEARS procedure, CT is currently the image modality of choice to accurately assess aortic root and ascending aorta diameters as well as origin of coronary arteries which is used to produce a bespoke personalised external arterial support mesh [22]. Images are ECG-gated, prospectively acquired in diastole unless heart rate is greater than 75 beats/min.

In older patients, TAVI can be an alternative procedure to bicuspid aortic valve dysfunction. CT is now the gold standard tool for annular sizing, determination of risk of annular injury and coronary occlusion, and to provide co-planar fluoroscopic angle prediction in advance of the procedure as well as visualising vascular accesses [48] (Fig. 13.6). Data acquisition strategies and scanning protocols vary depending on scanner manufacturer, system and institutional preferences [49]. All approaches share an ECG-gated computed tomographic angiography (CTA) data set that covers at least the aortic root in order to provide artefact-free anatomical information of the aortic root, followed by a commonly non-ECG-gated CTA data acquisition of the aorto/ilio/femoral vasculature for assessment of the access vasculature. Ideally, both acquisitions are combined in a comprehensive scanning protocol with a single contrast administration [48].

Longitudinal follow-up of aortopathies can be performed using CT when CMR is contra-indicated or if patients suffer from claustrophobia bearing in mind the cumulative radiation burden. Images should be acquired in the same cardiac phase to allow for reproducibility if heart rate allows.

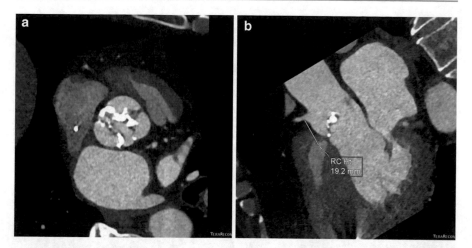

Fig. 13.6 CT images of bicuspid aortic valve. (**a**) Cross-sectional image of a functionally BAV showing heavy calcification of valve leaflets and fusion of the right and left coronary cusps; (**b**) Left ventricular outflow tract view used to measure distance between the right coronary artery and the aortic valve plane

13.4 Innovations Based on Multimodality Imaging

The rapidly advancing field of multimodality imaging represents several opportunities for innovations either in the actual imaging practice itself (e.g. introduction of new sequences, fast imaging, etc.) or in the use of computational modelling approaches that rely on imaging data for inputs and boundary conditions. These techniques have increasingly been used to provide valuable insights into key aspects of the aforementioned aortic diseases, and particularly haemodynamic, morphological and functional insights.

13.4.1 Four-Dimensional Flow Magnetic Resonance Imaging

Surgical and medical management of congenital aortic lesions and aortopathies has improved over the years, with improved survival and quality of life overall for patients with congenital heart disease (CHD) [50]. Cardiac MRI provides critical diagnostic data about cardiac anatomy and function, including haemodynamics. Three-dimensional cine phase-contrast (3D PC)-MRI also referred to as "4D flow" has emerged as a comprehensive tool for haemodynamic assessment over 2D PC-MRI, which is an established clinical tool for non-invasive evaluation of aortic blood flow [51]. The study of complex flow phenomena can benefit from the use of 4D flow, enabling the visualisation of complex flow patterns and the retrospective quantification of several flow parameters, including non-invasive pressure difference and kinetic energy (Fig. 13.7) [52–54]. Using 4D flow MRI, wall shear stress (WSS) on the arterial

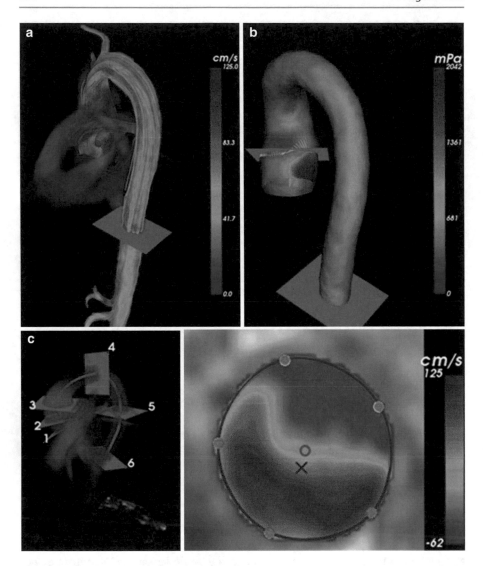

Fig. 13.7 Example of postprocessing of 4D flow data using commercial software (CAAS, Pie Medical Imaging, The Netherlands) in a BAV aorta, showing velocity streamlines (**a**), wall shear stress mapping on the aortic wall (**b**), and in-plane velocity distribution at multiple planes along the aortic centreline (**c**, showing in detail plane 1 as an example)

wall can be analysed in vivo [55]. Such haemodynamic force is exposed to modifications after cardiac contraction due to pulsatile pressure, as well as blood vessel geometry and mechanical properties [56]. Recent studies focus on accelerating aortic 4D flow acquisition (e.g. k-t accelerated aortic 4D flow MRI), as well as WSS computation (e.g. automated segmentation-free method) [51, 57] to improve the clinical applicability of the sequence by making it faster on the one hand, and to provide additional information in the form of new indices on the other hand.

13.4.1.1   4D Flow in Aortic Coarctation

Longitudinal studies reported decreased life expectancy in CoA patients associated with abnormal haemodynamics, the latter being a key factor in treatment decisions and successful long-term results [58]. Four-dimensional MRI can represent a clinically valuable tool for reliable evaluation of collateral blood flow, as well as demonstration of distorted flow patterns in patients with repaired and unrepaired aortic CoA [59] (Video 13.8). In a study analysing flow-derived vessel wall parameters, haemodynamic alterations in repaired CoA were identified along the entire aorta, independently of the region of repair, and were related to secondary complications, e.g. hypertension, aneurysm formation and re-stenosis [60]. In another study investigating the impact of inlet velocity profile on wall properties, helical flow at the aortic inlet was shown to substantially affect pressure drop and WSS, suggesting the interplay between valve function and vessel geometry on the resulting forcing acting on the aortic wall itself [58]. Pressure and energy loss estimates from 4D MRI can be affected by varying degrees of viscous dissipation and turbulent kinetic energy which can vary across different geometries and that, particularly in the case of viscous dissipation, can be substantially affected by image resolution [61].

13.4.1.2   4D Flow in BAV

Up to 70–80% of patients with BAV present with aortic root and ascending aorta dilatation. In some cases, the degree of dilatation and its progression are the reason for surgical referral. The mechanisms behind the aortic dilatations are still not clearly understood. There are two predominant theories behind BAV-associated aortopathy, the "genetic" and the "haemodynamic" theory. The genetic theory, as the widely accepted one, has been challenged or simply complemented by haemodynamic and anatomic observations, raising the possibility that abnormal flow patterns have an essential role in the development of aortic dilation in BAV patients [62–65]. Evidence shows that increased blood flow helicity and eccentricity contribute to increased WSS, leading to medial derangement in the greater aortic convexity, as well as higher growth rate and severity of ascending aorta (AAo) dilation [66–69]. On the other hand, a 3-year follow-up study showed WSS alterations in the absence of clinically relevant aortic anatomical remodelling [70]. According to observational studies including 4D flow and histological data analysis, there is an association between increased WSS and elastin dysregulation and higher concentration of mediators of extracellular matrix dysregulation (i.e. MMPs and TGF-β) [71, 72]. An association between increased WSS in the ascending aorta and the presence of aortic valve stenosis in the absence or early stages of aortic dilation has been reported in BAV patients [72, 73]. A recent pathology study investigating the effect on the aortic layers of jet and non-jet stream in BAV and TAV patients showed alterations in the intimal layer and inner media of all the jet specimens [74]. Longitudinal studies correlating haemodynamic with molecular mechanisms are required to risk-stratify patients with BAV aortopathy.

The use of 4D flow can facilitate the assessment of haemodynamic alterations in BAV aortopathogenesis and suggested the association of BAV fusion types with different dilation patterns, reinforced by in vitro observations and computational studies [75–77]. However, other studies report weak or no association between BAV morphotype and aneurysmal patterns [78, 79]. Four-dimensional MRI classification schemes considering BAV morphotypes and patterns of aortic flow in BAV aortopathy with good prognostic significance are still under investigation. Abnormal flow patterns can also be investigated following aortic valve replacement (AVR) in relation to progression of aortic dilation, with a study indicating different flow patterns following mechanical AVR or Ross vs. bioprosthetic AVR as partially explaining different aortic growth rates post-AVR [80]. Haemodynamics can also be linked to late post-AVR progression of BAV aortopathy [81].

An interesting technical development is the possibility of generating cohort averaged WSS maps using 4D flow, allowing the visualisation and identification of regionally altered WSS [82]. Such WSS atlases can identify regions of significantly altered WSS associated with differential expression of BAV aortopathy [83], comparing haemodynamic features between BAV patients and age-matched controls [84] or comparing BAV vs. TAV and dilated vs. non-dilated phenotypes [85] to further unravel the role of WSS in vessel wall remodelling.

13.4.1.3 4D Flow in Marfan Syndrome

Marfan patients typically show important aortic dilation resulting from cystic degeneration of the tunica media, with consequent flow alterations [86, 87]. An MRI study showed that Marfan patients have lower segmental WSS in the inner proximal descending aorta segment which links to increased vortex and helical flow patterns and enlarged diameter at sites of increased risk of aortic dissection [87], while it has been suggested that flow alterations originating from this site may explain (at least in part) the occurrence of Type-B dissection [88]. On the other hand, another study reported differences in WSS in Marfan aortas regardless of aortic dimensions [89], suggesting the need of aortic growth-WSS association studies in Marfan syndrome. Longitudinal studies with follow-up are required to enlighten the association between flow and aortic dilation patterns and relate haemodynamics with postoperative dissections [90].

Biomechanical characterisation has been performed in large cohorts, including BAV and Marfan patients, showing controversial results in terms of changes in aortic stiffness. In one study, Marfan patients showed to have stiffer aortas compared to BAV, with aortic stiffness strongly dependent on dilation severity [91] but aortic stiffness was reported as being greater in BAV compared to Marfan patients and being associated with slower aneurysm progression in another study [92]. Pulse wave velocity showed to be independently related to AAo dilation in BAV patients, but 4D flow MRI studies could contribute to assess aortic stiffness and pulse wave velocity in BAV and Marfan patients incorporating detailed haemodynamics information. A small 4D flow study including BAV and Marfan patients enabled to derive aortic relative pressure components and showed the potential of the technique to provide mechanistic information [93].

Whilst pathologies have been discussed here separately, future work should in general focus on standardising 4D flow MRI scan acquisition parameters and reporting of quantitative metrics, as well as developing automated analysis tools [94].

13.4.2 Computational Fluid Dynamics

While 4D flow is emerging as a single fast technique for comprehensive assessment of CHD [50], computational fluid dynamics (CFD) can also provide haemodynamic insights across different scenarios, based on computer simulations by solving mathematical equations in different geometries. Simulations of circulatory function can add to the knowledge of bio-fluid physiology, can investigate potential postoperative complications and can contribute to the development of medical devices [95].

Simulations based on CFD methodologies have been applied to the circulation for decades and can provide very valuable insights into aortic pathologies. Most of the imaging-based CFD studies in CoA patients (example in Fig. 13.8) focus on assessing the pressure difference across the CoA region, in order to potentially reduce the need for diagnostic catheterisation and optimise treatment [96–102]. The input geometry for the CFD simulations is typically derived from MRI or CT datasets, reconstructing the shape of the aortic arch and allowing to generate haemodynamic results pre- and post-CoA repair depending on the availability of clinical data or providing a virtual platform to evaluate surgical plans (e.g. simulating different

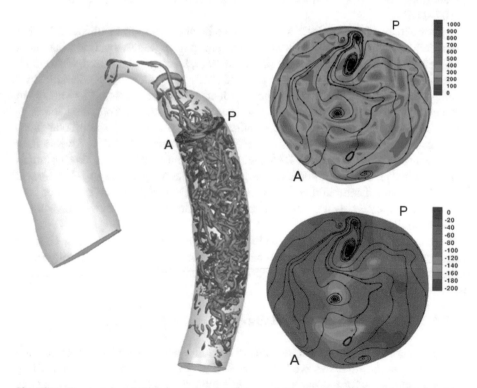

Fig. 13.8 Computational fluid dynamics simulations of flow across aortic coarctation showing detailed streamlines (black lines) on a plane distal from the COA site. Top right plane: velocity map. Bottom right plane: pressure map. *A* anterior, *P* posterior. (Courtesy of Vahid Goodarzi Ardakani (University of Bristol, UK))

repairs, surgical or interventional). Simulation-based haemodynamic analyses can thus contribute to the evaluation of therapeutic effects [103]. CFD can indeed also be used to simulate the effects of CoA stenting and provide information as to the correct stent type and size [104]. Whilst CoA repair can alleviate blood pressure gradients, long-term morbidity persists, and altered biomechanical indices such as averaged WSS and oscillatory shear index (OSI) derived from CFD simulations in CoA geometries can contribute to explain long-term morbidity [105]. A physiologically correct but time-consuming 4D MRI-based in vivo velocity profile merged with CFD studies could represent a crucial step towards patient-specific analysis of CoA haemodynamics. A new framework for estimation of lumped parameter models from uncertain clinical measurements with the aim to perform patient-specific haemodynamic analysis has been suggested and it was applied to CoA [106]. Extensive model validation in several clinical CoA cases is nonetheless required.

From a computational standpoint, more complex fluid-structure interaction (FSI) models can also generate WSS values and explore the possible cause-and-effect relationship between haemodynamics and tissue properties or aortic enlargement and progression, as well as performing a component-specific assessment of WSS magnitude, oscillatory and directional characteristics in BAV ascending aortas [107–110].

Comparisons between BAV and TAV have been carried out in silico, with CFD simulations showing that BAV was more prone to have jet flow/wall impingement against the greater curvature of the proximal AAo, leading to increased WSS [111]. Another study showed that the presence of aortic stenosis (AS), particularly in a right–non-coronary BAV morphotype, can lead to greater WSS and lower OSI in the greater curvature of the ascending aorta [66]. An attempt to compute haemodynamic alterations obtained after restoration of normal AAo and sinotubular junction geometry in a case of preserved BAV has been reported [112]. Adverse flow patterns were also observed in BAV patients with concomitant CoA, as a common comorbidity [113]. Better understanding of AAo haemodynamics in BAV disease could be obtained combining 4D flow MRI and CFD to help clinicians develop personalised risk assessment for aortic complications in BAV patients with or without comorbidities.

CFD studies can also yield valuable information as to aortic blood flow changes and variations in kinetic energy and energy loss as indicators of risk of rupture of aortic aneurysms in both BAV and Marfan patients [114].

13.4.3 Statistical Shape Modelling

Computational modelling can also aid in studying patient-specific anatomies and generating descriptive and predictive data, through a statistical shape modelling (SSM) framework for morphological assessment of cardiac and vascular structures [115]. The creation of image databases, such as the Cardiac Atlas Project [116], can allow population-based studies processing and analysing large amounts of 3D shape

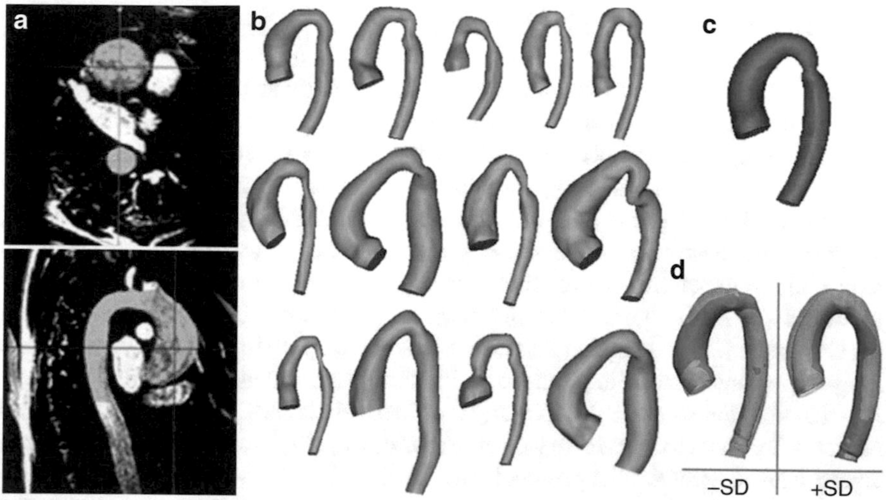

Fig. 13.9   Statistical shape modelling framework. (**a**) Segmentation of aortic arch anatomy from 3D MR angiogram. (**b**) Population of aortic arch anatomies from multiple patients, with varying arch morphology (all with aortic coarctation). (**c**) Average shape ("template") obtained from the population depicted in **b**. (**d**) Morphological variations around the mean (±1 standard deviation, SD)

information for the creation of average population shapes ("atlases") and calculating shape variability around such averages (Fig. 13.9) [117]. This approach yields the potential of identifying morphological biomarkers that can be related to the dynamic nature of the shape under investigation or to surgical/procedural decision-making and treatment personalisation [118].

Although SSM holds great potential for diagnosis and prognosis, not many studies have yet been performed to exploit the relation between shape and function in aortic diseases. For instance, two studies explored the association between aortic arch shape features late after successful aortic CoA repair and worse left ventricular function [119, 120] and another study explored differences in aortic arch architecture across BAV patients with/without repaired CoA identifying arch features in the repaired CoA subgroup associated with worse left ventricular function [121]. These studies, and future studies including follow-up information, could potentially have an impact on long-term risk assessment after CoA repair and risk stratification of patients, targeting treatment in the case of these two concomitant defects (BAV + COA).

As part of these analyses, morphological subgroups can be investigated using clustering techniques [122], and subsequent classification can be used for risk assessment. Furthermore, growth models and shape atlases could be used for device development. Merging imaging data from different sources, i.e. MRI, CT and 3D echocardiography, can lead to new models with functional and anatomical data from multiple sources.

13.4.4 Ventriculo-Vascular Coupling

Arterial vasculopathy and residual aortic obstruction can lead to left ventricular (LV) dysfunction in patients with aortic CoA related to adverse ventriculo-arterial (VA) coupling. A recent MRI follow-up study assessing the additive effect of hypertension to adverse VA coupling, considering aortic pulse wave velocity, aortic distensibility, global LV function, LV dimensions, and LV myocardial deformation, showed significantly increased aortic stiffness and hypertension in well-repaired CoA patients long term after repair, but preserved LV function [123]. Another study indicated abnormal arterial-left ventricular-left atrial interaction after intervention for CoA repair and interrupted aortic arch [124]. Computational fluid dynamics and lumped parameter modelling, based on imaging data, can also be used to estimate pre- and post-intervention VA coupling and haemodynamics [125]. As patients with repaired CoA tend to have increased afterload due to structural and functional aortic abnormalities, a novel MRI protocol was developed to allow for non-invasive haemodynamic assessment, showing abnormal conduit vessel function after coarctation of the aorta repair, including abnormal wave reflections associated with elevated LV mass [126]. Studies of vascular compliance and wave reflections may impact drug development in the future. Furthermore, it is known that wave reflection from CoA site creates a reflected backward compression wave that increases LV afterload; however not all reflected wave power will propagate back to the LV. Thus, according to a computational modelling study, wave transmission into supra-aortic branches may have an important impact on both cerebral haemodynamics and LV load in aortic CoA [127]. Another study exploring the link between cardiovascular and cerebrovascular disease showed an association between reduced aortic distensibility and higher aorto-carotid wave transmission and blood pressure in young adults having long-term repaired CoA [128].

Vascular coupling has been also studied in BAV disease. Impaired LV systolic mechanics in BAV patients appeared to be related only to the congenital abnormality of the aortic valve itself [129], while in another study no association was identified between myocardial function and distensibility and stiffness index of the ascending aorta [130]. Based on a retrospective MRI study, aortic stenosis and regurgitation in BAV are likely to significantly impact on elevated aortic peak velocities and WSS associated with parameters of LV remodelling (Fig. 13.5), albeit observed in a small population [131]. Comprehensive application of 4D MRI and other MRI sequences including T1-mapping techniques, providing comprehensive assessment of haemodynamics and possible LV remodelling, could shed more light on VA coupling in BAV patients. Feature tracking cardiac MRI (Fig. 13.10), allowing for strain analysis, has been reported to reveal LV abnormalities in BAV patients [132]; therefore it can also be used to unravel vascular coupling questions. These approaches are also intertwined with advancements in artificial intelligence and machine learning, as in the case of a proposed deep learning-based framework for automating the analysis of MRI analysis including volumes and strain without the need of clinician's oversight yet ensuring quality control [133]. These approaches warrant further exploration and certainly hold great potential for future applications

Fig. 13.10 Ventricular volumes curves: CMR feature tracking. The end-diastolic LV wall segmentations are used as the region of interest for the feature tracking (FT) algorithm. Global circumferential strain (ε_{circ}), radial strain (ε_{rad}) and longitudinal strain(εlong) are computed from the FT results. (Courtesy of Dr. Bram Ruijsink)

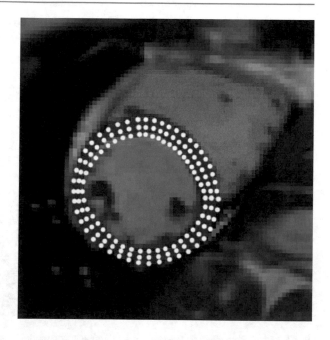

particularly in large-scale studies, from a research standpoint, and reduction of analysis time, from a clinical standpoint.

Ventricular contractility and VA coupling have also been shown to be impaired in patients with Marfan syndrome but preserved in non-syndromal thoracic aortic aneurysm and dissection patients [134]. Considering the aortic stiffness and intrinsic impairment of myocardial contractility in Marfan patients, more MRI and possibly also modelling studies should be performed to unravel vascular coupling impairment in this population.

13.4.5 Virtual Stenting

Data derived from multimodality imaging can also inform device selection for patient-specific virtual interventional planning. New methods have been described in the literature, including virtual deployment of stents or grafts into patient-specific geometries particularly of patients with CoA based on MRI data for personalised planning and including CFD [135]. Patient-specific models can be used to plan re-stenting for complex reCoA, showing the benefit of integrating computational techniques into patient management [104]. Such an approach can be applied to prospective model construction and incorporated in clinical use. CFD also facilitates virtual treatment of CoA for comparison of haemodynamic alterations between stents in the same vessel [136, 137]. In addition, modelling approaches allow to test modified/novel approaches, as in the case of a study comparing a conventional vs. a modified Cheatham-Platinum stent through biomechanical simulations in a virtual CoA environment, in this case

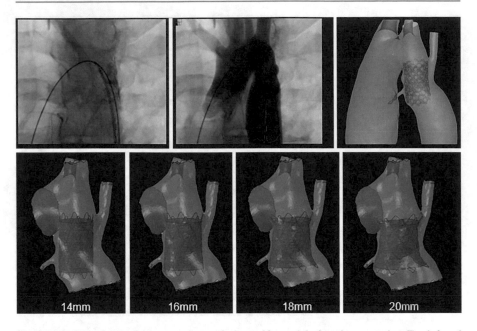

Fig. 13.11 Virtual stent deployment in a patient-specific model of aortic coarctation. Top left and middle panel: angiogram showing the catheter through existing stent and aortic arch anatomy. Top right panel: reconstruction of arch anatomy and existing stent from CT data revealing anterior wall aortic aneurysm and jailing of aberrant right subclavian artery. Bottom panels: simulations of deployment of covered stents of varying sizes (range: 14–20 mm) required to exclude the aortic aneurysm without blocking the flow in the right subclavian artery. (Courtesy of Silvia Schievano and Claudio Capelli (University College London, UK))

demonstrating similar results [138]. Quantitative techniques to assess turbulent kinetic energy and flow eccentricity can assess CoA severity and may improve the long-term outcome of CoA therapy, informing treatment choices. These CFD-derived parameters are included as part of simulations, like in the case of a patient-specific CoA model before and after a range of virtual interventions (Fig. 13.11) in order to non-invasively investigate the effect of different dilation options on the flow field and reach the least eccentric scenario with respect to neighbouring anatomical structures, such as an aberrant subclavian artery [139]. Intervention response maps could be established with CFD simulations, including also non-measurable haemodynamic metrics such as WSS, to better predict post-treatment outcome. Integration of MRI + CFD in a treatment predictive framework could result in establishing platforms for patient-specific planning and therapy.

13.4.6 Three-Dimensional Printing

Three-dimensional (3D) printing can be an extremely valuable technology in cardiology, as extensively reported in recent literature, with applications ranging

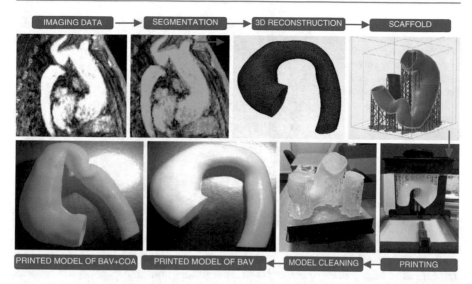

Fig. 13.12 Key steps in the 3D printing workflow (from top left): acquisition and segmentation of 3D MR data, 3D reconstruction and meshing, build of scaffold for model support, printing and cleaning. Examples of aortas with BAV with and without aortic coarctation

from patient/device selection to a better understanding of the pathophysiology and haemodynamics of the disease, from practising new procedures to testing new devices, from designing novel training interventions to counselling patients [140]. Importantly, 3D printing relies entirely on the availability of 3D imaging datasets and all modalities (echo, MRI, CT) are compatible with the process of generating 3D reconstructions and then printing the corresponding anatomical models. Key steps of the 3D printing workflow are schematically summarised in Fig. 13.12.

Three-dimensional printing has been used to plan percutaneous and surgical interventions, as in the case of an aortic arch with CoA where the model increased the safety and reduced the duration of the real-time procedure, as well as the radiation dose and contrast administration [141]. Stent grafting collapse is possible in the case of an excessive oversized device, and another interesting case study described a preoperative stent grafting simulation using a 3D-printed model for extensive aortic arch repair in a patient with CoA with multiple aneurysms [142]. CoA is often accompanied by transverse arch hypoplasia and 3D models with virtually repaired CoA can be printed and connected to an MRI-compatible experimental setups (pulse duplicator systems) to generate haemodynamic measurements and preoperatively assess the potential correction and quantify residual transverse arch obstruction [143]. 3D models have also been created for an aortic arch with type A dissection due to untreated CoA with concomitant BAV and arterial hypertension, for educational purposes [144]. Overall, 3D printing can be used in different clinical scenarios of CoA and can aid in patient evaluation and management, with studies having also evaluated and validated the accuracy of the technique [145].

Fig. 13.13 3D thermoplastic polymer models used to produce patients' specific polymer mesh sleeves for PEARS procedure. (Reproduced with permission and courtesy of Tal Golesworthy)

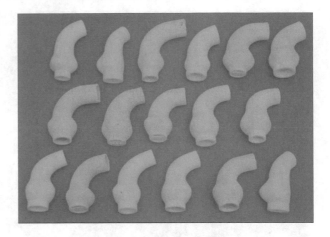

3D printing technology is also used in BAV to simulate transcatheter aortic valve implantation on a patient-specific 3D-printed model and predict paravalvular leak [146]. Three-dimensional printing has been also used in a follow-up study to assess the effectiveness of personalised external aortic root support (PEARS) for prevention of aortic root dilation in Marfan patients, by implanting a polymer mesh sleeve (Fig. 13.13) [147]. Finally, a study showed the possibility that a microporous fabric sleeve could be created on a 3D-printed aortic model and then incorporated to support the aortic root and allow recovery of the microstructure of the media [148]. Whilst larger studies are needed to demonstrate the undisputable benefit of such personalised approaches, increasing evidence suggests that 3D printing could positively impact on the prevention of aortic root dissection in Marfan patients [149]. In the future, the ability of designing and manufacturing personalised scaffolds could be integrated with the possibility of including personalised treatments, taking advantage of the therapeutic possibilities offered by 3D bio-printing technology.

13.5 Conclusions

Multimodality imaging today represents not only an integral element in the diagnosis and management of aortic disease, such as bicuspid aortic valve, Marfan syndrome and aortic coarctation, but also an invaluable source of data for more complex, often computer-based innovations that can contribute to our understanding of the underlying pathophysiology as well as to refining our ability of risk stratification, device selection and outcome prediction in the near future.

References

1. Hoffman JI, Kaplan S. The incidence of congenital heart disease. J Am Coll Cardiol. 2002;39(12):1890–900.
2. Fernandes SM, Sanders SP, Khairy P, Jenkins KJ, Gauvreau K, Lang P, et al. Morphology of bicuspid aortic valve in children and adolescents. J Am Coll Cardiol. 2004;44(8):1648–51.

3. Loeys BL, Chen J, Neptune ER, Judge DP, Podowski M, Holm T, et al. A syndrome of altered cardiovascular, craniofacial, neurocognitive and skeletal development caused by mutations in TGFBR1 or TGFBR2. Nat Genet. 2005;37(3):275–81.

4. Milewicz DM, Guo DC, Tran-Fadulu V, Lafont AL, Papke CL, Inamoto S, et al. Genetic basis of thoracic aortic aneurysms and dissections: focus on smooth muscle cell contractile dysfunction. Annu Rev Genomics Hum Genet. 2008;9:283–302.

5. Cedars A, Braverman AC. The many faces of bicuspid aortic valve disease. Progr Paediatr Cardiol. 2012;34(2):91–6.

6. Hor KN, Border WL, Cripe LH, Benson DW, Hinton RB. The presence of bicuspid aortic valve does not predict ventricular septal defect type. Am J Med Genet A. 2008;146A(24): 3202–5.

7. Treasure T, Pepper J, Golesworthy T, Mohiaddin R, Anderson RH. External aortic root support: NICE guidance. Heart. 2012;98(1):65–8.

8. Treasure T, Pepper J. Personalised external aortic root support (PEARS) compared with alternatives for people with life-threatening genetically determined aneurysms of the aortic root. Diseases. 2015;3(1):2–14.

9. Nishimura RA, Otto CM, Bonow RO, Carabello BA, Erwin JP 3rd, Guyton RA, et al. 2014 AHA/ACC guideline for the Management of Patients with Valvular Heart Disease: a report of the American College of Cardiology/American Heart Association task force on practice guidelines. Circulation. 2014;129(23):e521–643.

10. American College of Cardiology/American Heart Association Task Force on Practice G, Society of Cardiovascular A, Society for Cardiovascular A, Interventions, Society of Thoracic S, Bonow RO, et al. ACC/AHA 2006 guidelines for the management of patients with valvular heart disease: a report of the American College of Cardiology/American Heart Association Task Force on Practice Guidelines (writing committee to revise the 1998 Guidelines for the Management of Patients With Valvular Heart Disease): developed in collaboration with the Society of Cardiovascular Anesthesiologists: endorsed by the Society for Cardiovascular Angiography and Interventions and the Society of Thoracic Surgeons. Circulation. 2006;114(5): e84–231.

11. Detaint D, Michelena HI, Nkomo VT, Vahanian A, Jondeau G, Sarano ME. Aortic dilatation patterns and rates in adults with bicuspid aortic valves: a comparative study with Marfan syndrome and degenerative aortopathy. Heart. 2014;100(2):126–34.

12. Della Corte A, Bancone C, Buonocore M, Dialetto G, Covino FE, Manduca S, et al. Pattern of ascending aortic dimensions predicts the growth rate of the aorta in patients with bicuspid aortic valve. JACC Cardiovasc Imaging. 2013;6(12):1301–10.

13. Michelena HI, Prakash SK, Della Corte A, Bissell MM, Anavekar N, Mathieu P, et al. Bicuspid aortic valve: identifying knowledge gaps and rising to the challenge from the international bicuspid aortic valve consortium (BAVCon). Circulation. 2014;129(25):2691–704.

14. Pape LA, Tsai TT, Isselbacher EM, Oh JK, O'Ggara PT, Evangelista A, et al. Aortic diameter >or = 5.5 cm is not a good predictor of type A aortic dissection: observations from the international registry of acute aortic dissection (IRAD). Circulation. 2007;116(10):1120–7.

15. Kang JW, Song HG, Yang DH, Baek S, Kim DH, Song JM, et al. Association between bicuspid aortic valve phenotype and patterns of valvular dysfunction and bicuspid aortopathy comprehensive evaluation using MDCT and echocardiography. JACC Cardiovasc Imag. 2013;6(2):150–61.

16. Hiratzka LF, Bakris GL, Beckman JA, Bersin RM, Carr VF, Casey DE, et al. 2010 ACCF/AHA/AATS/ACR/ASA/SCA/SCAI/SIR/STS/SVM Guidelines for the Diagnosis and Management of Patients With Thoracic Aortic Disease—A Report of the American College of Cardiology Foundation/American Heart Association Task Force on Practice Guidelines, American Association for Thoracic Surgery, American College of Radiology, American Stroke Association, Society of Cardiovascular Anesthesiologists, Society for Cardiovascular Angiography and Interventions, Society of Interventional Radiology, Society of Thoracic Surgeons, and Society for Vascular Medicine. Circulation. 2010;121(13):E266–369.

17. Mc KV. The cardiovascular aspects of Marfan's syndrome: a heritable disorder of connective tissue. Circulation. 1955;11(3):321–42.

18. De Paepe A, Devereux RB, Dietz HC, Hennekam RC, Pyeritz RE. Revised diagnostic criteria for the Marfan syndrome. Am J Med Genet. 1996;62(4):417–26.

19. Erbel R, Aboyans V, Boileau C, Bossone E, Bartolomeo RD, Eggebrecht H, et al. 2014 ESC guidelines on the diagnosis and treatment of aortic diseases: document covering acute and chronic aortic diseases of the thoracic and abdominal aorta of the adult. The task force for the diagnosis and treatment of aortic diseases of the European Society of Cardiology (ESC). Eur Heart J. 2014;35(41):2873–926.

20. Bin Mahmood SU, Velasquez CA, Zafar MA, Saeyeldin AA, Brownstein AJ, Ziganshin BA, et al. Medical management of aortic disease in Marfan syndrome. Ann Cardiothorac Surg. 2017;6(6):654–61.

21. Hiratzka LF, Bakris GL, Beckman JA, Bersin RM, Carr VF, Casey DE Jr, et al. 2010 ACCF/AHA/AATS/ACR/ASA/SCA/SCAI/SIR/STS/SVM Guidelines for the diagnosis and management of patients with thoracic aortic disease. A Report of the American College of Cardiology Foundation/American Heart Association Task Force on Practice Guidelines, American Association for Thoracic Surgery, American College of Radiology, American Stroke Association, Society of Cardiovascular Anesthesiologists, Society for Cardiovascular Angiography and Interventions, Society of Interventional Radiology, Society of Thoracic Surgeons, and Society for Vascular Medicine. J Am Coll Cardiol. 2010;55(14): e27–e129.

22. Treasure T, Petrou M, Rosendahl U, Austin C, Rega F, Pirk J, et al. Personalized external aortic root support: a review of the current status. Eur J Cardiothorac Surg. 2016;50(3):400–4.

23. Perloff JK. The clinical recognition of congenital heart disease. 4th ed. Philadelphia: WB Saunders; 1994.

24. Niwa K, Perloff JK, Bhuta SM, Laks H, Drinkwater DC, Child JS, et al. Structural abnormalities of great arterial walls in congenital heart disease: light and electron microscopic analyses. Circulation. 2001;103(3):393–400.

25. Campbell M. Natural history of coarctation of the aorta. Br Heart J. 1970;32(5):633–40.

26. Connelly MS, Webb GD, Somerville J, Warnes CA, Perloff JK, Liberthson RR, et al. Canadian consensus conference on congenital heart defects in the adult 1996. Can J Cardiol. 1998;14(4):533–97.

27. Kvitting JP, Olin CL. Clarence Crafoord: a giant in cardiothoracic surgery, the first to repair aortic coarctation. Ann Thorac Surg. 2009;87(1):342–6.

28. Bambul Heck P, Pabst von Ohain J, Kaemmerer H, Ewert P, Hager A. Survival and cardiovascular events after coarctation-repair in long-term follow-up (COAFU): predictive value of clinical variables. Int J Cardiol. 2017;228:347–51.

29. Konen E, Merchant N, Provost Y, McLaughlin PR, Crossin J, Paul NS. Coarctation of the aorta before and after correction: the role of cardiovascular MRI. Am J Roentgenol. 2004;182(5):1333–9.

30. Valsangiacomo Buechel ER, Grosse-Wortmann L, Fratz S, Eichhorn J, Sarikouch S, Greil GF, et al. Indications for cardiovascular magnetic resonance in children with congenital and acquired heart disease: an expert consensus paper of the imaging working group of the AEPC and the cardiovascular magnetic resonance section of the EACVI. Eur Heart J Cardiovasc Imaging. 2015;16(3):281–97.

31. Babu-Narayan SV, Giannakoulas G, Valente AM, Li W, Gatzoulis MA. Imaging of congenital heart disease in adults. Eur Heart J. 2016;37(15):1182–95.

32. Burchill LJ, Huang J, Tretter JT, Khan AM, Crean AM, Veldtman GR, et al. Noninvasive imaging in adult congenital heart disease. Circ Res. 2017;120(6):995–1014.

33. Orwat S, Diller GP, Baumgartner H. Imaging of congenital heart disease in adults: choice of modalities. Eur Heart J Cardiovasc Imaging. 2014;15(1):6–17.

34. Lancellotti P, Tribouilloy C, Hagendorff A, Moura L, Popescu BA, Agricola E, et al. European Association of Echocardiography recommendations for the assessment of valvular regurgitation. Part 1: aortic and pulmonary regurgitation (native valve disease). Eur J Echocardiogr. 2010;11(3):223–44.

35. Baumgartner H, Hung J, Bermejo J, Chambers JB, Evangelista A, Griffin BP, et al. Echocardiographic assessment of valve stenosis: EAE/ASE recommendations for clinical practice. Eur J Echocardiogr. 2009;10(1):1–25.

36. Lang RM, Badano LP, Mor-Avi V, Afilalo J, Armstrong A, Ernande L, et al. Recommendations for cardiac chamber quantification by echocardiography in adults: an update from the American Society of Echocardiography and the European Association of Cardiovascular Imaging. J Am Soc Echocardiogr. 2015;28(1):1–39 e14.

37. Nagueh SF, Smiseth OA, Appleton CP, Byrd BF 3rd, Dokainish H, Edvardsen T, et al. Recommendations for the evaluation of left ventricular diastolic function by echocardiography: an update from the American Society of Echocardiography and the European Association of Cardiovascular Imaging. Eur Heart J Cardiovasc Imaging. 2016;17(12):1321–60.

38. Lang RM, Badano LP, Mor-Avi V, Afilalo J, Armstrong A, Ernande L, et al. Recommendations for cardiac chamber quantification by echocardiography in adults: an update from the American Society of Echocardiography and the European Association of Cardiovascular Imaging. Eur Heart J Cardiovasc Imaging. 2015;16(3):233–70.

39. Simpson J, Lopez L, Acar P, Friedberg MK, Khoo NS, Ko HH, et al. Three-dimensional echocardiography in congenital heart disease: an expert consensus document from the European Association of Cardiovascular Imaging and the American Society of Echocardiography. J Am Soc Echocardiogr. 2017;30(1):1–27.

40. Sicari R, Nihoyannopoulos P, Evangelista A, Kasprzak J, Lancellotti P, Poldermans D, et al. Stress echocardiography expert consensus statement—European Association of Echocardiography (EAE) (a registered branch of the ESC). Eur J Echocardiogr. 2008;9(4):415–37.

41. Park JH, Woo JS, Ju S, Jung SW, Lee I, Kim JB, et al. Layer-specific analysis of dobutamine stress echocardiography for the evaluation of coronary artery disease. Medicine (Baltimore). 2016;95(32):e4549.

42. Maintz D, Seifarth H, Raupach R, Flohr T, Rink M, Sommer T, et al. 64-slice multidetector coronary CT angiography: in vitro evaluation of 68 different stents. Eur Radiol. 2006;16(4):818–26.

43. Yang WJ, Chen KM, Pang LF, Guo Y, Li JY, Zhang H, et al. High-definition computed tomography for coronary artery stent imaging: a phantom study. Korean J Radiol. 2012;13(1):20–6.

44. den Harder AM, Sucha D, van Hamersvelt RW, Budde RP, de Jong PA, Schilham AM, et al. Imaging of pediatric great vessel stents: computed tomography or magnetic resonance imaging? PLoS One. 2017;12(1):e0171138.

45. Rigsby CK, McKenney SE, Hill KD, Chelliah A, Einstein AJ, Han BK, et al. Radiation dose management for pediatric cardiac computed tomography: a report from the image gently 'Have-A-Heart' campaign. Pediatr Radiol. 2018;48(1):5–20.

46. Barrera CA, Otero HJ, White AM, Saul D, Biko DM. Image quality and radiation dose of ECG-triggered high-pitch dual-source cardiac computed tomography angiography in children for the evaluation of central vascular stents. Int J Cardiovasc Imaging. 2019;35(2):367–74.

47. Nordmeyer J, Gaudin R, Tann OR, Lurz PC, Bonhoeffer P, Taylor AM, et al. MRI may be sufficient for noninvasive assessment of great vessel stents: an in vitro comparison of MRI, CT, and conventional angiography. Am J Roentgenol. 2010;195(4):865–71.

48. Blanke P, Weir-McCall JR, Achenbach S, Delgado V, Hausleiter J, Jilaihawi H, et al. Computed tomography imaging in the context of transcatheter aortic valve implantation (TAVI) / transcatheter aortic valve replacement (TAVR): an expert consensus document of the Society of Cardiovascular Computed Tomography. J Cardiovasc Comput Tomogr. 2019;13(1):1–20.

49. Abbara S, Blanke P, Maroules CD, Cheezum M, Choi AD, Han BK, et al. SCCT guidelines for the performance and acquisition of coronary computed tomographic angiography: a report of the society of cardiovascular computed tomography guidelines committee: endorsed by the north American Society for Cardiovascular Imaging (NASCI). J Cardiovasc Comput Tomogr. 2016;10(6):435–49.

50. Vasanawala SS, Hanneman K, Alley MT, Hsiao A. Congenital heart disease assessment with 4D flow MRI. J Magn Reson Imaging. 2015;42(4):870–86.

51. Bollache E, Barker AJ, Dolan RS, Carr JC, van Ooij P, Ahmadian R, et al. K-t accelerated aortic 4D flow MRI in under two minutes: feasibility and impact of resolution, k-space sampling patterns, and respiratory navigator gating on hemodynamic measurements. Magn Reson Med. 2018;79(1):195–207.
52. Donati F, Figueroa CA, Smith NP, Lamata P, Nordsletten DA. Non-invasive pressure difference estimation from PC-MRI using the work-energy equation. Med Image Anal. 2015;26(1):159–72.
53. Stankovic Z, Allen BD, Garcia J, Jarvis KB, Markl M. 4D flow imaging with MRI. Cardiovasc Diagn Ther. 2014;4(2):173–92.
54. Lantz J, Ebbers T, Engvall J, Karlsson M. Numerical and experimental assessment of turbulent kinetic energy in an aortic coarctation. J Biomech. 2013;46(11):1851–8.
55. Randles A, Frakes DH, Leopold JA. Computational fluid dynamics and additive manufacturing to diagnose and treat cardiovascular disease. Trends Biotechnol. 2017;35(11):1049–61.
56. Secomb TW. Hemodynamics. Compr Physiol. 2016;6(2):975–1003.
57. Masutani EM, Contijoch F, Kyubwa E, Cheng J, Alley MT, Vasanawala S, et al. Volumetric segmentation-free method for rapid visualization of vascular wall shear stress using 4D flow MRI. Magn Reson Med. 2018;80(2):748–55.
58. Goubergrits L, Mevert R, Yevtushenko P, Schaller J, Kertzscher U, Meier S, et al. The impact of MRI-based inflow for the hemodynamic evaluation of aortic coarctation. Ann Biomed Eng. 2013;41(12):2575–87.
59. Hope MD, Meadows AK, Hope TA, Ordovas KG, Saloner D, Reddy GP, et al. Clinical evaluation of aortic coarctation with 4D flow MR imaging. J Magn Reson Imaging. 2010;31(3);711–8.
60. Frydrychowicz A, Markl M, Hirtler D, Harloff A, Schlensak C, Geiger J, et al. Aortic hemodynamics in patients with and without repair of aortic coarctation in vivo analysis by 4D flow-sensitive magnetic resonance imaging. Invest Radiol. 2011;46(5):317–25.
61. Casas B, Lantz J, Dyverfeldt P, Ebbers T. 4D flow MRI-based pressure loss estimation in stenotic flows: evaluation using numerical simulations. Magn Reson Med. 2016;75(4):1808–21.
62. Cicek MS. Altered hemodynamics in bicuspid aortic valve disease: leaning more toward nurture! J Thorac Cardiovasc Surg. 2017;153(4):S63–S4.
63. Sophocleous F, Milano EG, Pontecorboli G, Chivasso P, Caputo M, Rajakaruna C, et al. Enlightening the association between bicuspid aortic valve and aortopathy. J Cardiovasc Dev Dis. 2018;5(2):21.
64. Maredia AK, Greenway SC, Verma S, Fedak PWM. Bicuspid aortic valve-associated aortopathy: update on biomarkers. Curr Opin Cardiol. 2018;33(2):134–9.
65. Forte A, Della Corte A. Editorial: the pathogenetic mechanisms at the basis of aortopathy associated with bicuspid aortic valve: insights from "omics", models of disease and emergent technologies. Front Physiol. 2017;8.
66. Youssefi P, Gomez A, He TG, Anderson L, Bunce N, Sharma R, et al. Patient-specific computational fluid dynamics-assessment of aortic hemodynamics in a spectrum of aortic valve pathologies. J Thorac Cardiovasc Surg. 2017;153(1):8.
67. den Reijer PM, Sallee D, van der Velden P, Zaaijer ER, Parks WJ, Ramamurthy S, et al. Hemodynamic predictors of aortic dilatation in bicuspid aortic valve by velocity-encoded cardiovascular magnetic resonance. J Cardiovasc Magn Reson. 2010;12:4.
68. Hope MD, Hope TA, Crook SES, Ordovas KG, Urbania TH, Alley MT, et al. 4D flow CMR in assessment of valve-related ascending aortic disease. JACC Cardiovasc Imag. 2011;4(7):781–7.
69. DeCampli WM. Ascending aortopathy with bicuspid aortic valve: more, but not enough, evidence for the hemodynamic theory. J Thorac Cardiovasc Surg. 2017;153(1):6–7.
70. Piatti F, Sturla F, Bissell MM, Pirola S, Lombardi M, Nesteruk I, et al. 4D flow analysis of BAV-related fluid-dynamic alterations: evidences of wall shear stress alterations in absence of clinically-relevant aortic anatomical remodeling. Front Physiol. 2017;8.
71. Guzzardi DG, Barker AJ, van Ooij P, Malaisrie SC, Puthumana JJ, Belke DD, et al. Valve-related hemodynamics mediate human bicuspid aortopathy insights from wall shear stress mapping. J Am Coll Cardiol. 2015;66(8):892–900.

72. Bollache E, Guzzardi DG, Sattari S, Olsen KE, Di Martino ES, Malaisrie SC, et al. Aortic valve-mediated wall shear stress is heterogeneous and predicts regional aortic elastic fiber thinning in bicuspid aortic valve-associated aortopathy. J Thorac Cardiovasc Surg. 2018;156(6):2112.
73. Farag ES, van Ooij P, Planken RN, Dukker KCP, de Heer F, Bouma BJ, et al. Aortic valve stenosis and aortic diameters determine the extent of increased wall shear stress in bicuspid aortic valve disease. J Magn Reson Imaging. 2018;48(2):522–30.
74. Grewal N, Girdauskas E, DeRuiter M, Goumans MJ, Poelmann RE, Klautz RJM, et al. The role of hemodynamics in bicuspid aortopathy: a histopathologic study. Cardiovasc Pathol. 2019;41:29–37.
75. McNally A, Madan A, Sucosky P. Morphotype-dependent flow characteristics in bicuspid aortic valve ascending aortas: a benchtop particle image velocimetry study. Front Physiol. 2017;8.
76. Rodriguez-Palomares JF, Dux-Santoy L, Guala A, Kale R, Maldonado G, Teixido-Tura G, et al. Aortic flow patterns and wall shear stress maps by 4D-flow cardiovascular magnetic resonance in the assessment of aortic dilatation in bicuspid aortic valve disease. J Cardiovasc Magn Reson. 2018;20.
77. Cao K, Atkins SK, McNally A, Liu J, Sucosky P. Simulations of morphotype-dependent hemodynamics in non-dilated bicuspid aortic valve aortas. J Biomech. 2017;50:63–70.
78. Sievers HH, Stierle U, Hachmann RMS, Charitos EI. New insights in the association between bicuspid aortic valve phenotype, aortic configuration and valve haemodynamics. Eur J Cardiothorac Surg. 2016;49(2):439–46.
79. Habchi KM, Ashikhmina E, Vieira VM, Shahram JT, Isselbacher EM, Sundt TM, et al. Association between bicuspid aortic valve morphotype and regional dilatation of the aortic root and trunk. Int J Cardiovasc Imaging. 2017;33(3):341–9.
80. Bissell MM, Loudon M, Hess AT, Stoll V, Orchard E, Neubauer S, et al. Differential flow improvements after valve replacements in bicuspid aortic valve disease: a cardiovascular magnetic resonance assessment. J Cardiovasc Magn Reson. 2018;20.
81. Naito S, Gross T, Disha K, von Kodolitsch Y, Reichenspurner H, Girdauskas E. Late post-AVR progression of bicuspid aortopathy: link to hemodynamics. Gen Thorac Cardiovasc Surg. 2017;65(5):252–8.
82. van Ooij P, Potters WV, Nederveen AJ, Allen BD, Collins J, Carr J, et al. A methodology to detect abnormal relative wall shear stress on the full surface of the thoracic aorta using four-dimensional flow MRI. Magn Reson Med. 2015;73(3):1216–27.
83. van Ooij P, Potters W, Nederveen A, Collins J, Carr J, Malaisrie S, et al. Thoracic aortic wall shear stress atlases in patients with bicuspid aortic valves. J Cardiovasc Magn Reson. 2014;16:161.
84. van Ooij P, Garcia J, Potters WV, Malaisrie SC, Collins JD, Carr JC, et al. Age-related changes in aortic 3D blood flow velocities and wall shear stress: implications for the identification of altered hemodynamics in patients with aortic valve disease. J Magn Reson Imaging. 2016;43(5):1239–49.
85. van Ooij P, Markl M, Collins JD, Carr JC, Rigsby C, Bonow RO, et al. Aortic valve stenosis alters expression of regional aortic wall shear stress: new insights from a 4-dimensional flow magnetic resonance imaging study of 571 subjects. J Am Heart Assoc. 2017;6(9): e005959.
86. Wang HH, Chiu HH, Tseng WYI, Peng HH. Does altered aortic flow in Marfan syndrome relate to aortic root dilatation? J Magn Reson Imaging. 2016;44(2):500–8.
87. Geiger J, Hirtler D, Gottfried K, Rahman O, Bollache E, Barker AJ, et al. Longitudinal evaluation of aortic hemodynamics in Marfan syndrome: new insights from a 4D flow cardiovascular magnetic resonance multi-year follow-up study. J Cardiovasc Magn Reson. 2017;19.
88. Geiger J, Markl M, Herzer L, Hirtler D, Loeffelbein F, Stiller B, et al. Aortic flow patterns in patients with Marfan syndrome assessed by flow-sensitive four-dimensional MRI. J Magn Reson Imaging. 2012;35(3):594–600.
89. Geiger J, Arnold R, Herzer L, Hirtler D, Stankovic Z, Russe M, et al. Aortic wall shear stress in Marfan syndrome. Magn Reson Med. 2013;70(4):1137–44.

90. Hope TA, Kvitting JPE, Hope MD, Miller DC, Markl M, Herfkens RJ. Evaluation of Marfan patients status post valve-sparing aortic root replacement with 4D flow. Magn Reson Imaging. 2013;31(9):1479–84.
91. Guala A, Rodriguez-Palomares J, Dux-Santoy L, Teixido-Tura G, Maldonado G, Galian L, et al. Influence of aortic dilation on the regional aortic stiffness of bicuspid aortic valve assessed by 4-dimensional flow cardiac magnetic resonance comparison with Marfan syndrome and degenerative aortic aneurysm. JACC Cardiovasc Imag. 2019;12(6): 1020–9.
92. de Wit A, Vis K, Jeremy RW. Aortic stiffness in heritable aortopathies: relationship to aneurysm growth rate. Heart Lung Circ. 2013;22(1):3–11.
93. Lamata P, Pitcher A, Krittian S, Nordsletten D, Bissell MM, Cassar T, et al. Aortic relative pressure components derived from four-dimensional flow cardiovascular magnetic resonance. Magn Reson Med. 2014;72(4):1162–9.
94. Lewandowski AJ, Raman B, Banerjee R, Milanesi M. Novel insights into complex cardiovascular pathologies using 4D flow analysis by cardiovascular magnetic resonance imaging. Curr Pharm Des. 2017;23(22):3262–7.
95. Lee BK. Computational fluid dynamics in cardiovascular disease. Korean Circ J. 2011;41(8): 423–30.
96. Riesenkampff E, Fernandes JF, Meier S, Goubergrits L, Kropf S, Schubert S, et al. Pressure fields by flow-sensitive, 4D, velocity-encoded CMR in patients with aortic coarctation. JACC Cardiovasc Imaging. 2014;7(9):920–6.
97. Bruning J, Hellmeier F, Yevtushenko P, Kuhne T, Goubergrits L. Uncertainty quantification for non-invasive assessment of pressure drop across a coarctation of the aorta using CFD. Cardiovasc Eng Technol. 2018;9(4):582–96.
98. Rengier F, Delles M, Eichhorn J, Azad YJ, von Tengg-Kobligk H, Ley-Zaporozhan J, et al. Noninvasive pressure difference mapping derived from 4D flow MRI in patients with unrepaired and repaired aortic coarctation. Cardiovasc Diagn Ther. 2014;4(2):97–103.
99. Rengier F, Delles M, Eichhorn J, Azad YJ, von Tengg-Kobligk H, Ley-Zaporozhan J, et al. Noninvasive 4D pressure difference mapping derived from 4D flow MRI in patients with repaired aortic coarctation: comparison with young healthy volunteers. Int J Cardiovasc Imaging. 2015;31(4):823–30.
100. Ralovich K, Itu L, Vitanovski D, Sharma P, Ionasec R, Mihalef V, et al. Noninvasive hemodynamic assessment, treatment outcome prediction and follow-up of aortic coarctation from MR imaging. Med Phys. 2015;42(5):2143–56.
101. Rinaudo A, D'Ancona G, Baglini R, Amaducci A, Follis F, Pilato M, et al. Computational fluid dynamics simulation to evaluate aortic coarctation gradient with contrast-enhanced CT. Comput Methods Biomech Biomed Engin. 2015;18(10):1066–71.
102. Goubergrits L, Riesenkampff E, Yevtushenko P, Schaller J, Kertzscher U, Hennemuth A, et al. MRI-based computational fluid dynamics for diagnosis and treatment prediction: clinical validation study in patients with coarctation of aorta. J Magn Reson Imaging. 2015;41(4):909–16.
103. Yang F, Zhai B, Hou LG, Zhang Q, Wang J. Computational fluid dynamics in the numerical simulation analysis of end-to-side anastomosis for coarctation of the aorta. J Thorac Dis. 2018;10(12):6578–84.
104. Cosentino D, Capelli C, Derrick G, Khambadkone S, Muthurangu V, Taylor AM, et al. Patient-specific computational models to support interventional procedures: a case study of complex aortic re-coarctation. EuroIntervention. 2015;11(6):669–72.
105. LaDisa JF, Figueroa CA, Vignon-Clementel IE, Kim HJ, Xiao N, Ellwein LM, et al. Computational simulations for aortic coarctation: representative results from a sampling of patients. J Biomech Eng Trans ASME. 2011;133(9):091008.
106. Pant S, Fabreges B, Gerbeau JF, Vignon-Clementel IE. A methodological paradigm for patient-specific multi-scale CFD simulations: from clinical measurements to parameter estimates for individual analysis. Int J Numer Method Biomed Eng. 2014;30(12): 1614–48.

107. Atkins SK, Cao K, Rajamannan NM, Sucosky P. Bicuspid aortic valve hemodynamics induces abnormal medial remodeling in the convexity of porcine ascending aortas. Biomech Model Mechanobiol. 2014;13(6):1209–25.
108. Atkins SK, Moore AN, Sucosky P. Bicuspid aortic valve hemodynamics does not promote remodeling in porcine aortic wall concavity. World J Cardiol. 2016;8(1):89–97.
109. Oliveira D, Rosa SA, Tiago J, Ferreira RC, Agapito AF, Sequeira A. Bicuspid aortic valve aortopathies: an hemodynamics characterization in dilated aortas. Comput Methods Biomech Biomed Engin. 2019;22:815.
110. Liu J, Shar JA, Sucosky P. Wall shear stress directional abnormalities in BAV aortas: toward a new hemodynamic predictor of aortopathy? Front Physiol. 2018;9:993.
111. Kimura N, Nakamura M, Komiya K, Nishi S, Yamaguchi A, Tanaka O, et al. Patient-specific assessment of hemodynamics by computational fluid dynamics in patients with bicuspid aortopathy. J Thorac Cardiovasc Surg. 2017;153(4):S52.
112. Condemi F, Campisi S, Viallon M, Croisille P, Fuzelier JF, Avril S. Ascending thoracic aorta aneurysm repair induces positive hemodynamic outcomes in a patient with unchanged bicuspid aortic valve. J Biomech. 2018;81:145–8.
113. Wendell DC, Samyn MM, Cava JR, Ellwein LM, Krolikowski MM, Gandy KL, et al. Including aortic valve morphology in computational fluid dynamics simulations: initial findings and application to aortic coarctation. Med Eng Phys. 2013;35(6):723–35.
114. Gulan U, Calen C, Duru F, Holzner M. Blood flow patterns and pressure loss in the ascending aorta: a comparative study on physiological and aneurysmal conditions. J Biomech. 2018;76:152–9.
115. Lamata P, Casero R, Carapella V, Niederer SA, Bishop MJ, Schneider JE, et al. Images as drivers of progress in cardiac computational modelling. Prog Biophys Mol Biol. 2014;115(2–3):198–212.
116. Fonseca CG, Backhaus M, Bluemke DA, Britten RD, Chung JD, Cowan BR, et al. The cardiac atlas project—an imaging database for computational modeling and statistical atlases of the heart. Bioinformatics. 2011;27(16):2288–95.
117. Durrleman S, Pennec X, Trouve A, Ayache N. Statistical models of sets of curves and surfaces based on currents. Med Image Anal. 2009;13(5):793–808.
118. Biglino G, Capelli C, Bruse J, Bosi GM, Taylor AM, Schievano S. Computational modelling for congenital heart disease: how far are we from clinical translation? Heart. 2017;103(2):98–103.
119. Bruse JL, Khushnood A, McLeod K, Biglino G, Sermesant M, Pennec X, et al. How successful is successful? Aortic arch shape after successful aortic coarctation repair correlates with left ventricular function. J Thorac Cardiovasc Surg. 2017;153(2):418–27.
120. Bruse JL, McLeod K, Biglino G, Ntsinjana HN, Capelli C, Hsia TY, et al. A statistical shape modelling framework to extract 3D shape biomarkers from medical imaging data: assessing arch morphology of repaired coarctation of the aorta. BMC Med Imaging. 2016;16(1):40.
121. Sophocleous F, Biffi B, Milano EG, Bruse J, Caputo M, Rajakaruna C, et al. Aortic morphological variability in patients with bicuspid aortic valve and aortic coarctation. Eur J Cardiothorac Surg. 2018;55(4):704–13.
122. Bruse JL, Zuluaga MA, Khushnood A, McLeod K, Ntsinjana HN, Hsia TY, et al. Detecting clinically meaningful shape clusters in medical image data: metrics analysis for hierarchical clustering applied to healthy and pathological aortic arches. IEEE Trans Biomed Eng. 2017;64(10):2373–83.
123. Dijkema HJ, Slieker MG, Leiner T, Grotenhuis HB. Arterioventricular interaction after coarctation repair. Am Heart J. 2018;201:49–53.
124. Li VWY, Cheung YF. Arterial-left ventricular-left atrial coupling late after repair of aortic coarctation and interruption. Eur Heart J Cardiovasc Imag. 2015;16(7):771–80.
125. Keshavarz-Motamed Z, Nezami FR, Partida RA, Nakamura K, Staziaki PV, Ben-Assa E, et al. Elimination of transcoarctation pressure gradients has no impact on left ventricular function or aortic shear stress after intervention in patients with mild coarctation. JACC Cardiovasc Interv. 2016;9(18):1953–65.

126. Quail MA, Short R, Pandya B, Steeden JA, Khushnood A, Taylor AM, et al. Abnormal wave reflections and left ventricular hypertrophy late after coarctation of the aorta repair. Hypertension. 2017;69(3):501–9.
127. Mynard JP, Kowalski R, Cheung MMH, Smolich JJ. Beyond the aorta: partial transmission of reflected waves from aortic coarctation into supra-aortic branches modulates cerebral hemodynamics and left ventricular load. Biomech Model Mechanobiol. 2017;16(2):635–50.
128. Kowalski R, Lee MGY, Doyle LW, Cheong JLY, Smolich JJ, d'Udekem Y, et al. Reduced aortic distensibility is associated with higher Aorto-carotid wave transmission and central aortic systolic pressure in young adults after Coarctation repair. J Am Heart Assoc. 2019;8(7):e011411.
129. Nucifora G, Miller J, Gillebert C, Shah R, Perry R, Raven C, et al. Ascending aorta and myocardial mechanics in patients with "clinically normal" bicuspid aortic valve insights from cardiovascular magnetic resonance tissue-tracking imaging. Int Heart J. 2018;59(4):741–9.
130. Ekici F, Uslu D, Bozkurt S. Elasticity of ascending aorta and left ventricular myocardial functions in children with bicuspid aortic valve. Echocardiography. 2017;34(11):1660–6.
131. Geiger J, Rahsepar AA, Suwa K, Powell A, Ghasemiesfe A, Barker AJ, et al. 4D flow MRI, cardiac function, and T1-mapping: association of valve-mediated changes in aortic hemodynamics with left ventricular remodeling. J Magn Reson Imaging. 2018;48(1):121–31.
132. Burris NS, Lima APS, Hope MD, Ordovas KG. Feature tracking cardiac MRI reveals abnormalities in ventricular function in patients with bicuspid aortic valve and preserved ejection fraction. Tomography. 2018;4(1):26–32.
133. Ruijsink B, Puyol-Anton E, Oksuz I, Sinclair M, Bai W, Schnabel JA, et al. Fully automated, quality-controlled cardiac analysis from CMR: validation and large-scale application to characterize cardiac function. JACC Cardiovasc Imaging. 2019;13(3):684–95.
134. Loeper F, Oosterhof J, van den Dorpel M, van der Linde D, Lu YX, Robertson E, et al. Ventricular-vascular coupling in Marfan and non-Marfan aortopathies. J Am Heart Assoc. 2016;5(11):e003705.
135. Xiong GL, Choi G, Taylor CA. Virtual interventions for image-based blood flow computation. Comput Aided Des. 2012;44(1):3–14.
136. Kwon S, Feinstein JA, Dholakia RJ, LaDisa JF. Quantification of local hemodynamic alterations caused by virtual implantation of three commercially available stents for the treatment of aortic coarctation. Pediatr Cardiol. 2014;35(4):732–40.
137. Gundert TJ, Shadden SC, Williams AR, Koo BK, Feinstein JA, LaDisa JF. A rapid and computationally inexpensive method to virtually implant current and next-generation stents into subject-specific computational fluid dynamics models. Ann Biomed Eng. 2011;39(5):1423–37.
138. Burkhardt BEU, Byrne N, Forte MNV, Iannaccone F, De Beule M, Morgan GJ, et al. Evaluation of a modified Cheatham-platinum stent for the treatment of aortic coarctation by finite element modelling. JRSM Cardiovasc Dis. 2018;7:204800401877395.
139. Andersson M, Lantz J, Ebbers T, Karlsson M. Quantitative assessment of turbulence and flow eccentricity in an aortic coarctation: impact of virtual interventions (vol 6, pg 281, 2015). Cardiovasc Eng Technol. 2015;6(4):577–89.
140. Biglino G, Capelli C, Taylor AM, Schievano S. 3D printing cardiovascular anatomy: a single-centre experience. In: New trends in 3D printing. London: IntechOpen; 2016.
141. Ghisiawan N, Herbert CE, Zussman M, Verigan A, Stapleton GE. The use of a three-dimensional print model of an aortic arch to plan a complex percutaneous intervention in a patient with coarctation of the aorta. Cardiol Young. 2016;26(8):1568–72.
142. Shijo T, Shirakawa T, Yoshitatsu M, Iwata K. Stent grafting simulation using a three-dimensional printed model for extensive aortic arch repair combined with coarctation. Eur J Cardiothorac Surg. 2018;54(3):593–5.
143. Whitehead K, Gralewski K, Dori Y. Abstract 18738: using 3D printing with virtual surgery to identify residual transverse arch obstruction in coarctation correction. Circulation. 2016;134:A18738.

144. Meyer-Szary J, Waldoch A, Sabiniewicz R, Wozniak-Mielczarek L, Brzezinski M, Kwiatkowska J. Life-threatening complication of untreated coarctation of the aorta in a teenager solidified in a three-dimensional printed cardiovascular model. Cardiol J. 2018;25(3): 420–1.
145. Parimi M, Buelter J, Thanugundla V, Condoor S, Parkar N, Danon S, et al. Feasibility and validity of printing 3D heart models from rotational angiography (vol 39, pg 653, 2018). Pediatr Cardiol. 2018;39(4):659.
146. Lee APW, Leong CWM, Kwok KW, Fan YT. Using 3D printed models for planning transcatheter aortic valve implantation in patients with bicuspid aortic valve. J Am Coll Cardiol. 2018;71(11):1130.
147. Izgi C, Newsome S, Alpendurada F, Nyktari E, Boutsikou M, Pepper J, et al. External aortic root support to prevent aortic dilatation in patients with Marfan syndrome. J Am Coll Cardiol. 2018;72(10):1095–105.
148. Pacini D. Re: histology of a Marfan aorta 4.5 years after personalized external aortic root support. Eur J Cardiothorac Surg. 2015;48(3):505–6.
149. Pepper J, Petrou M, Rega F, Rosendahl U, Golesworthy T, Treasure T. Implantation of an individually computer-designed and manufactured external support for the Marfan aortic root. Multimed Man Cardiothorac Surg. 2013;2013:mmt004.

Transposition of the Great Arteries Repaired by Arterial Switch Operation

14

Magalie Ladouceur, Gilles Soulat, and Elie Mousseaux

14.1 Long-Term Results and Surveillance After Arterial Switch Operation

In 1975, Jatene et al. [1] performed the first successful arterial switch operation (ASO). During the ASO, the great arteries are transected and "switched" to the other semilunar valve, and the coronary arteries are translocated to the "neo-aorta." The LeCompte maneuver [2] is also performed during such operation to avoid distortion of the branch pulmonary arteries in the process of switching the great vessels. The LeCompte maneuver relocates the aorta posterior to the pulmonary artery such that both branch pulmonary arteries extend anteriorly to the aorta (Fig. 14.1). However, patients can have residual lesions and/or sequelae from interventions that require lifelong surveillance and care. Survival into adulthood after ASO is excellent and the risk of reoperation seems to be low [3]. Nevertheless, long-term outcomes in adults with ASO are scarce [4, 5] and some results suggest a significant proportion

M. Ladouceur (✉)
Université de Paris, PARCC, INSERM, Paris, France

Medico-Surgical Unit of Adult Congenital Heart Disease, Assistance Publique Hôpitaux de Paris, Hôpital Européen Georges Pompidou-AP-HP, Paris University, Paris, France

Adult Congenital Heart Disease Unit, Centre de référence des Malformations Cardiaques Congénitales Complexes, M3C, Paris, France
e-mail: magalie.ladouceur@aphp.fr

G. Soulat · E. Mousseaux
Université de Paris, PARCC, INSERM, Paris, France

Medico-Surgical Unit of Adult Congenital Heart Disease, Assistance Publique Hôpitaux de Paris, Hôpital Européen Georges Pompidou-AP-HP, Paris University, Paris, France

Cardiovascular Imaging Department, Paris, France
e-mail: gilles.soulat@aphp.fr; elie.mousseaux@aphp.fr

© Springer Nature Switzerland AG 2021
P. Gallego, I. Valverde (eds.), *Multimodality Imaging Innovations In Adult Congenital Heart Disease*, Congenital Heart Disease in Adolescents and Adults,
https://doi.org/10.1007/978-3-030-61927-5_14

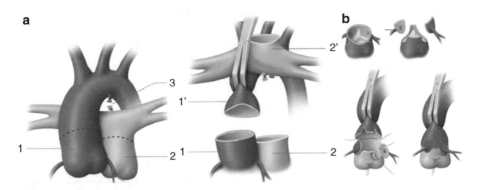

Fig. 14.1 Description of arterial switch procedure with LeCompte maneuver. After initiating extracorporeal circulation and clamping the aorta, the ascending aorta (1) and the pulmonary artery (2) are sectioned above the sinotubular junction (Panel **a**). The coronary ostia are detached from the aortic root, with surrounding aortic wall, and then mobilized and reimplanted at the level of the pulmonary root (Panel **b**). After section of the ductus arteriosus (3) and mobilization of the pulmonary artery branches, the pulmonary bifurcation is transposed anteriorly to the ascending aorta (Lecompte maneuver, Panel **a**). The native pulmonary root (which becomes the neo-aortic root arising from the left ventricle) is anastomosed to the proximal ascending aorta. The loss of aortic wall created by excision of the coronary ostia is compensated by an autologous pericardium patch. The native aortic root (which becomes the pulmonary neo-root arising from the right ventricle) is anastomosed to the pulmonary artery trunk just before the pulmonary bifurcation. From Vouhé et al. [6]

of re-interventions. ASO may have lifelong consequences, some of which may still be unrecognized, requiring ongoing medical surveillance.

Myocardial ischemia is the most feared complication. Indeed, during ASO, coronary arteries are transferred to the neo-aorta, which may be a difficult step in the case of particular abnormalities of origin or distribution of these arteries. Obstructed coronary arteries are present in 5–7% of survivors [3, 7, 8] and remain the most common cause of morbidity and mortality following ASO. The incidence of coronary events is most prevalent in the first 3 months after ASO and has bimodal pattern. Indeed, a high early incidence was first observed, even if such incidence tends to decrease with surgical experience, followed by a low occurrence of coronary events. Furthermore, such coronary events at long term, was rarely reported in adult population. The prevalence is estimated between 0.7% and 2.1% [5, 7], but detection of subclinical myocardial ischemia after the ASO remains a challenge.

Risk of myocardial ischemia is closely associated with a risk of life-threatening ventricular tachyarrhythmia including sudden cardiac death (SCD). Studies have reported a 0.3 to 0.8% incidence of SCD [3–5, 9, 10]. Such incidence seems to decrease in adulthood reaching 1.8/1000 patient-year [11]. Early SCD (after ASO) is frequently associated with technical difficulties during coronary artery transfer [7]. Whether this is associated with atypical or intramural coronary arteries or exercise-induced external compression of unusually distributed coronary arteries, is unclear [9, 12, 13]. As consequence, high-risk patients with a history of atypical, intramural or problematic coronary reimplantation may require in depth screening prior to engaging in high-level physical activity [14, 15].

Other events concern lesions of the great arteries. Neo-aortic valve regurgitation (AR) is common after ASO. Freedom from AR of Grades IV, III, and II at 23 years was 90.2 ± 6.6, 70.9 ± 9.6, and $20.3 \pm 5.5\%$, respectively. Older age at time of ASO, presence of VSD, bicuspid pulmonic valve, previous PA banding, perioperative mild AR and higher neo-aortic root/ascending aorta ratio were all identified as risk factors for AR [16–18]. Neo-aortic root dilation is common [19, 20], especially if there is size discrepancy of the great arteries [18]. Aortic root dilatation is moderately progressive during follow-up with an average increase rate of 0.03 points per year of the root Z-score [17]. Of note, none aortic dissection has been described after ASO, but the duration of the monitoring proposed in the published studies was limited and it is currently difficult to anticipate the very long-term outcome of this lesion.

Finally, amongst vascular sequelae after ASO, the neopulmonary root and pulmonary artery branches are commonly involved. Pulmonary branch stenosis was observed in two third of patients after ASO and was the most common reason for reintervention [21]. Abnormal pulmonary artery stretch, decreased pulmonary artery distensibility because of scar and overt stenosis of the neopulmonary root and branch pulmonary arteries may result in right ventricular hypertrophy, right ventricular relaxation disturbances, and right ventricular dilatation. Smaller size and reduced distensibility of the neopulmonary root has been recognized as an important and common determinant of reduced exercise capacity after the ASO at long-term follow-up [22].

Cardiovascular magnetic resonance (CMR) and computed tomography (CT) have been shown to be robust imaging modalities in adolescents and adult patients with a wide variety of congenital heart disease. These modalities have a major role in screening for residual lesions after ASO, particularly in adult patients.

14.2 Cardiac Magnetic Resonance Imaging

Cardiac magnetic resonance imaging (CMR) provides information of great vessels anatomy, intracardiac volumes and function, as well as eventually stress imaging in addition to myocardial fibrosis. As for other congenital heart disease, CMR should be always preferred over CT to avoid ionizing radiation as much as possible, and therefore would be the preferred imaging modality to follow these patients [23, 24].

Beyond the standards assessment of cardiac cavities volumes and function, specific goals of CMR in the follow-up after an arterial switch are the assessment of the aortic root dilatation, right ventricle outflow track imaging looking for stenosis, and if needed perfusion stress imaging. A CMR acquisition protocol is proposed in Table 14.1 and a summary of the main elements for reporting is provided in Table 14.2.

Table 14.1 Proposed CMR protocol

Localizer
Cine SSFP in axial plane
2D Cine SSFP, 2, 3 and 4 chambers, short axis stack
Contrast Enhanced MRA
"Whole heart" 4D flow
LGE; short axis and long axis
3D SSFP
Optional: • Perfusion stress protocol instead of contrast enhanced MRA if there is concern about ischemia   • 2D PC plane orthogonal to the main, left and right pulmonary arteries and the ascending aorta   • 2D SSFP short axis or long axis on the aortic root and RV outflow track

Table 14.2 CMR reporting elements

Left and right ventricle   • LV and RV volumes, mass, ejection fraction, wall motion analysis   • Myocardial perfusion if stress perfusion imaging was performed   • Presence of myocardial fibrosis/ sequelae of myocardial infarction
Pulmonary pathway   • Location and grading of RV outflow track and pulmonary artery obstruction   • Flow distribution in the pulmonary arteries   • Quantification of neo-pulmonary valve regurgitation
Aorta   • Size of the aortic root   • Quantification of the neo aortic valve regurgitation
Look for residual septal defects. Report QP/QS
Coronary arteries   • Origins and courses in relation with pulmonary arteries   • If possible, description of the degree of obstruction

14.2.1 Evaluation of Aortic Root Dilatation and Biomechanics

Dilatation of the aortic root is common and should be carefully monitored. 3D SSFP with an isotropic resolution is probably the best way to measure the aortic root. It can be performed without contrast administration and is usually done in free breathing using an echo navigator. Alternatively, contrast enhancement magnetic resonance angiography (CE-MRA) could be used during gadolinium chelate contrast administration. CE-MRA is less sensitive to susceptibly artifacts and therefore is more useful at 3-tesla magnetic field or in case of metallic implants. Thanks to these volumetric acquisitions, and following guidelines on aortic imaging, measurement should be done using multiplanar reformatting in order to be perpendicular to the center line [25, 26]. An example of aortic root dilatation is illustrated in Fig. 14.2.

Aortic biomechanics, usually impaired after ASO, can be assessed with CMR. Pulse wave velocity can be measured between 2 locations of the large vessel of interest. The distance between the 2 locations (in m) along the vessel of interest

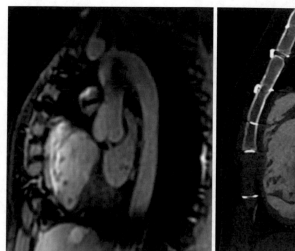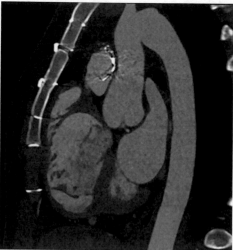

Fig. 14.2 Aorta in arterial switch. CMR on the left using SSFP 3D sequence (without gadolinium injection) and CT at the arterial phase on the right in the same patient; showing a dilatation of the neo aortic root as well as an angulation of the aortic arch. Sternotomy wires and stent in the pulmonary arteries are responsible of susceptibility artifacts in MRI, however evaluation of aortic dimension is still feasible

is divided by the difference in arrival time (in s) to calculate the pulse wave velocity (expressed in meters per second) as a marker of vessel stiffness. Distensibility is measured from the local vessel area change between systole and diastole corrected for pulse pressure. Pulse wave velocity and distensibility are inversely related. The proximal aorta and aortic arch act as a buffer for left ventricular systolic load, modulating ventricular–aortic coupling between the left ventricle and elastic proximal aorta. Aortic stiffening in ASO patients may contributes to the occurrence of aortic regurgitation and left ventricular dysfunction. Many possible other contributing factors to aortic stiffening in ASO patients have been suggested, including abnormal aorticopulmonary septation, damage to the vasa vasorum, surgical manipulation, inherited intrinsic wall abnormalities, and adaptation of the former pulmonary arterial wall to higher systemic pressures. Moreover, a gothic shape of the aortic arch due to a marked angulation has been described [27]. As illustrated in Fig. 14.2, this shape results from the aorta mobilization during Lecompte maneuver causing a central position of the ascending aorta and creating a kind of plicature between the ascending and descending aorta. Acute aortic angles are more frequently associated with neo-aortic root dilatation and higher incidence of regurgitation [28]. Reduced aortic bioelasticity and aortic arch angulation are likely to contribute to LV remodeling and diastolic dysfunction [27, 29]. Impaired aortic elasticity is strongly associated with age in patients after ASO [30]. These measurements are not routinely performed but may become useful in the follow-up studies for better understanding the early onset of degenerative cardiovascular disease.

14.2.2 Evaluation of the Right Ventricle Outflow Track and Pulmonary Arteries

RVOT and neopulmonary root just located behind the sternum have limiting acoustic windows during echocardiography evaluation, especially in adults [31]. 3D SSFP of CE-MRA can be used to detect anatomical stenosis and to eventually precise the relationship with coronary arteries before an invasive procedure. More interestingly, several recent works have emphasized the ability of 4D flow to assess peak velocities in this setting [31–33]. Even if there is small trend to underestimate peak velocities, likely due to both spatial and temporal averaging, 4D flow has the advantage of analyzing velocities in the entire acquired volume and is not dependent on the orientation of the flow and the changes in direction of the flow that may occur in space and over time. This technique may be well suited to detect, locate, and quantify the area of maximal velocities. In addition, 4D flow can be further used to assess the flow ratio between the left or the right lung or detect small defects or leaks [34, 35]. An example of pulmonary arteries stenosis assess by 4D flow is provided in Fig. 14.3.

14.2.3 Evaluation of Myocardial Perfusion

CMR is increasingly used in stress perfusion imaging outside of congenital heart diseases. Magnetic resonance coronary angiography provides accurate information on coronary anatomy, ostial stenosis, and proximal coronary artery kinking in

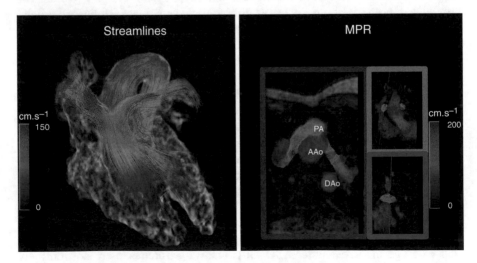

Fig. 14.3 4D flow. On the left, streamlines at systole peak showing acceleration in the pulmonary arteries. On the right, multiplanar reformatting showing a superimposition of velocity absolute values over modulus imaging, with a velocity in the right pulmonary artery >2 m s^{-1}. *AAo* ascending aorta, *DAo* descending aorta, *MPR* multiplanar reconstruction, *PA* pulmonary artery

patients after ASO. Furthermore, late gadolinium enhancement is also a useful CMR technique to identify myocardial infarcts and viability when coronary occlusion has occurred. Late gadolinium enhancement combined with stress perfusion CMR has been used to detect coronary involvement after the ASO [36, 37]. However, this approach seems to be weak for detecting myocardial ischemia during a pharmacological stress. Thus, it has been suggested that CMR is not routinely indicated to evaluate possible myocardial ischemic damage in asymptomatic and clinically stable adult patients after the ASO given the low probability of proximal coronary stenosis. In the presence of a detected or known proximal stenosis, the usefulness of this method in asymptomatic patients may be considered. Furthermore, in case of anteriorly reimplanted left coronary artery, due to the high proportion of patients with perfusion abnormality [37] and the high risk for early stenosis after ASO, the potential interest of stress CMR has to discuss in such patients [12]. Therefore, stress perfusion imaging is indicated only in selected cases, usually in case of coronary artery disease symptoms [24] and can also be considered in patients with anteriorly reimplanted left coronary artery. The perfusion protocols follow the general adults' protocols. Regadenoson stress can be used to implement the perfusion stress test in a more easy way to the rest of the CMR examination with a total acquisition time that remains reasonable [38] (Fig. 14.4).

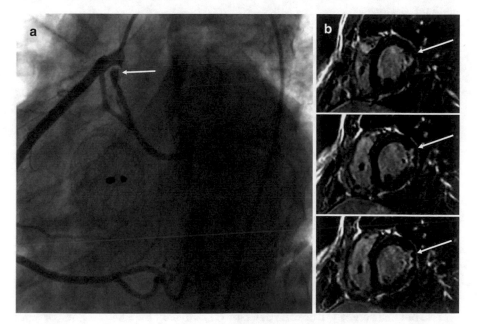

Fig. 14.4 Example of coronary arteries complications in arterial switch operation. On the left, Invasive coronary angiogram showing an occlusion of the circumflex artery rising from the right coronary ostia (white arrow). On the right, late gadolinium enhancement sequence in the same patient showing a subendocardial myocardial infarction on the anterolateral wall with myocardial viability (white arrow)

14.2.4 Follow-up Interval

In case of asymptomatic patient with no sequelae, CMR should be performed every 3 to 5 years. In case of symptoms or residual lesions, imaging should be performed every 1 to 3 years [24].

14.3 Computed Tomography

With high temporal and spatial resolutions on the total acquired volume, CT can comprehensively evaluate anatomical characteristics in ASO patients. Thanks to the past decade improvement, CT currently provides a good quality imaging at a lower radiation dose regardless of the heart rate (<1 mSv).

14.3.1 CT Acquisition Protocol

CT protocol for the follow-up of TGA after arterial switch is highly dependent of the clinical question and/or contraindication to MRI, of the type of CT scanner and finally of the assessment strategy implemented in a center specialized in adult congenital heart disease.

14.3.1.1 Contrast Injection
Timing of the injection and ECG gated scan should allow the examination of both right and left side of the heart. To achieve this biventricular opacification, a longer contrast injection is needed as well as a flush by a saline injection, but due to fast acquisition time of recent CT system, less than 70 mL of contrast medium volume are often sufficient. According to the experience of center a two or triphasic injection can be used.

14.3.1.2 Gating Management
– Retrospectively gated scan should be used only for patient in whom a multiphasic analysis of the heart is needed, mainly for cardiac function calculation in case of contraindication to MRI.
– Prospectively gated scan should be always preferred to minimize ionizing radiation: exposure to less than 1 mSv. A systolic prospective gated scan may be useful in case of high heart rate, as well as an absolute timing period after the R wave in case of arrhythmia. Use of Beta Blockers and nitrate can be considered accordingly in the absence of contraindication.
– Use of Dual source CT or wide detector CT, allowing high helical pitch or axial acquisition, should be preferred to improve image quality with a lower ionizing radiation level.

14.3.1.3   Dose Management

- Low KV imaging should be preferred for the arterial phase of the scan in order to decrease both the radiation dose and the contrast medium volume.
- Integrative reconstruction and automated tube current/ voltage selection depending on patient morphology should be used if available.
- Acquisition coverage should be also adapted to the clinical question, because only the heart or the heart and the all-thoracic great vessels can be included in the all-acquired CT volume.

14.3.2   Indication and Reporting Elements

CT is mainly indicated when CMR is contraindicated or in case of poor image quality. Reporting elements are similar to CMR (Table 14.2).

14.3.2.1   Coronary Arteries

CT provide a much better anatomical analysis of the coronary arteries compared to CMR, and CT is mainly used for this purpose with a low dose strategy.

A comprehensive evaluation of coronary arteries after ASO should include several features:

- 3D reconstruction (volume rendering) of the coronary arteries with the assessment of their pattern and relationship to the surrounding structures
- 2D curved multiplanar reconstructions of the main coronary arteries
- Localization of the origin of the coronary arteries in the neo-aortic sinus and the level of coronary reimplantation (distance between the plane of the neo-aortic valve and the origin of the main coronary arteries (methods proposed by Szymczyk et al. [39] and Ou et al. [12]).
- Spatial relationships between the coronaries and the adjacent great arteries (aorta and pulmonary artery).
- Branching angle of the coronary ((methods proposed by Szymczyk et al. [39] and Ou et al. [12]).
- Lowest diameters of the coronary artery cross-sectional areas in their proximal sections.

Proximal coronary artery stenosis can be well detected by using CT as well as the origins, the course of the coronary arteries and their relationships with other cardiovascular structures (Fig. 14.5).

Abnormal coronary origin and coronary artery complication after ASO is closely related to the initial coronary arteries pattern [7]. Yacoub and Radley-Smith classification is usually used for the description of coronary pattern [40]. Type A is the normal distribution; type B is characterized by the presence of a single orifice; type C shows two coronary orifices originating close to each other at the facing

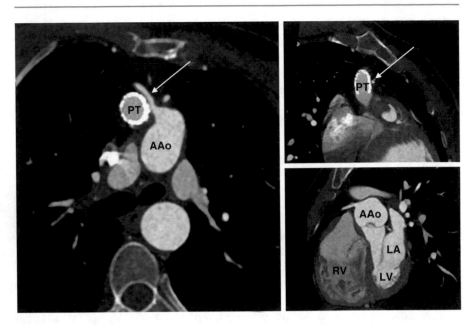

Fig. 14.5 Evaluation of coronary arteries by CT. Multiplanar reformatting showing the right coronary artery rising close to the stent of the pulmonary trunk (PT) without any stenosis. Note that the stent is responsible for minimal artifacts

commissure; type D is similar to type A with the exception that the circumflex artery arises from the right artery and curves posteriorly around the pulmonary trunk; and type E is defined by origin of the circumflex artery from the right posterior sinus. Types B and C are characterized by artery coursing between the aorta and the pulmonary trunk, usually with an intramural course and imply surgical difficulties. They seem to be more frequently associated with late coronary complication after ASO [7]. Types D and E are characterized by an abnormal looping of one or both arteries. Another classification of the coronary pattern is based on coronary looping side. Figure 14.6 illustrates the different coronary pattern in D-transposition of the great arteries.

There is not clear consensus regarding postoperative evaluation of coronary arteries in adults with TGA after an ASO. In a pediatric population, including 190 consecutive patients, coronary lesion defined by >30% up to occlusion were diagnosed in 8.9% of patients [12]. Other authors proposed to routinely perform coronary computed tomography angiography on patients with initial unusual coronary arteries pattern (excluding patients with circumflex coronary artery branching from the right coronary artery anomaly, which is considered to be mild) [39]. All the patients included in this study were asymptomatic, albeit a quarter had significant coronary abnormalities, including acute proximal angulation and stenosis, intra-arterial course, muscular bridge and coronary fistulas to pulmonary arteries. Half of them had acute angulation of at least one coronary artery. Most of the potentially severe anatomical features were related to the left coronary artery or the left anterior descending artery.

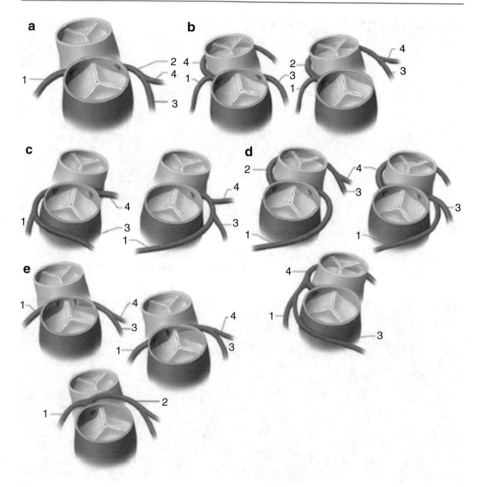

Fig. 14.6 Different coronary patterns in transposition of the great arteries. *1*: right coronary artery; *2*: Left main coronary artery; *3*: left anterior descending coronary artery; *4*: circumflex coronary artery. (**a**) Usual pattern; (**b**) coronary pattern with posterior loop; (**c**) coronary pattern with anterior loop; (**d**) coronary pattern with anterior and posterior loop; (**e**) coronary pattern with course between the pulmonary artery and aorta. From Vouhe et al. [6]

Ou et al. studied mechanisms involved in coronary abnormalities after ASO using CT [12]. For the left main and left anterior descending artery, anterior positioning of the transferred left coronary artery appeared to predispose to a tangential course of the proximal left coronary artery promoting stenosis (Fig. 14.7). The same authors showed this coronary abnormality was associated with impaired myocardial perfusion on stress CMR study [37]. Circumflex lesions occurred in Yacoub type D coronaries where a long initially retroaortic artery was stretched by its new positioning behind an enlarged neo-aorta. Right coronary artery lesions occurred only in cases in which the reimplantation site was very high above the right coronary sinus with potential compression from the main pulmonary artery bifurcation immediately above.

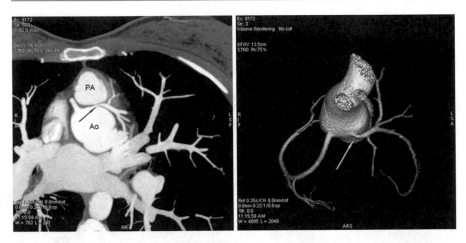

Fig. 14.7 Significant stenosis of the ostium of the left coronary artery by anterior compression by the pulmonary artery. The reimplantation is here too anterior. *PA* pulmonary artery, *Ao* neo-aorta

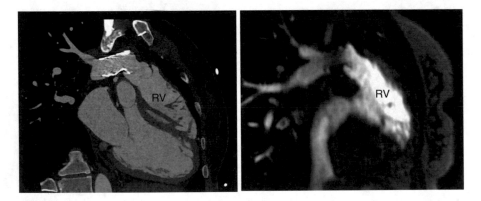

Fig. 14.8 Example of pulmonary stenting follow-up CT at the arterial phase on the left and Angio-MRA on the right (with gadolinium injection) showing a stent in the right pulmonary artery. Artifacts are lower on CT compared to MRA even if the lumen of the vessel is still analyzable on the MRA. *RV* right ventricle

Impact of these coronary abnormalities in asymptomatic patients (including negative stress test) on postoperative follow-up remains unknown. However, imaging of coronary arteries after ASO should be known in every patient.

14.3.2.2   RVOT and Great Vessels
CT can also be particularly useful in case of metallic stent and before reintervention for neopulmonary root or pulmonary arteries stenosis, and in case of suspected endocarditis. Notably, CT can also provide relationship with coronary arteries and sternum in case of planed RVOT intervention. CT is also a very reliable method to depict the anatomy and estimate diameter of the aorta and pulmonary arteries (Figs. 14.2 and 14.8).

References

1. Jatene AD, Fontes VF, Paulista PP, de Souza LC, Neger F, Galantier M, et al. Successful anatomic correction of transposition of the great vessels. A preliminary report. Arq Bras Cardiol. 1975;28(4):461–4.
2. Lecompte Y, Zannini L, Hazan E, Jarreau MM, Bex JP, Tu TV, et al. Anatomic correction of transposition of the great arteries. J Thorac Cardiovasc Surg. 1981;82(4):629–31.
3. Khairy P, Clair M, Fernandes SM, Blume ED, Powell AJ, Newburger JW, et al. Cardiovascular outcomes after the arterial switch operation for D-transposition of the great arteries. Circulation. 2013;127(3):331–9.
4. Tobler D, Williams WG, Jegatheeswaran A, Van Arsdell GS, McCrindle BW, Greutmann M, et al. Cardiac outcomes in young adult survivors of the arterial switch operation for transposition of the great arteries. J Am Coll Cardiol. 2010;56(1):58–64.
5. Kempny A, Wustmann K, Borgia F, Dimopoulos K, Uebing A, Li W, et al. Outcome in adult patients after arterial switch operation for transposition of the great arteries. Int J Cardiol. 2013;167(6):2588–93.
6. Vouhe P, et al. Traitement chirurgical de la transposition des gros vaisseaux. EMC - Techniques chirurgicales. Thorax. 2018;13(3):1–19. [Article 42–817].
7. Legendre A, Losay J, Touchot-Koné A, Serraf A, Belli E, Piot JD, et al. Coronary events after arterial switch operation for transposition of the great arteries. Circulation. 2003;108(Suppl 1):186–90.
8. Raisky O, Bergoend E, Agnoletti G, Ou P, Bonnet D, Sidi D, et al. Late coronary artery lesions after neonatal arterial switch operation: results of surgical coronary revascularization. Eur J Cardio Thorac Surg. 2007;31(5):894–8.
9. Fricke TA, d'Udekem Y, Richardson M, Thuys C, Dronavalli M, Ramsay JM, et al. Outcomes of the arterial switch operation for transposition of the great arteries: 25 years of experience. Ann Thorac Surg. 2012;94(1):139–45.
10. Losay J, Touchot A, Serraf A, Litvinova A, Lambert V, Piot JD, et al. Late outcome after arterial switch operation for transposition of the great arteries. Circulation. 2001;104(12 Suppl 1):I121–6.
11. van Wijk SWH, van der Stelt F, Ter Heide H, Schoof PH, Doevendans PAFM, Meijboom FJ, et al. Sudden death due to coronary artery lesions long-term after the arterial switch operation: a systematic review. Can J Cardiol. 2017;33(9):1180–7.
12. Ou P, Khraiche D, Celermajer DS, Agnoletti G, Le Quan Sang K-H, Thalabard JC, et al. Mechanisms of coronary complications after the arterial switch for transposition of the great arteries. J Thorac Cardiovasc Surg. 2013;145(5):1263–9.
13. Gatlin S, Kalynych A, Sallee D, Campbell R. Detection of a coronary artery anomaly after a sudden cardiac arrest in a 17 year-old with D-transposition of the great arteries status post arterial switch operation: a case report. Congenit Heart Dis. 2011;6(4):384–8.
14. Pizzi MN, Franquet E, Aguadé-Bruix S, Manso B, Casaldáliga J, Cuberas-Borrós G, et al. Long-term follow-up assessment after the arterial switch operation for correction of dextro-transposition of the great arteries by means of exercise myocardial perfusion-gated SPECT. Pediatr Cardiol. 2014;35(2):197–207.
15. Tanel RE, Wernovsky G, Landzberg MJ, Perry SB, Burke RP. Coronary artery abnormalities detected at cardiac catheterization following the arterial switch operation for transposition of the great arteries. Am J Cardiol. 1995;76(3):153–7.
16. Lo Rito M, Fittipaldi M, Haththotuwa R, Jones TJ, Khan N, Clift P, et al. Long-term fate of the aortic valve after an arterial switch operation. J Thorac Cardiovasc Surg. 2015;149(4):1089–94.
17. Losay J, Touchot A, Capderou A, Piot J-D, Belli E, Planché C, et al. Aortic valve regurgitation after arterial switch operation for transposition of the great arteries: incidence, risk factors, and outcome. J Am Coll Cardiol. 2006;47(10):2057–62.
18. Lim H-G, Kim W-H, Lee JR, Kim YJ. Long-term results of the arterial switch operation for ventriculo-arterial discordance. Eur J Cardio Thorac Surg. 2013;43(2):325–34.

19. Michalak KW, Moll JA, Moll M, Dryzek P, Moszura T, Kopala M, et al. The neoaortic root in children with transposition of the great arteries after an arterial switch operation. Eur J Cardio Thorac Surg. 2013;43(6):1101–8.
20. Shepard CW, Germanakis I, White MT, Powell AJ, Co-Vu J, Geva T. Cardiovascular magnetic resonance findings late after the arterial switch operation. Circ Cardiovasc Imaging. 2016;9(9):e004618.
21. Angeli E, Raisky O, Bonnet D, Sidi D, Vouhé PR. Late reoperations after neonatal arterial switch operation for transposition of the great arteries. Eur J Cardio Thorac Surg. 2008;34(1):32–6.
22. Baggen VJM, Driessen MMP, Meijboom FJ, Sieswerda GT, Jansen NJG, van Wijk SWH, et al. Main pulmonary artery area limits exercise capacity in patients long-term after arterial switch operation. J Thorac Cardiovasc Surg. 2015;150(4):918–25.
23. Cohen MS, Eidem BW, Cetta F, Fogel MA, Frommelt PC, Ganame J, et al. Multimodality imaging guidelines of patients with transposition of the great arteries: a report from the American Society of Echocardiography developed in collaboration with the Society for Cardiovascular Magnetic Resonance and the Society of Cardiovascular Computed Tomography. J Am Soc Echocardiogr. 2016;29(7):571–621.
24. Stout KK, Daniels CJ, Aboulhosn JA, Bozkurt B, Broberg CS, Colman JM, et al. 2018 AHA/ACC guideline for the Management of Adults with Congenital Heart Disease: executive summary. J Am Coll Cardiol. 2019;73(12):1494–563.
25. Baumgartner H, Falk V, Bax JJ, De Bonis M, Hamm C, Holm PJ, et al. 2017 ESC/EACTS Guidelines for the management of valvular heart disease. Eur Heart J. 2017;38:2739–91. http://academic.oup.com/eurheartj/article/doi/10.1093/eurheartj/ehx391/4095039/2017-ESCEACTS-Guidelines-for-the-management-of.
26. Authors/Task Force members, Erbel R, Aboyans V, Boileau C, Bossone E, Bartolomeo RD, et al. 2014 ESC guidelines on the diagnosis and treatment of aortic diseases: document covering acute and chronic aortic diseases of the thoracic and abdominal aorta of the adult * the Task Force for the diagnosis and treatment of aortic diseases of the European Society of Cardiology (ESC). Eur Heart J. 2014;35(41):2873–926.
27. Ladouceur M, Boutouyrie P, Boudjemline Y, Khettab H, Redheuil A, Legendre A, et al. Unknown complication of arterial switch operation: resistant hypertension induced by a strong aortic arch angulation. Circulation. 2013;128(25):e466–8.
28. Martins D, Khraiche D, Legendre A, Boddaert N, Raisky O, Bonnet D, Raimondi F. Aortic angle is associated with neo-aortic root dilatation and regurgitation following arterial switch operation. Int J Cardiol. 2019;280:53–6. https://pubmed.ncbi.nlm.nih.gov/30660585/?from_term=Raimondi+arterial+switch+transposition&from_pos=2. Accessed 7 Jun 2020.
29. Grotenhuis HB, Cifra B, Mertens LL, Riessenkampff E, Manlhiot C, Seed M, et al. Left ventricular remodelling in long-term survivors after the arterial switch operation for transposition of the great arteries. Eur Heart J Cardiovasc Imaging. 2019;20(1):101–7.
30. Voges I, Jerosch-Herold M, Hedderich J, Hart C, Petko C, Scheewe J, et al. Implications of early aortic stiffening in patients with transposition of the great arteries after arterial switch operation. Circ Cardiovasc Imaging. 2013;6(2):245–53.
31. Belhadjer Z, Soulat G, Ladouceur M, Pitocco F, Legendre A, Bonnet D, et al. Neopulmonary outflow tract obstruction assessment by 4D flow MRI in adults with transposition of the great arteries after arterial switch operation. J Magn Reson Imaging. 2019;51(6):1699–705.
32. Rose MJ, Jarvis K, Chowdhary V, Barker AJ, Allen BD, Robinson JD, et al. Efficient method for volumetric assessment of peak blood flow velocity using 4D flow MRI: peak velocity assessment with 4D flow. J Magn Reson Imaging. 2016;44(6):1673–82. Accessed 4 Oct 2016. https://doi.org/10.1002/jmri.25305.
33. Jarvis K, Vonder M, Barker AJ, Schnell S, Rose M, Carr J, et al. Hemodynamic evaluation in patients with transposition of the great arteries after the arterial switch operation: 4D flow and 2D phase contrast cardiovascular magnetic resonance compared with Doppler echocardiography. J Cardiovasc Magn Reson. 2016;18(1):59. https://doi.org/10.1186/s12968-016-0276-8.
34. Valverde I, Nordmeyer S, Uribe S, Greil G, Berger F, Kuehne T, et al. Systemic-to-pulmonary collateral flow in patients with palliated univentricular heart physiology: measurement using

cardiovascular magnetic resonance 4D velocity acquisition. J Cardiovasc Magn Reson. 2012;14(25):10–1186.

35. Hsiao A, Lustig M, Alley MT, Murphy MJ, Vasanawala SS. Evaluation of valvular insufficiency and shunts with parallel-imaging compressed-sensing 4D phase-contrast MR imaging with stereoscopic 3D velocity-fusion volume-rendered visualization. Radiology. 2012;265(1):87–95.

36. Tobler D, Motwani M, Wald RM, Roche SL, Verocai F, Iwanochko RM, et al. Evaluation of a comprehensive cardiovascular magnetic resonance protocol in young adults late after the arterial switch operation for d-transposition of the great arteries. J Cardiovasc Magn Reson. 2014;16:98.

37. Raimondi F, Aquaro GD, De Marchi D, Sandrini C, Khraiche D, Festa P, et al. Cardiac magnetic resonance myocardial perfusion after arterial switch for transposition of great arteries. JACC Cardiovasc Imaging. 2018;11(5):778–9.

38. Noel CV, Krishnamurthy R, Masand P, Moffett B, Schlingmann T, Cheong BY, et al. Myocardial stress perfusion MRI: experience in pediatric and young-adult patients following arterial switch operation utilizing Regadenoson. Pediatr Cardiol. 2018;39(6):1249–57.

39. Szymczyk K, Moll M, Sobczak-Budlewska K, Moll JA, Stefańczyk L, Grzelak P, et al. Usefulness of routine coronary CT angiography in patients with transposition of the great arteries after an arterial switch operation. Pediatr Cardiol. 2018;39(2):335–46.

40. Yacoub MH, Radley-Smith R. Anatomy of the coronary arteries in transposition of the great arteries and methods for their transfer in anatomical correction. Thorax. 1978;33(4):418–24.

The Systemic Right Ventricle

Craig S. Broberg and Abigail Khan

15.1 Introduction

Dysfunction of the systemic right ventricle (RV) is prevalent in patients with transposition of the great arteries (TGA). Dysfunction and heart failure are expected, yet there is wide variation in their progression. Imaging may improve understanding of the systemic RV's vulnerability and the pathogenesis of RV dysfunction. The goal of this chapter is to explore the current experience of systemic RV imaging and discuss the use of newer and emerging imaging tools with potential applications. General guidelines for TGA imaging have been published [1], and the reader is guided elsewhere for a thorough discussion of clinical imaging applications for these patients.

15.2 Imaging Goals

Today's imaging techniques, whether echocardiography or cardiac magnetic resonance (CMR), often focus on volume quantification for assessment of ventricular function. The lack of meaningful associations with ejection fraction may partly stem from the difficulties in its quantification. Even with CMR, which is considered the most accurate method, different techniques can be used for volume quantification (Fig. 15.1), either including or excluding the trabeculations [2, 3]. Measured ejection fractions may vary by 10% between methods. D and L loop ventricles are generally similar in shape, though systolic function tends to be lower in DTGA [4]. Axial plane vs. short axis plane acquisitions for volume quantification give largely

C. S. Broberg (✉) · A. Khan
Adult Congenital Heart Program, Knight Cardiovascular Institute, Oregon Health and Science University, Portland, OR, USA
e-mail: brobergc@ohsu.edu; khaab@ohsu.edu

© Springer Nature Switzerland AG 2021
P. Gallego, I. Valverde (eds.), *Multimodality Imaging Innovations In Adult Congenital Heart Disease*, Congenital Heart Disease in Adolescents and Adults, https://doi.org/10.1007/978-3-030-61927-5_15

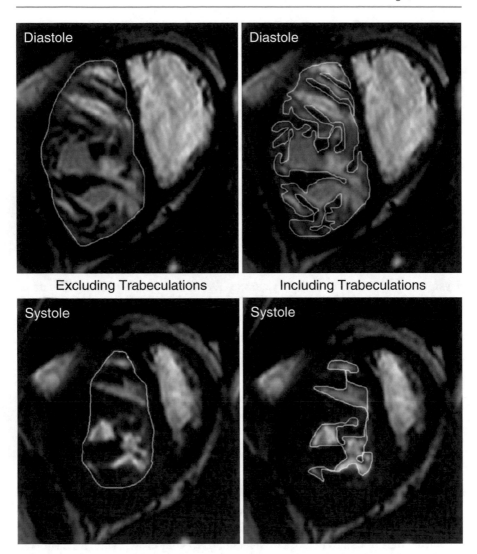

Fig. 15.1 Trabeculation contouring methods that are used. One involves contouring along the compacted areas of myocardium only (left panels), which is simpler in diastole but more arbitrary in systole. The other accounts for the trabeculations as part of the myocardial mass (right panels). Contouring can be difficult in diastole but more simple in systole. The former method gives larger ventricular volumes and hence lower ejection fraction than the later. Both are acceptable, but serial comparisons should take methodology into account

similar results [5]. Imaging goals in TGA also include assessment of systemic atrio-ventricular valve function (Fig. 15.2), the venous pathways in D-loop transposition, and the subpulmonic left ventricle [6], since an enlarged LV may be a sign of adverse volume or pressure loading, such as baffle leak or pulmonary hypertension (Fig. 15.3).

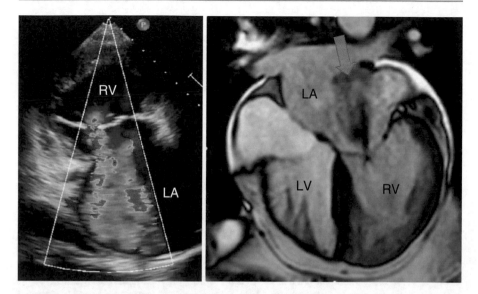

Fig. 15.2 Tricuspid regurgitation by Echo (right) and CMR (left). The degree of dephasing by CMR varies; therefore, subjective interpretation of the jet size etc. is not a reliable means of quantifying regurgitation. Instead, the regurgitant volume can be quantified with CMR

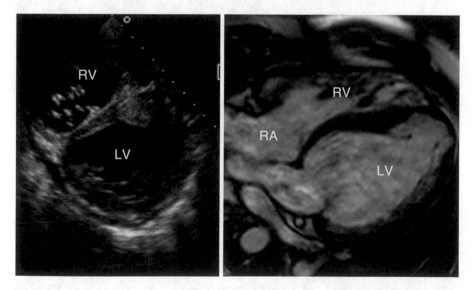

Fig. 15.3 DTGA with prior atrial switch palliation, with an abnormally enlarged, hypertrophied subpulmonic left ventricle in the setting of coexisting pulmonary arterial hypertension

But there is a need to move beyond the standard goal of assessing ventricular volume and function, as these have only weak associations with adverse events and prognosis [7]. Two other myocardial imaging techniques beyond simple volume quantification are now becoming mainstream have a role in the assessment of the systemic RV as well, broadening our understanding of its behavior over time. Their emerging applications will be discussed below.

15.3   Strain

Systemic RV strain can be measured with speckle-tracking echocardiography, which tracks acoustic signals throughout the cardiac cycle and detects subclinical cardiac dysfunction (Fig. 15.4). Strain imaging requires a high frame rate and good image quality, which can be challenging especially for the D-looped systemic RV which can be more retrosternal than the L-looped RV. It generally tracks only the thinner, compacted layer of RV myocardium, thus not the trabeculations, even though these may also contribute to overall ejection. Strain can be quantified as radial, circumferential, or longitudinal deformation. The latter is generally favored for left ventricle mechanics.

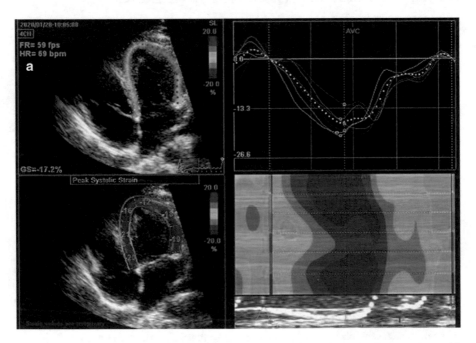

Fig. 15.4 (a) Longitudinal strain by speckle-tracking echocardiography in a patient with L-transposition of the great arteries and preserved systolic function. Note the fairly uniform motion of the myocardium with each segment across time (lower right panel). (b) Strain mapping from a different vendor in a patient with severely reduced RV systolic function. Global 2D strain measured was very abnormal at −2.6%

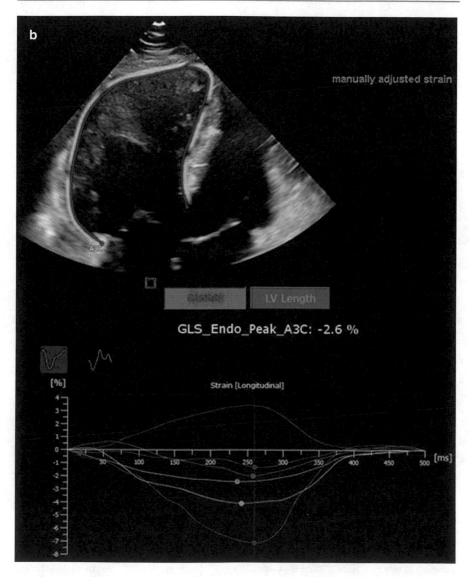

Fig. 15.4 (continued)

Global RV longitudinal strain (GLS) has been shown to correlate with CMR-derived RV ejection fraction, which makes it an appealing measure for use in clinical practice. RV GLS of ≥ -10 (example shown, Fig. 15.4b) is associated with a significantly higher risk of clinical events [8]. GLS is lower in those with poor exercise capacity, and may predict clinical status and events. Another disadvantage is that there are multiple strain algorithms, and results vary across vendors. A summary of published studies using strain in systemic RV patients is presented (Table 15.1). Strain by echo, which its high temporal resolution gives segmental

Table 15.1 Summary of studies using strain quantification on the systemic right ventricle

Reference	Year	N	Subtype	Imaging	Key findings
Bos et al. [30]	2006	13	ccTGA	Echo	Peak systolic strain lower than controls
Pettersen et al. [31]	2007	14	DTGA	Echo	Circumferential strain was greater than longitudinal. Torsion absent in systemic RV
Kalogeropoulos et al. [32]	2009	27	DTGA	Echo	Strain differs from controls
Becker et al. [33]	2010	31	Mixed	Echo	Circumferential greater than longitudinal, pattern different from normal RV
Di Salvo et al. [34]	2010	26	DTGA	Echo	Segmental strain pattern differed from controls, transverse strain correlated with exercise capacity
Chow et al. [35]	2011	29	DTGA	Echo	Lower diastolic strain values compared to controls, correlating with LV diastolic function
Kalogeropoulos et al. [10]	2012	64	DTGA	Echo	RV GLS was associated with clinical events in follow up
Diller et al. [36]	2012	129	Mixed	Echo	RV GLS abnormal vs. controls, and similar between ventricles. RV GLS related to clinical events
Thattaliyah et al. [12]	2015	20	DTGA	CMR	GLS and circumferential strain were reduced
Lipczynska et al. [37]	2015	40	DTGA	Echo	RV GLS associated with other functional parameters but not TAPSE, and predicted ejection fraction by CMR
Eindhoven et al. [38]	2015	42	Mixed	Echo	RV GLS lower than controls, DTGA worse than ccTGA, and correlated with NTproBNP and QRS duration
Burkhardt et al. [39]	2016	29	DTGA	CMR	RV GLS is reduced, RV circumferential strain is preserved
Tutarel et al. [11]	2016	91	DTGA	CMR	Strain parameters correlate with ejection fraction for both ventricles
Kowalik et al. [40]	2016	33	ccTGA	Echo	RV GLS correlated with RV ejection fraction by MRI
Ladouceur et al. [41]	2016	47	DTGA	Echo	RV GLS correlated with VO_2, not RV ejection fraction
Storsten et al. [42]	2018	14	DTGA	Echo	Abnormal septal circumferential strain
Timoteo et al. [43]	2018	26	Mixed	Echo	Abnormal RV GLS
Helsen et al. [44]	2018	105	Mixed	Echo	Strain parameters did not correlate with exercise capacity
Shiina et al. [2]	2018	71	Mixed	CMR	Longitudinal early diastolic strain rate and intra- and inter-ventricular dyssynchrony were predictive of major cardiac events
Geenen et al. [45]	2019	86	Mixed	Echo	Only septal strain was associated with clinical outcomes

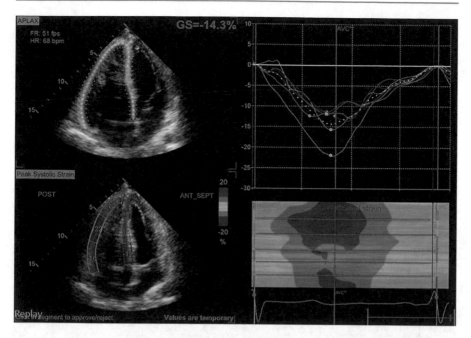

Fig. 15.5 Global longitudinal strain in a patient with an atrial switch palliation and coexistent pulmonary hypertension. Note the relatively lower systolic strain along the septum (lower rows of the display in lower right corner), since pulmonary hypertension may affect septal motion

time to peak strain, which can be useful in assessing synergy, and/or utility of biventricular pacing strategies. Strain patterns may be altered by coexistent pulmonary hypertension (Fig. 15.5).

Strain can also be measured using feature-tracking methods by CMR [9, 10] which overcomes the limitations posed by poor acoustic windows. Strain maps can be displayed on the acquired cine image (Fig. 15.6). It also provides, due to more reliable spatial resolution, additional metrics such as differentiation of function of the subendocardial from the epicardial layers, or individual vector tracking (Fig. 15.7) though the clinical relevance of these features is unknown. Feature tracking with strain has demonstrated that ventricular dysynchrony is associated with adverse clinical events [7], demonstrating the potential to become a tool to identify at-risk patients in the future. For today, its utility comes through in informing our understanding of the patterns of systemic RV failure over time. It should be noted that echo and CMR strain values will differ; significant differences in temporal resolution, frame rate, and algorithms hamper comparisons across modalities. Hence, echo strain and CMR strain should not be assumed to be equitable.

Fig. 15.6 Feature-tracking radial strain by CMR in a patient with L-transposition of the great arteries. The color values show relative strain at each pixel. Note that strain near the outflow tract is beginning to reverse late in systole earlier than other segments

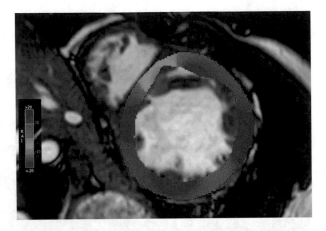

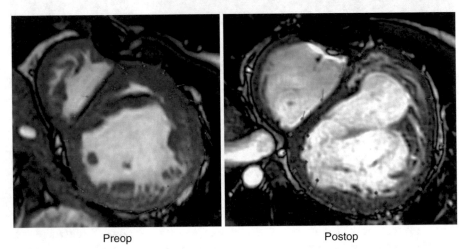

Preop   Postop

Fig. 15.7 Point vector plot by CMR strain analysis in a patient with L-transposition of the great arteries before and after tricuspid valve surgery. Green dots/lines represent motion of points along the epicardial surface of the RV, red dots/lines represent endocardial motion. Notice how the length of the lines is significantly lower following surgery, wherein systolic function had declined

15.4   Myocardial Fibrosis

Much imaging interest has focused on myocardial fibrosis, spurred by noninvasive detection and quantification techniques that have reached widespread use across cardiology, particularly the application of CMR, and this has become an established method for studying cardiomyopathic processes. There are two main techniques for fibrosis imaging: late gadolinium enhancement (LGE) and quantification of the extracellular volume. Existing studies, though limited, collectively demonstrate that myocardial fibrosis is associated with clinical deterioration.

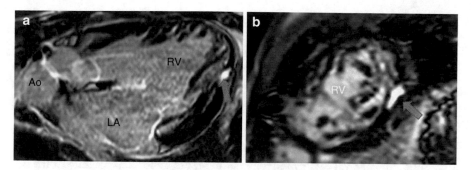

Fig. 15.8 Focal plaque of myocardial fibrosis demonstrated by late gadolinium enhancement (yellow arrow) seen in the apical inferior free wall of a patient with congenitally corrected transposition of the great arteries (Long axis view, 8A, short axis view, 8B)

15.4.1 Late Gadolinium Enhancement

LGE, or delayed gadolinium enhancement, is based on the fact that areas of myocardium with dense extracellular space, when compared to normal myocardium, will show persistently higher signal several minutes after gadolinium contrast administration (Fig. 15.8). In TGA, LGE has demonstrated systemic RV fibrosis in up to 61% of patients [11]. Affected patients are older and have worse systemic RV function than unaffected patients. They also have more arrhythmia and syncope, adding credibility as a marker of myocardial damage [11]. Others have reported similar results and associations [12], including with wall stress and collagen biomarkers [13, 14]. This later association importantly supports the hypothesis that LGE represents true myocardial fibrosis. LGE extent is associated with dyssynchrony in addition to lower exercise capacity and prior arrhythmia, implying a link between the fibrotic process, electromechanical delay, and clinical events [15].

Research suggests that myocardial fibrosis is part of the natural history pathway of the systemic RV, yet not all studies show a similar prevalence of LGE, and some show none [16–18]. The discrepancy may reflect the subjective nature of LGE, especially amongst dense trabeculations. Alternatively, patient age or surgical techniques may vary, reflecting inherent heterogeneity. Additionally, most studies were done exclusively in DTGA.

Only limited studies address whether detecting fibrosis can alter prognosis. The largest included 55 patients, 56% with LGE [19]. RV LGE was independently associated with adverse outcome after 7.8 years (combined endpoint of sustained tachyarrhythmia, heart failure admission, transplantation, or death). In addition, there was a clinical-pathologic correlation with an explanted heart after transplantation. Though this supports the idea that fibrosis is an important mediator of cardiovascular dysfunction and clinical events, there are still questions whether the presence of LGE should direct patient care.

15.4.2 Extracellular Volume Fraction

Fibrosis is likely diffused throughout the myocardium, and LGE may be insensitive in areas of less dense fibrosis [20]. Hence, the detection of diffuse fibrosis as a scalable quantity is potentially valuable, namely using T1 mapping techniques which generate an extracellular volume fraction (ECV). The process has been discussed earlier in this volume (Chapter Ref). T1 times alone, measured from otherwise normal myocardial segments, have been shown to be prognostic in certain conditions including coronary artery disease. In the systemic RV, these times are usually higher than for a normal LV, possibly reflective of the more trabeculated nature of the RV myocardium. The behavior of T1 after gadolinium contrast is shown (Fig. 15.9). The T1 values fall, with lower values wherever gadolinium contrast concentration is highest, notably in the blood pool more than the myocardium. Gradually, as contrast is cleared from the circulation, the T1 values return to normal, a process that is usually complete by about 30 min. The relative change in myocardium compared to blood pool allows for quantification of ECV. An area with less fibrosis will have higher T1 times after gadolinium compared to areas with fibrosis (Fig. 15.9). Most scanners will allow for a T1 map to be produced, an image where each pixel's value (grayscale or other color spectrum) represents the T1 time (Fig. 15.10). Inspection of such a map obtained 10–15 min after contrast can sometimes demonstrate areas of abnormal myocardium, much like LGE, where the T1 value is darker (i.e., lower T1, more approximate to the value for the blood pool). ECV utilizes these measures of T1 before and after administration of gadolinium, and plots the change against

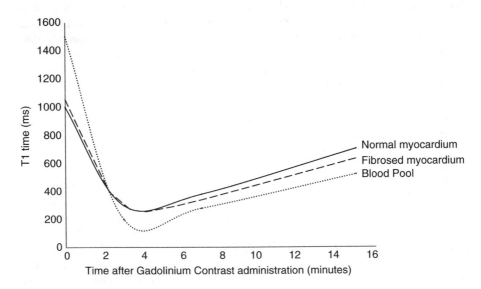

Fig. 15.9 Relative T1 times of myocardium and blood pool before and at certain time points after gadolinium contrast administration. Areas of fibrosed myocardium will have T1 times that more approximate that of the blood pool. This difference is utilized in quantification of the extracellular volume fraction

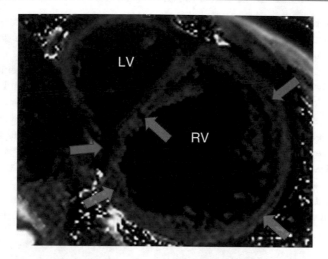

Fig. 15.10 T1 pixel mapping in a patient with congenitally corrected transposition of the great arteries. Dark areas indicate lower T1 values, usually from focal fibrosis (yellow arrows) including focal transmural foci in the septum, diffuse foci in the inferior wall, and mid wall areas of the lateral free wall. Lower T1 values are also commonly seen at the inferior RV-LV junction (blue arrow). Dark areas along the dense trabeculations (green arrow) reflect blood pool signal rather than true myocardial fibrosis

that of the blood pool [21]. This requires careful contouring to avoid extracellular fat or myocardial trabeculations that are extensive in the systemic RV. ECV demonstrates diffuse fibrosis in ACHD patients with various lesions, and correlates with ventricular size and function [21].

The first study to explore this method in the systemic RV was done using an equilibrium contrast method, involving a constant infusion of gadolinium [18]. The study highlighted the difficulties of measuring T1 in the RV, and found that ECV quantification for the RV free wall was not feasible with the method. However, septal ECV was measured, and found to be higher than the septum in controls. ECV did not correlate with RV volume or ejection fraction, reminiscent of other studies wherein the RV EF was less predictive of function or outcome than might be expected.

Using more traditional methods, the second study to study ECV in the systemic RV included 53 patients with both D- and congenitally corrected TGA as well as a smaller cohort of controls [22]. ECV was "abnormal" meaning higher than the LV in controls in 29% of those studied. Unlike in other conditions, typical associations between ECV and other clinical parameters indicating worse clinical function were not found. This included no association with RV volume or function, tricuspid regurgitation severity, prior arrhythmia, collagen byproducts in serum, or serum aldosterone. Those with abnormal ECV did have a higher median B-type natriuretic peptide levels however, as well as an intriguing longer 6-min walk time. The later finding raises questions about whether fibrosis may be favorable for exercise response, though this needs to be confirmed in other studies. In follow up (median 4.4 years) ECV was associated with clinical heart failure end-points such as arrhythmia, hospitalization, transplant, or death. Thus ECV again seems to point to a process within the myocardium that is related to gradual functional deterioration and manifestations of clinical heart failure.

However, RV ECV quantification can be complicated by trabecular contrast pooling (Fig. 15.10), which can lower post-contrast T1 values and artificially increase ECV quantification. ECV may actually be less sensitive to small amounts of fibrosis because of smaller sampling; LGE is usually assessed over the entire heart whereas ECV is only assessed over 1–3 short axis planes. Small amounts of fibrosis, though present, may not be enough to increase the ECV above a "normal" value and hence may not be detected. Furthermore, the variance between measurements over time is not well known. Still, the method is growing more ubiquitous in many imaging laboratories and may in the future play a more substantial role as an objective measure of myocardial change that could prompt certain management decisions.

15.4.3 Other Emerging Techniques

Looking forward, there are emerging imaging applications now that may have potential value in understanding the fate of the systemic RV. Using four-dimensional flow quantification (Fig. 15.11), investigators have studied diastolic fluid dynamics, defining flow energetics into and through the normal subpulmonic RV, by tracking multidimensional flow velocities [23]. Such studies have collectively demonstrated the contribution of RV volume and geometry to diastolic filling [24]. The technique is non-invasive but requires significant offline analysis, and such methods have not yet been applied to the systemic RV. In time, however, these flow maps may eventually provide better understanding of how the systemic RV adapts to its unusual loading conditions, namely the systemic level pressure-loading present since birth and the adjacent pressure-unloaded morphologic LV.

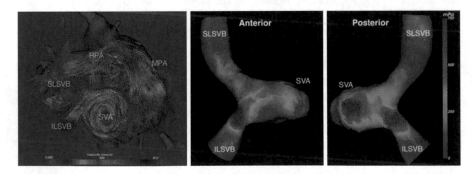

Fig. 15.11 4D flow mapping used to quantify flow energetics through the venous pathways of a patient with D-transposition of the great arteries after atrial switch palliation. (Reprint with permission)

Flow dynamics in diastole are also significantly affected by venous baffles in the setting of a systemic RV. The use of 4D flow as a tool for evaluation of intra-atrial baffle flow has been demonstrated [25]. Recognizing that the venous pathways affect biventricular filling and stroke volume augmentation during exercise [26], it is foreseeable that 4D flow techniques will be applied to atrial flow in atrial switch patients to further elucidate how venous flow energetics alter ventricular mechanics, and vice versa.

The normal RV has two fiber layers, and its contraction is usually longitudinal. CMR diffusion tensor imaging (DTI) is a technique used to demonstrate velocity of tissue within the myocardial wall, giving insight into fiber architecture and showing adaptation to its unique loading conditions [27] (Fig. 15.12). DTI may be a tool for furthering our understanding of not only how the ventricle adapts, but what leads to its failure.

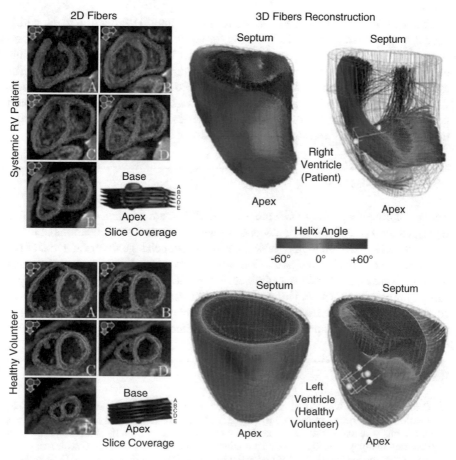

Fig. 15.12 An example of diffusion tensor imaging (DTI) applied to the systemic RV of a patient with congenitally corrected transposition. The imaging demonstrates augmentation of a mid-myocardial fiber layer contributing to myocardial motion. (Reprint with permission)

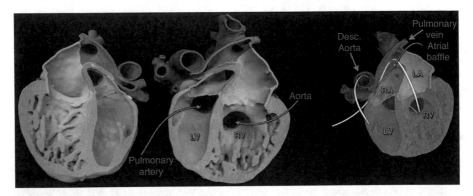

Fig. 15.13 3D model print of the atrial baffle and venous pathways in a patient with D-transposition of the great arteries. (Reprint with permission)

Finally, CMR or CT imaging can be formatted into 3D printed models, which have been shown to have application both for education and, at times, clinical care particularly for intervention planning [28] (Fig. 15.13). This can be a boon for surgeons and proceduralists for understanding the complexities of the atrial switch, for example. It is also possible to create virtual, functional three-dimensional models that can be viewed via virtual/augmented reality methods [29]. This in theory could provide detailed inspection of baffles and tricuspid valve function, though whether this will have any real-world application for patient care remains to be seen.

15.5 Conclusions

The major imaging goals in TGA are to assess RV size and function, tricuspid valve regurgitation, and baffle leak or stenosis. However, the newest applications of imaging offer more understanding of how the myocardium changes over time and of the pathogenesis of ventricular dysfunction, which is an integral determinant of clinical outcome. Research using these techniques has painted a convincing picture of myocardial fibrosis as a linchpin in the gradual deterioration of ventricular function and adverse clinical outcomes. Other techniques emerging may also have widening application to the systemic RV and continue to offer further clarity on its fate.

References

1. Cohen MS, Eidem BW, Cetta F, Fogel MA, Frommelt PC, Ganame J, Han BK, Kimball TR, Johnson RK, Mertens L, Paridon SM, Powell AJ, Lopez L. Multimodality Imaging Guidelines of Patients with Transposition of the Great Arteries: A Report from the American Society of Echocardiography Developed in Collaboration with the Society for Cardiovascular Magnetic Resonance and the Society of Cardiovascular Computed Tomography. J Am Soc Echocardiogr. 2016;29:571–621.

2. Winter MM, Bouma BJ, van Dijk AP, Groenink M, Nieuwkerk PT, van der Plas MN, Sieswerda GT, Konings TC, Mulder BJ. Relation of physical activity, cardiac function, exercise capacity, and quality of life in patients with a systemic right ventricle. Am J Cardiol. 2008;102:1258–62.

3. Driessen MM, Baggen VJ, Freling HG, Pieper PG, van Dijk AP, Doevendans PA, Snijder RJ, Post MC, Meijboom FJ, Sieswerda GT, Leiner T, Willems TP. Pressure overloaded right ventricles: a multicenter study on the importance of trabeculae in RV function measured by CMR. Int J Cardiovasc Imaging. 2014;30:599–608.

4. Morcos M, Kilner PJ, Sahn DJ, Litt HI, Valsangiacomo-Buechel ER, Sheehan FH. Comparison of systemic right ventricular function in transposition of the great arteries after atrial switch and congenitally corrected transposition of the great arteries. Int J Cardiovasc Imaging. 2017;33:1993–2001.

5. Jimenez-Juan L, Joshi SB, Wintersperger BJ, Yan AT, Ley S, Crean AM, Nguyen ET, Deva DP, Paul NS, Wald RM. Assessment of right ventricular volumes and function using cardiovascular magnetic resonance cine imaging after atrial redirection surgery for complete transposition of the great arteries. Int J Cardiovasc Imaging. 2013;29:335–42.

6. Stauber A, Wey C, Greutmann M, Tobler D, Wustmann K, Wahl A, Valsangiacomo Buechel ER, Wilhelm M, Schwerzmann M. Left ventricular outflow tract obstruction and its impact on systolic ventricular function and exercise capacity in adults with a subaortic right ventricle. Int J Cardiol. 2017;244:139–42.

7. Shiina Y, Inai K, Takahashi T, Taniguchi K, Watanabe E, Fukushima K, Niwa K, Nagao M. Inter- and intra-ventricular dyssynchrony in the systemic right ventricle is a surrogate marker of major cardiac events in mildly symptomatic patients. Heart Vessels. 2018;33:1086–93.

8. Kalogeropoulos AP, Deka A, Border W, Pernetz MA, Georgiopoulou VV, Kiani J, McConnell M, Lerakis S, Butler J, Martin RP, Book WM. Right ventricular function with standard and speckle-tracking echocardiography and clinical events in adults with D-transposition of the great arteries post atrial switch. J Am Soc Echocardiogr. 2012;25:304–12.

9. Tutarel O, Orwat S, Radke RM, Westhoff-Bleck M, Vossler C, Schulke C, Baumgartner H, Bauersachs J, Rontgen P, Diller GP. Assessment of myocardial function using MRI-based feature tracking in adults after atrial repair of transposition of the great arteries: reference values and clinical utility. Int J Cardiol. 2016;220:246–50.

10. Thattaliyath BD, Forsha DE, Stewart C, Barker PC, Campbell MJ. Evaluation of right ventricular myocardial mechanics using velocity vector imaging of cardiac MRI cine images in transposition of the great arteries following atrial and arterial switch operations. Congenit Heart Dis. 2015;10:371–9.

11. Babu-Narayan SV, Goktekin O, Moon JC, Broberg CS, Pantely GA, Pennell DJ, Gatzoulis MA, Kilner PJ. Late gadolinium enhancement cardiovascular magnetic resonance of the systemic right ventricle in adults with previous atrial redirection surgery for transposition of the great arteries. Circulation. 2005;111:2091–8.

12. Giardini A, Lovato L, Donti A, Formigari R, Oppido G, Gargiulo G, Picchio FM, Fattori R. Relation between right ventricular structural alterations and markers of adverse clinical outcome in adults with systemic right ventricle and either congenital complete (after Senning operation) or congenitally corrected transposition of the great arteries. Am J Cardiol. 2006;98:1277–82.

13. Ladouceur M, Baron S, Nivet-Antoine V, Maruani G, Soulat G, Pereira H, Blanchard A, Boutouyrie P, Paul JL, Mousseaux E. Role of myocardial collagen degradation and fibrosis in right ventricle dysfunction in transposition of the great arteries after atrial switch. Int J Cardiol. 2018;258:76–82.

14. Lipczynska M, Szymanski P, Kumor M, Klisiewicz A, Hoffman P. Collagen turnover biomarkers and systemic right ventricle remodeling in adults with previous atrial switch procedure for transposition of the great arteries. PLoS One. 2017;12:e0180629.

15. Babu-Narayan SV, Prati D, Rydman R, Dimopoulos K, Diller GP, Uebing A, Henein MY, Kilner PJ, Gatzoulis MA, Li W. Dyssynchrony and electromechanical delay are associated with focal fibrosis in the systemic right ventricle - insights from echocardiography. Int J Cardiol. 2016;220:382–8.

16. Fratz S, Hauser M, Bengel FM, Hager A, Kaemmerer H, Schwaiger M, Hess J, Stern HC. Myocardial scars determined by delayed-enhancement magnetic resonance imaging and positron emission tomography are not common in right ventricles with systemic function in long-term follow up. Heart. 2006;92:1673–7.

17. Preim U, Hoffmann J, Lehmkuhl L, Kehrmann J, Riese F, Daehnert I, Kostelka M, Gutberlet M, Grothoff M. Systemic right ventricles rarely show myocardial scars in cardiac magnetic resonance delayed-enhancement imaging. Clin Res Cardiol. 2013;102:337–44.

18. Plymen CM, Sado DM, Taylor AM, Bolger AP, Lambiase PD, Hughes M, Moon JC. Diffuse myocardial fibrosis in the systemic right ventricle of patients late after mustard or Senning surgery: an equilibrium contrast cardiovascular magnetic resonance study. Eur Heart J Cardiovasc Imaging. 2013;14:963–8.

19. Rydman R, Gatzoulis MA, Ho SY, Ernst S, Swan L, Li W, Wong T, Sheppard M, McCarthy KP, Roughton M, Kilner PJ, Pennell DJ, Babu-Narayan SV. Systemic right ventricular fibrosis detected by cardiovascular magnetic resonance is associated with clinical outcome, mainly new-onset atrial arrhythmia, in patients after atrial redirection surgery for transposition of the great arteries. Circ Cardiovasc Imaging. 2015;8:e002628.

20. Ladouceur M, Bruneval P, Mousseaux E. Cardiovascular flashlight. Magnetic resonance assessment of fibrosis in systemic right ventricle after atrial switch procedure. Eur Heart J. 2009;30:2613.

21. Broberg CS, Chugh SS, Conklin C, Sahn DJ, Jerosch-Herold M. Quantification of diffuse myocardial fibrosis and its association with myocardial dysfunction in congenital heart disease. Circ Cardiovasc Imaging. 2010;3:727–34.

22. Broberg CS, Valente AM, Huang J, Burchill LJ, Holt J, Van Woerkom R, Powell AJ, Pantely GA, Jerosch-Herold M. Myocardial fibrosis and its relation to adverse outcome in transposition of the great arteries with a systemic right ventricle. Int J Cardiol. 2018;271:60–5.

23. Carlsson M, Heiberg E, Toger J, Arheden H. Quantification of left and right ventricular kinetic energy using four-dimensional intracardiac magnetic resonance imaging flow measurements. Am J Physiol Heart Circ Physiol. 2012;302:H893–900.

24. Barker N, Fidock B, Johns CS, Kaur H, Archer G, Rajaram S, Hill C, Thomas S, Karunasaagarar K, Capener D, Al-Mohammad A, Rothman A, Kiely DG, Swift AJ, Wild JM, Garg P. A systematic review of right ventricular diastolic assessment by 4D flow CMR. Biomed Res Int. 2019;2019:6074984.

25. van der Palen RL, Westenberg JJ, Hazekamp MG, Kuipers IM, Roest AA. Four-dimensional flow cardiovascular magnetic resonance for the evaluation of the atrial baffle after mustard repair. Eur Heart J Cardiovasc Imaging. 2016;17:353.

26. Winter MM, van der Plas MN, Bouma BJ, Groenink M, Bresser P, Mulder BJ. Mechanisms for cardiac output augmentation in patients with a systemic right ventricle. Int J Cardiol. 2010;143:141–6.

27. Harmer J, Pushparajah K, Toussaint N, Stoeck CT, Chan R, Atkinson D, Razavi R, Kozerke S. In vivo myofibre architecture in the systemic right ventricle. Eur Heart J. 2013;34:3640.

28. Anwar S, Singh GK, Varughese J, Nguyen H, Billadello JJ, Sheybani EF, Woodard PK, Manning P, Eghtesady P. 3D printing in complex congenital heart disease: across a Spectrum of age, pathology, and imaging techniques. JACC Cardiovasc Imaging. 2017;10:953–6.

29. Butera G, Sturla F, Pluchinotta FR, Caimi A, Carminati M. Holographic augmented reality and 3D printing for advanced planning of sinus Venosus ASD/partial anomalous pulmonary venous return percutaneous management. JACC Cardiovasc Interv. 2019;12:1389–91.

30. Bos JM, Hagler DJ, Silvilairat S, Cabalka A, O'Leary P, Daniels O, Miller FA, Abraham TP. Right ventricular function in asymptomatic individuals with a systemic right ventricle. J Am Soc Echocardiogr. 2006;19:1033–7.

31. Pettersen E, Helle-Valle T, Edvardsen T, Lindberg H, Smith HJ, Smevik B, Smiseth OA, Andersen K. Contraction pattern of the systemic right ventricle shift from longitudinal to circumferential shortening and absent global ventricular torsion. J Am Coll Cardiol. 2007;49:2450–6.

32. Kalogeropoulos AP, Georgiopoulou VV, Giamouzis G, Pernetz MA, Anadiotis A, McConnell M, Lerakis S, Butler J, Book WM, Martin RP. Myocardial deformation imaging of the systemic right ventricle by two-dimensional strain echocardiography in patients with d-transposition of the great arteries. Hellenic J Cardiol. 2009;50:275–82.

33. Becker M, Humpel C, Ocklenburg C, Muehler E, Schroeder J, Eickholt C, Hoffmann R, Marx N, Franke A. The right ventricular response to high afterload: comparison between healthy persons and patients with transposition of the great arteries: a 2D strain study. Echocardiography (Mount Kisco, NY). 2010;27:1256–62.

34. Di Salvo G, Pacileo G, Rea A, Limongelli G, Baldini L, D'Andrea A, D'Alto M, Sarubbi B, Russo MG, Calabro R. Transverse strain predicts exercise capacity in systemic right ventricle patients. Int J Cardiol. 2010;145:193–6.

35. Chow PC, Liang XC, Cheung YF. Diastolic ventricular interaction in patients after atrial switch for transposition of the great arteries: a speckle tracking echocardiographic study. Int J Cardiol. 2011;152:28–34.

36. Diller GP, Radojevic J, Kempny A, Alonso-Gonzalez R, Emmanouil L, Orwat S, Swan L, Uebing A, Li W, Dimopoulos K, Gatzoulis MA, Baumgartner H. Systemic right ventricular longitudinal strain is reduced in adults with transposition of the great arteries, relates to subpulmonary ventricular function, and predicts adverse clinical outcome. Am Heart J. 2012;163:859–66.

37. Lipczynska M, Szymanski P, Kumor M, Klisiewicz A, Mazurkiewicz L, Hoffman P. Global longitudinal strain may identify preserved systolic function of the systemic right ventricle. Can J Cardiol. 2015;31:760–6.

38. Eindhoven JA, Menting ME, van den Bosch AE, McGhie JS, Witsenburg M, Cuypers JA, Boersma E, Roos-Hesselink JW. Quantitative assessment of systolic right ventricular function using myocardial deformation in patients with a systemic right ventricle. Eur Heart J Cardiovasc Imaging. 2015;16:380–8.

39. Burkhardt BEU, Kellenberger CJ, Franzoso FD, Geiger J, Oxenius A, Valsangiacomo Buechel ER. Right and left ventricular strain patterns after the atrial switch operation for D-transposition of the great arteries-a magnetic resonance feature tracking study. Front Cardiovasc Med. 2019;6:39.

40. Kowalik E, Mazurkiewicz L, Kowalski M, Klisiewicz A, Marczak M, Hoffman P. Echocardiography vs magnetic resonance imaging in assessing ventricular function and systemic atrioventricular valve status in adults with congenitally corrected transposition of the great arteries. Echocardiography (Mount Kisco, NY). 2016;33:1697–702.

41. Ladouceur M, Redheuil A, Soulat G, Delclaux C, Azizi M, Patel M, Chatellier G, Legendre A, Iserin L, Boudjemline Y, Bonnet D, Mousseaux E, Investigators S. Longitudinal strain of systemic right ventricle correlates with exercise capacity in adult with transposition of the great arteries after atrial switch. Int J Cardiol. 2016;217:28–34.

42. Storsten P, Eriksen M, Remme EW, Boe E, Erikssen G, Smiseth OA, Skulstad H. Dysfunction of the systemic right ventricle after atrial switch: physiological implications of altered septal geometry and load. J Appl Physiol (1985). 2018;125:1482–9.

43. Timoteo AT, Branco LM, Rosa SA, Galrinho A, Sousa L, Oliveira JA, Pinto MF, Agapito AF, Ferreira RC. Longitudinal strain by two-dimensional speckle tracking to assess ventricular function in adults with transposition of the great arteries: can serial assessment be simplified? Rev Port Cardiol. 2018;37:739–45.

44. Helsen F, De Meester P, Van De Bruaene A, Gabriels C, Santens B, Claeys M, Claessen G, Goetschalckx K, Buys R, Gewillig M, Troost E, Voigt JU, Claus P, Bogaert J, Budts W. Right ventricular systolic dysfunction at rest is not related to decreased exercise capacity in patients with a systemic right ventricle. Int J Cardiol. 2018;260:66–71.

45. Geenen LW, van Grootel RWJ, Akman K, Baggen VJM, Menting ME, Eindhoven JA, Cuypers J, Boersma E, van den Bosch AE, Roos-Hesselink JW. Exploring the prognostic value of novel markers in adults with a systemic right ventricle. J Am Heart Assoc. 2019;8:e013745.

Univentricular Heart: Staged Palliation

16

Emanuela R. Valsangiacomo Buechel

16.1 Basic Principles of Staged Palliation in Univentricular Hearts

The concept of univentricular heart (UVH) is rather a functional than a merely ana-tomical definition. The term UVH is referred to all conditions in which the two ventricles are unable to sustain separately the systemic and the pulmonary circula-tion, and therefore are not eligible for biventricular repair [1]. UVH occur in about 10% of all congenital heart disease [2], and include diagnoses such as tricuspid atresia, pulmonary atresia with intact ventricular septum, unbalanced atrioventricu-lar septal defect, double inlet left ventricle, hypoplastic left heart syndrome, double outlet right ventricle with hypoplastic left ventricle, and others. Substantially the dominant ventricle can be of a right or left morphology.

The current available treatment strategy for patients with an UVH is a staged surgical path with the ultimate goal of having the available ventricular mass (single ventricle) pumping into the systemic circulation, and the pulmonary circulation being supplied by passive inflow from the systemic veins into the pulmonary arter-ies. The Fontan circulation represents a highly abnormal physiology, since a single pump is the driving force for both, the systemic and the pulmonary circulation. Thus this staged treatment has to be considered a palliation [3].

16.1.1 Surgical Palliation for UVH

Stage one. The goal of the first intervention is to achieve a balance between the pulmonary (Qp) and the systemic (Qs) circulation. Is the pulmonary blood supply

E. R. Valsangiacomo Buechel (✉)
Pediatric Heart Centre, University Children's Hospital Zurich, Zurich, Switzerland
e-mail: Emanuela.valsangiacomo@kispi.uzh.ch

© Springer Nature Switzerland AG 2021   309
P. Gallego, I. Valverde (eds.), *Multimodality Imaging Innovations In Adult Congenital Heart Disease*, Congenital Heart Disease in Adolescents and Adults,
https://doi.org/10.1007/978-3-030-61927-5_16

insufficient, then an aortopulmonary connection (shunt) needs to be created. In case of poor systemic perfusion, usually a Damus–Kaye–Stancel operation/shunt, with or without aortic arch reconstruction (Norwood) is the operation of choice. In case of an unprotected pulmonary circulation, a pulmonary banding is performed for protecting the pulmonary vascular bed from overcirculation (Figs. 16.1a, b).

Stage two. As a second step the superior vena cava is surgically anastomosed to the pulmonary arteries—the so-called cavopulmonary connection. At time of this intervention the shunt is ligated and/or the pulmonary artery resected. This operation is usually performed at the age of 4–6 months (Fig. 16.2).

Stage three. The Fontan operation consists in channeling the inferior vena cava, including the hepatic vein, to the pulmonary arteries—the total cavopulmonary connection (TCPC); nowadays this is performed using a goretex extracardiac conduit [4]. Since its first description [5] the Fontan operation has changed considerably, and in the last decades various techniques have been applied, including the atriopulmonary connection, the intracardiac lateral tunnel, and the extracardiac lateral tunnel. The ultimate goal of this surgical evolvement has been to prevent the observed complications and to improve outcome. When imaging adult patients after a Fontan operation, knowledge of all these different postsurgical anatomies is mandatory (Fig. 16.3a–c).

Survival rate after the Fontan procedure have substantially improved over the last decades, however mid-and long-term morbidity remains substantial [6–8]. Multimodality imaging with its recent developments plays an important role in managing these patients throughout the stages of treatment and during long-term follow-up [9–11].

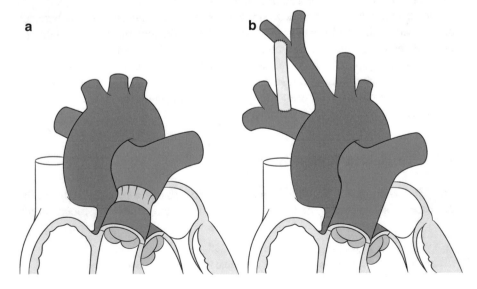

Fig. 16.1 Initial palliation in univentricular defects. (**a**) Pulmonary banding for reduction of a pulmonary hypercirculation. (**b**) Blalock–Taussig shunt for increasing pulmonary circulation

Fig. 16.2 Cavopulmonary anastomosis redirecting the flow from the superior caval vein into the pulmonary arteries

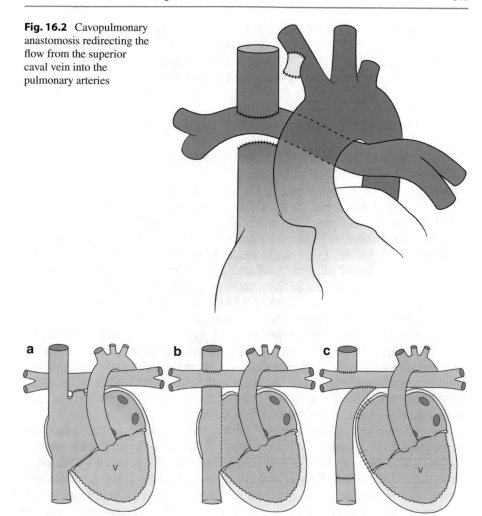

Fig. 16.3 Different techniques used for the Fontan operation. (**a**) Fontan–Kreutzer anastomosis. (**b**) Lateral intra-atrial conduit. (**c**) Extracardial conduit

During the stepwise treatment the single ventricle and its myocardium is exposed to different loading conditions, with an initial volume loading (stage 1) and a subsequent staged volume unloading (stage 2 and 3). If a residual obstruction is present, such as in the reconstructed aortic arch, an additional pressure overload may challenge myocardial performance. During the stages the single ventricle is undergoing different phases of remodeling. Moreover due to myocardial hypertrophy and stiffness, UVH are at risk for diastolic dysfunction. Importantly in addition to contractility, ventricular relaxation is a major determinant of global ventricular function. Ventricular performance is one crucial determinant of outcome in UVH patients, in whom the entire cardiovascular system is required to perform energetically as efficiently as possible.

This chapter will discuss the clinical application of different advanced imaging modalities throughout the surgical stages for treatment of UVH. This will include the initial stage before BCPC, the stage before and after Fontan completion and follow-up. The available imaging data on outcome will be discussed as well.

16.2 Imaging Modalities and Their Applications

16.2.1 Three-Dimensional Echocardiography

Three-dimensional echocardiography (3D echo) is commonly used for measurement of the volume of the single ventricle. Particularly in young pediatric patients with UVH and with the use of new matrix-array 3D echo probe, a good accuracy of 3D echo measurements of mass and volumes have been reported compared to CMR as the reference modality [12, 13]. The restricted acoustic window in adults and the limited visualization of all contours of the single ventricle may represent a limitation for a broader clinical use of 3D echo in all patients. The relatively low frame rate often requires acquisition of multiple beats, which can lead to significant artifacts in patients who are unable to hold their breath.

Nevertheless 3D echo has the potential of becoming an important modality for the serial analysis of ventricular size and performance in selected UVH patients. 3D echo has been used for describing the changes in ventricular volume during remodeling throughout the stages [14]. Volume measurements obtained by 3D echo are significantly lower than those obtained by CMR, and limits of agreement are wide, so that the two modalities are not interchangeable [13].

The presence of atrioventricular (AV) valve regurgitation is a well-known risk factor for adverse outcome in UVH patients [15]. By using 3D echo at the neonatal age and before any interventions, it has been shown that the geometry of the tricuspid valve (TV) is intrinsically abnormal in patients with HLHS [16, 17]. Additionally during the treatment stages the shape of the TV is adapting to the new hemodynamic conditions (Fig. 16.4) [18]. After Fontan completion the dynamic changes of the valve annulus have been studied by 3D echo. The annular dimensions and shape, as well as the angle of the papillary muscle, vary throughout the cardiac cycle and are associated with TR. These observations are important for planning surgical annuloplasty and/or design novel subvalvar interventions [19].

The use of 3D echo has also been described in single cases for detecting the presence of a thrombus in the Fontan conduit [20], or as 3D TEE for guiding percutaneous Fontan fenestration closure [21].

16.2.2 Speckle Tracking Echocardiography

Speckle tracking is an established echocardiographic application for assessing and quantifying strain and strain rate as parameters of myocardial deformation.

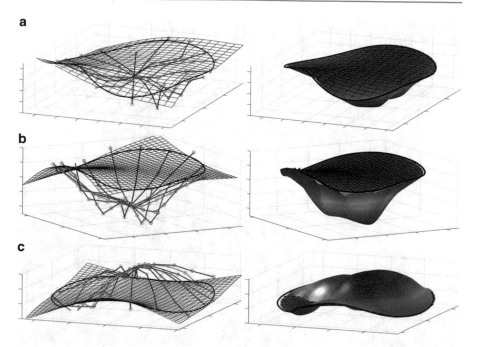

Fig. 16.4 The shape of the tricuspid valve in patients with HLHS assessed by 3D echocardiography. The raw leaflet coordinates and the best-fit annulus are shown on the left panels. The best-fit leaflet surface and the annular plane are shown on the right panels. (**a**) Tricuspid leaflet and annulus geometry demonstrating minimal tethering or prolapse. (**b**) Tricuspid valve with a large tethering volume. (**c**) Tricuspid valve with a large prolapse volume. (From [18])

The LV has another fiber orientation than a RV, which needs to be taken into account when interpreting results from myocardial deformation imaging. In single ventricles the myocardial arrangement is even more variable, due to the different myocyte size, myocyte disarray and an increase in connective tissue/fibrosis. The interventricular interaction may be completely different in presence of a dominant ventricle and a hypoplastic ventricle, or in a completely alone single ventricle [22].

Speckle tracking measurements of global strain in UVH have a good reproducibility and accuracy. In contrast regional strain measurements have been shown to have a wide variability; therefore global strain is considered a more robust technique and should be used for evaluation of UVH [23]. Speckle tracking studies have shown that myocardial deformation in UVH, single RV or single LV, is reduced compared to the normal RV and LV (Fig. 16.5) [24, 25]. After the Fontan operation similar global longitudinal strain (GLS) has been described for the single LV and the single RV; no association has been found between GLS and ejection fraction measured by CMR [26].

Speckle tracking can also be used for assessing the rotation and torsion particularly of the single LV. Lopez et al. described pattern of reduced basal circumferential strain and rotation and an augmented apical rotation and torsion; they explain the findings with the differences in myocardial fiber orientation, increased fibrosis,

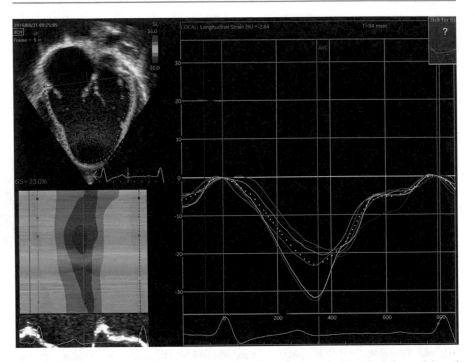

Fig. 16.5 Speckle tracking from the apical four-chamber view in a double inlet left ventricle and the resultant longitudinal strain deformation curve. Global longitudinal strain is calculated as −23%

and with the altered loading conditions throughout the phases of palliation. In specific lesions, such as pulmonary atresia with intact ventricular septum a reduced GLS may also result from an unfavorable interventricular interaction [27].

Strain rate (SR) are considered to be less loading-dependent conditions than strain. In Fontan patients with HLHS SR has been demonstrated to be a good noninvasive surrogate for the end systolic elastance, which is a load-independent parameter of systolic function, but requires invasive catheterization [28]. Thus changes in SR may detect early RV dysfunction.

In patients with HLHS longitudinal data on myocardial deformation have been obtained throughout the stages [29, 30]. In healthy children GLS and GCS improve during time, from neonate to the age of 3.5 years. In patients with a single RV strain values tend to remain at the neonatal level, therefore are decreasing during time. During the stages of palliation, GLS was at highest at stage 1 (Pre-Norwood); at the next stage (pre-BCPC) a decreases GLS but a maintained GCS were observed. This may reflect an adaptive process of the single RV, and a relative shift from longitudinal to circumferential contraction (Fig. 16.6). In spite of this mild remodeling, there is an overall progressive reduction of both, the RV longitudinal and circumferential deformation. This suggests that the single RV may have a mechanical disadvantage from birth and a further progressive impairment with age, with an intrinsic inability of the RV myocardium to fully adapt to chronic systemic pressures [30, 31].

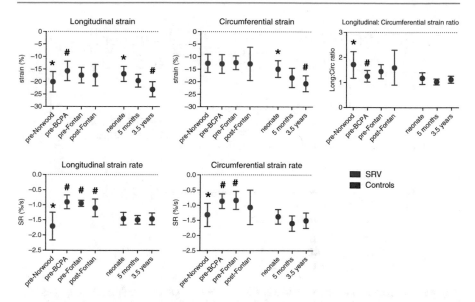

Fig. 16.6 Trends in longitudinal and circumferential strain and strain rate and ratio of longitudinal to circumferential strain throughout the UVH treatment stages. Patients with single right ventricles (blue) and normal controls (red) are compared. Asterisks indicate significant differences from pound signs on post hoc testing. (From [30])

Similarly a decline of SR in HLHS patients during follow-up after the Fontan palliation has been described [32]. More data are required to understand the clinical impact of these observations.

The most robust outcome data using speckle tracking in UVH patients, are those reported by Ghelani et al., who used advanced imaging in a large cohort of 127 Fontan patients for predicting outcome during long-term follow-up, consisting in death, transplantation, exercise capacity, postoperative metrics, arrhythmias and composite endpoints of them. CMR determined ventricle volumes combined with speckle tracking GCS were clear-cut predictors of prognosis (Fig. 16.7) [33]. Other data from a single-center retrospective study have shown that circumferential SR together with the pulmonary venous resistance were the only independent variables associated with a prolonged length of hospitalization >14 days at time of Fontan completion [34].

16.2.3 Feature Tracking CMR

Since the development of feature tracking CMR (FT-CMR) this technique is increasingly used for assessing myocardial deformation in UVH patients. FT-CMR presents some advantages compared to other modalities; the images are independent from the quality and the field of view of the acoustic windows; FT is applied on the Steady State Free Precession (SSFP) cine images routinely acquired for

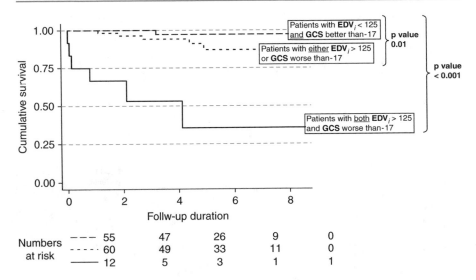

Fig. 16.7 Kaplan-Meier survival estimates in 127 Fontan patients. Echocardiography-derived GCS lower than −17% and CMR-derived EDV$_I$ >125 mL/BSA are strong predictor for worse prognosis. (From [33])

ventricular measurement and does not require any additional image acquisition (Fig. 16.8) [35, 36]. If assessment of FT is planned, than SSFP acquisition parameters should be optimized to obtain sufficient spatial and temporal (< 25 ms) resolution. FT-CMR in UVH patients is highly reproducible and can be performed with low inter- and intraobserver variability [37].

Even though the values obtained by speckle tracking and by feature tracking are not interchangeable [38, 39], similar trends have been found in UVH patients.

By using FT-CMR several authors described than UVH after Fontan present decreased GCS compared to normal hearts; in contrast only a small difference was found for GLS [37, 40]. Similarly to the results reported for speckle tracking, GLS values measured by FT-CMR in UVH were not correlated with ejection fraction; a weak correlation was found between GCS and ejection fraction [37]. By using FT-CMR Ghelani et al. could demonstrate that ventricular morphology has an influence on fiber stress and strain; so patients with a dominant RV tended to show higher fiber stress, higher rate of ventricular dilation and lower circumferential fiber shortening. Again, these findings suggest that the myocardial fiber architecture may contribute to the suboptimal adaptation of the RV to function as a systemic ventricle [40].

Regarding prognosis, reduced GCS at FT-CMR and ventricular dilation were found to be risk factors for death or heart transplantation in a cohort of 193 UVH patients [40]. Another study has shown that reduced GLS (<11.8%) and a higher dyssynchrony index (>63.5 ms) are independent predictors of major adverse events in adolescents and young adult Fontan patients, and can be used as parameters for risk stratification [41].

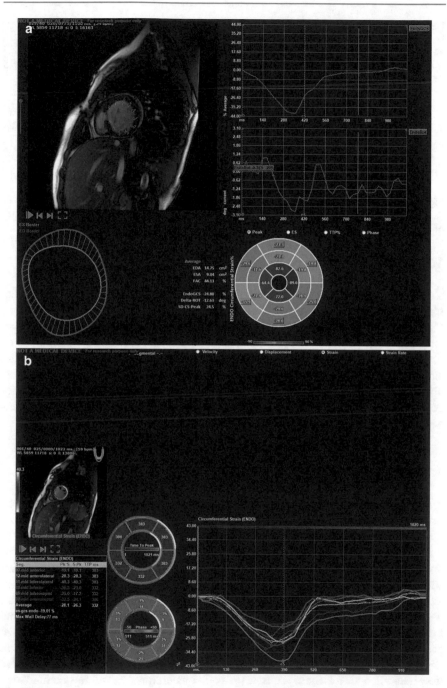

Fig. 16.8 CMR Feature tracking analysis in UVH (Medis® Software). (**a**) Measurement of global circumferential strain. (**b**) Measure of time to peak in the different myocardial segments

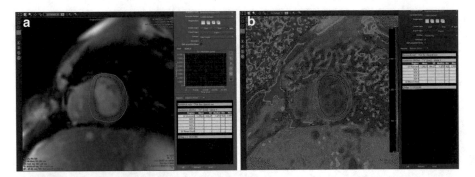

Fig. 16.9 CMR T1 measurement in a Fontan patient. (**a**) The T1 relaxation curve provides the T1 value of the region of interest, in this case a mid-ventricular slice on the left ventricle. (**b**) T1 map of the same subject

16.2.4 CMR T1 Mapping

T1 mapping is a specific CMR technique used for assessment of diffuse myocardial fibrosis. The value of T1 mapping has been shown in several acquired heart disease. However reports on its use are still limited in congenital heart disease and particularly in Fontan patients. In a small cohort of 21 patients elevated T1 values and an increased extracellular volume have been described for the single RV but not for the single LV in comparison with normal subjects. These findings suggest an unfavorable fibrotic remodeling of the single RV in systemic position. Increased T1 values correlated with worse GLS, but a correlation with ventricular volume, EF% or ventricular mass/volume ratio could not be demonstrated (Fig. 16.9) [42].

16.2.5 CMR 4D Flow

The study of the intracardiac and intravascular blood flow in Fontan patients is an important aspect of non-invasive hemodynamics assessment. The dynamic three-dimensional characteristics of the 4D flow technique makes this modality particularly suitable for the evaluation and quantification of intraventricular and vascular flow pattern in UVH (Fig. 16.10) [43]. The use of 4D flow overcomes the cumbersome acquisition of many 2D PC images in several locations. With one single acquisition during free-breathing, all data are available for post-processing and flow can be measured in every desired location. In case of unexpected findings additional locations of measurements can be added, or measurement repeated for increased accuracy [44]. Thus 4D flow can be considered reliable, less operator-dependent and more time-efficient than 2D flow acquisition. 4D flow with its retrospective flow tracking option is more accurate than other techniques for inflow quantification through the AV valve and therefore for the ventricular filling volume (Fig. 16.11) [45].

In UVH 4D flow enables noninvasive assessment of the energetic efficacy of the myocardial pump. Kinetic energy (KE) is dependent on the morphology of the

Fig. 16.10 Flow dynamics in a Fontan patient with double outflow tracts. Particle pathlines demonstrate the pulmonary vein and ventricle flow paths (blue). The ejection flow paths are shown as red and orange. Flow streams through each outflow tract remain independent with the more anterior outflow tract supplying the aortic branch vessels and the more posterior outflow tract supplying the descending aorta

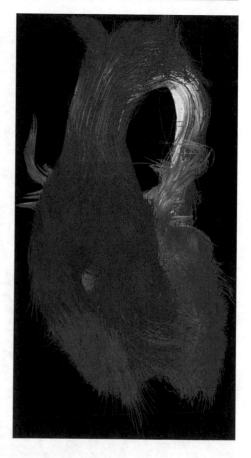

ventricle, and diastolic KE indexed to stroke volume in Fontan patients is decreased compared to controls [46]. The decreased KE in Fontan patients may be a result of impaired ventricular filling [47]. Kamphuis et al. studied the intraventricular viscous energy loss (EL) in proportion to KE in 30 Fontan patients and reported that UVH present a disproportionate intraventricular EL relative to KE; the amount of intraventricular EL was related to the intracardiac anatomy and highest if the blood entering the ventricle is ejected through a ventricular septal defect to the aorta (Fig. 16.12) [48]. Under dobutamin stress intraventricular KE, EL and flow vorticity increase; the difference of this parameters at rest compared to stress is correlated to clinical parameters such as VO_2max and exercise capacity [49].

Another important application of 4D flow is assessment of the flow within the vascular structures of the TCPC. Particularly the distribution of flow from the inferior vena cava (IVC) into the right and left pulmonary artery is of great interest. Ideally the IVC, i.e., hepatic, flow should be equally distributed to both lungs; IVC blood contains the so-called "hepatic factor," which is thought to prevent the formation of arteriovenous malformations in the lungs and cyanosis. By using particle tracing analysis, 4D CMR studies have demonstrated that within the TCPC blood

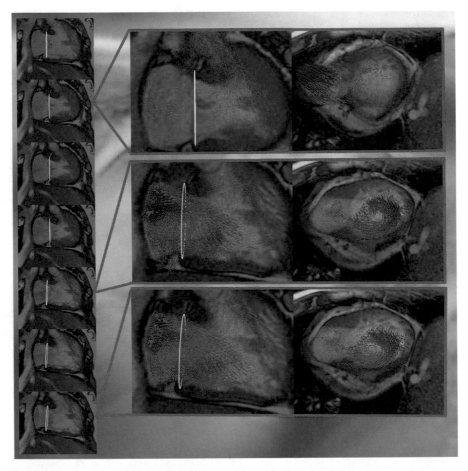

Fig. 16.11 4D flow—valve motion tracking. Tracking of the atrioventricular valve from cine images is shown on the left at selected time points throughout the cardiac cycle. At three time points, velocity vectors are shown in long-axis and in short-axis views illustrating the complex flow dynamics both through the valve and within the single ventricle

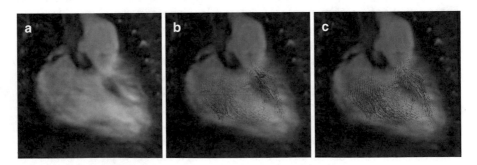

Fig. 16.12 Velocity dynamics and energy loss in the single ventricle. (**a**) Long-axis view of the single right ventricle. (**b**) Velocity vectors show ventricle inflow and outflow dynamics with an accelerated flow in the subaortic (neo-aorta) ejecting portion. (**c**) Corresponding high viscous energy losses (red) in the turbulent flow of the outflow tract

Fig. 16.13 TCPC flow dynamics. Flow stream analysis show that the IVC and SVC connections are orientated so that the IVC flow (blue) is directed to the left pulmonary artery and the SVC flow (purple) toward the right pulmonary artery

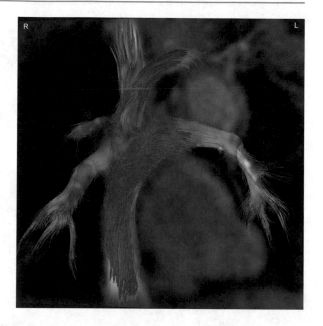

flow from the SVC flows preferentially into the RPA, while flow from the IVC (with the hepatic factor) is directed mainly into the LPA (Fig. 16.13) [50, 51]. In case of clinical deterioration during follow-up and for pre-surgical planning before Fontan revision 4D flow and computational dynamics can be used as advanced noninvasive diagnostic tools to study this complex hemodynamics [52].

When working with 4D flow, critical appraisal of the results obtained is crucial. Potential sources of error have been analyzed and described in a small cohort of Fontan patients. So flow distribution errors were as high as 22.5%; the described potential reasons for errors consisted of noise, low spatial resolution, eddy currents, and inaccurate segmentation. Whereas it is unlikely that severe flow distribution asymmetry may be missed, these observations suggest a clear necessity for eddy current correction and accurate segmentation to minimize errors when assessing Fontan patients [50].

16.3   Computational Fluid Dynamics

Recently increasing evidence has been gained, suggesting a critical influence of energy efficiency and power loss (Ploss) respectively, on the hemodynamics of the Fontan circulation. In addition to inside the ventricular cavity, Ploss can occur along the TCPC vascular pathway [53, 54]. Knowledge about the correlation between Ploss and the geometry of the TCPC has been gained by using CMR based computational fluid dynamics [55]. In a large cohort of 100 Fontan patients Haggerty et al. performed computational analysis of the Fontan connection (Fig. 16.14). Their results suggest some clinically relevant insights, which include (1) a large

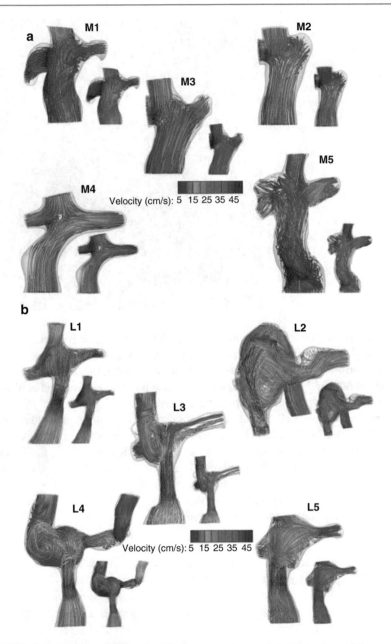

Fig. 16.14 3D velocity streamlines in different cavopulmonary morphologies with low and high energy dissipation. (**a**) 3D velocity streamlines color coded by local velocity magnitude and vessel of origin (blue, IVC; red, SVC) for the 5 TCPC with lowest energy dissipation. (**b**) Elevated energy dissipation is observed in TCPC with turbulent high velocity flow due to abrupt changes in diameter. (From [53])

Fig. 16.15 SSFP image of the extracardiac Fontan conduit. In the growing patient, there is a mismatch between the diameter of the inferior caval vein and the conduit; in addition with the growth of the patient there is a traction of the conduit on the inferior caval vein (arrow). *AO* Neo-aorta (dilated), *IVC* inferior vena cava, *SVC* superior vena cava

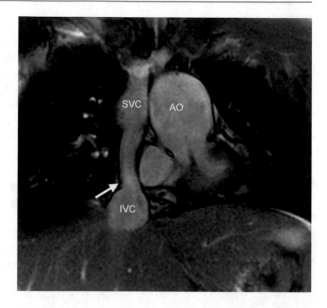

variability of Ploss among patients independently from age and development; (2) an inverse correlation between indexed Ploss and Qs supporting the hypothesis that TCPC hemodynamics directly influence ventricular preload and filling; (3) small pulmonary arteries or stenosis in the Fontan pathway have a detrimental effect on Ploss; (4) intra-atrial and extracardiac Fontan connections do not show any energetic difference [53]. In Fontan patients the pulmonary arteries are not growing in proportion to somatic growth; this mismatch can potentially cause an increasing Ploss in the Fontan circulation over time [56]. Other authors suggest the inferior vena cava junction to the extracardiac conduit to be a critical location for Ploss, with some evidence that a 16 mm Conduit may not be adequate in the adult patients (Fig. 16.15) [57]. Similarly to the intraventricular EL, Ploss in the TCPC also increases under exercise [58, 59].

Computational fluid dynamics has the potential to be used for the geometrical surgical planning of the TCPC, with particular focus on the hepatic flow distribution and therefore to help improving patient outcome. Prediction of hepatic flow distribution can be performed accurately for specific graft types, however some methodological improvements and more follow-up and outcome data are still needed [60, 61]. The effects of aortopulmonary collateral flow on the net vascular resistance of the Fontan circulation, as well as the prediction of the effects of interventions such as a y-graft implementation and stent dilatation in TCPC vessels have also been studied with computational fluid dynamics [62]. The dramatic improvements in noninvasive imaging modalities, including 3D echo and 4D flow, that can be integrated in computational models, as well as in the modeling algorithms themselves, directs computer modeling more and more toward being a tool for personalized medicine and shifts their role from understanding physiology to predicting the results of interventions and outcome. Nevertheless large validation studies and larger series correlating computer fluid dynamics-derived parameters to clinical outcomes are needed before clinical implementation can be considered [63].

There are some known challenges of Ploss quantification by computational fluid dynamics [54]; these include an accurate assessment of boundary conditions, the assumption of a rigid vessel wall and steady versus pulsatile flow conditions. The influence of respiration on blood flow within the Fontan pathway has been widely discussed. During inspiration the venous flow can increase up to 87% [64]. Even though clear differences has been observed throughout the respiratory cycle, the calculated average differences on Ploss and hepatic flow distribution are minimal and do not significantly influence clinically relevant parameters. These observations validate the routine use of breath-holding techniques for measuring the mean flows in Fontan patients. As an additional internal validation the mean flows in the IVC and descending aorta can be taken, as they are interchangeable [64, 65]. Most recently 4D flow has been increasingly used for evaluating TCPC flow as described above; in contrast to computational fluid dynamics 4D flow is an in vivo technique and reduces the number of assumptions needed for calculation of Ploss [46, 54].

16.4 3D Printing

3D data set amenable for 3D printing can be obtained by CMR, CT, or even by 3D echo.

3D printing is a very useful technique for advanced visualization and diagnosis, for planning and simulation of surgery and interventions, for research, education and communication [66]. A multicenter international study recently demonstrated that in 48% of the cases the visualization of a 3D model of the lesion helped redefining the surgical approach [67]. In complex lesions 3D printing is particularly valuable in the decision process if biventricular repair is feasible or palliation with a Fontan approach may be a safer treatment option [68] (Fig. 16.16). In complex congenital heart disease such as UVH 3D models are helpful for education of trainees, cardiac nurses and for facilitating communication with parents during clinical consultation [69, 70].

3D printing combined with 4D flow has been utilized for planning Fontan revision [71, 72]. Particularly in patients with pulmonary arteriovenous malformations, Fontan takedown and redirection of the hepatic venous flow may result in a significant clinical improvement [72].

A specific research application of 3D dataset and printing is the combination of the 3D Fontan geometry with computational fluid modeling of flow for developing new intravascular pumping devices that could be placed in the TCPC [73]. Such devices could be applied in a failing Fontan circulation and have the potential to improve survival in failure patients; their survival is currently totally dependent on organ availability for transplantation.

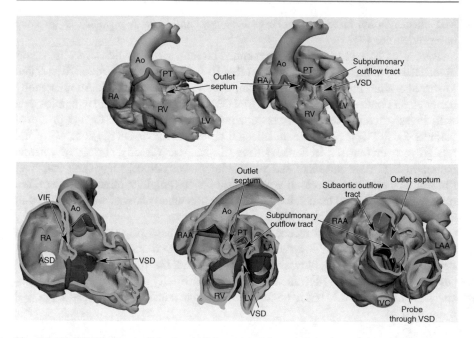

Fig. 16.16 3D Printing model of a double outlet right ventricle. In complex lesions such as DORV, understanding the connections between the ventricle and the outflow tracts may help surgical decision about biventricular or univentricular repair. Upper Panel: external view. Lower Panel: intracardiac view from 3 different projections. *Ao* Aorta, *ASD* atrial septal defect, *IVC* inferior vena cava, *LA* left atrium, *LAA* left atrial appendage, *LV* left ventricle, *PT* pulmonary trunk, *RA* right atrium, *RAA* right atrial appendage, *RV* right ventricle, *VSD* ventricular septal defect. (Courtesy of Dr. Yoo, Hospital for Sick Children, Toronto, Canada)

16.5 Imaging of Liver Fibrosis

Fontan-associated liver disease (FALD) is a well-known long-term sequela in Fontan patients. Liver fibrosis and eventually cirrhosis are the major structural finding and represent a complication of chronic increased hepatic venous pressure [74–76]. Noninvasive assessment of liver fibrosis can be performed by ultrasound transient elastography or by MR/CT techniques [77].

Post-contrast MR/CT images show abnormal enhancement of the liver parenchyma, with zonal or reticular enhancement pattern. During progression of the disease benign hypervascular regenerative nodules has to be differentiated from hepatocellular carcinomas [78]. Recently MR elastography has been developed for detecting liver stiffness and fibrosis [79]. Diagnostic performance of MR elastography is acceptable, but is diminished in patients with concomitant liver steatosis [80]. Moreover in Fontan patients liver stiffness may be increased not only because of fibrosis, but also due to venous congestion. Nevertheless in a cohort of 49 Fontan patients a good correlation has been described among liver stiffness at

MR elastography, histology scoring at biopsy, and Fontan pressure at invasive hemodynamics [81].

Recently CMR T1 mapping demonstrated an increased hepatic extracellular volume. These preliminary results suggest that liver fibrosis is not necessarily related to the age after Fontan nor to the central venous pressure [82]. Another study included 33 Fontan patients and compared CMR computational fluid dynamics data with invasive catheterization measurements and liver biopsies. In this group of patients local TCPC hemodynamics, such as resistance or energy loss, were not related to liver fibrosis; in contrast liver fibrosis was directly correlated with an increased IVC flow and increased ventricular power output, suggesting that liver fibrosis may cause an increased volume load for the single ventricle and therefore represent an additional burden for cardiac function when patients are entering adult age [83].

Disappointingly a most recent prospective study assessing the combination of several modalities for noninvasive screening of FALD found a lack of correlation between the obtained noninvasive parameters and the histologically confirmed severity of liver fibrosis [84]. In summary, the sensitivity and accuracy of noninvasive screening for FALD has to be further investigated and its clinical use supported by more data.

References

1. Frescura C, Thiene G. The new concept of univentricular heart. Front Pediatr. 2014;2:62.
2. Khairy P, Poirier N, Mercier L-A. Univentricular heart. Circulation. 2007;115(6):800–12.
3. Gewillig M, Brown SC. The Fontan circulation after 45 years: update in physiology. Heart. 2016;102(14):1081.
4. Marcelletti C, et al. Inferior vena cava-pulmonary artery extracardiac conduit. A new form of right heart bypass. J Thorac Cardiovasc Surg. 1990;100(2):228–32.
5. Fontan F, Baudet E. Surgical repair of tricuspid atresia. Thorax. 1971;26(3):240–8.
6. Khairy P, et al. Long-term survival, modes of death, and predictors of mortality in patients with Fontan surgery. Circulation. 2008;117(1):85–92.
7. d'Udekem Y, et al. Redefining expectations of long-term survival after the Fontan procedure. Circulation. 2014;130(11_suppl_1):S32–8.
8. Pundi KN, et al. 40-year follow-up after the Fontan operation: long-term outcomes of 1,052 patients. J Am Coll Cardiol. 2015;66(15):1700–10.
9. Di Salvo G, et al. Imaging the adult with congenital heart disease: a multimodality imaging approach—position paper from the EACVI. Eur Heart J Cardiovasc Imaging. 2018;19(10):1077–98.
10. Valsangiacomo Buechel ER, et al. Indications for cardiovascular magnetic resonance in children with congenital and acquired heart disease: an expert consensus paper of the imaging working group of the AEPC and the cardiovascular magnetic resonance section of the EACVI. Eur Heart J Cardiovasc Imaging. 2015;16(3):281–97.
11. Ginde S, Goot BH, Frommelt PC. Imaging adult patients with Fontan circulation. Curr Opin Cardiol. 2017;32(5):521–8.
12. Soriano BD, et al. Matrix-Array 3-dimensional echocardiographic assessment of volumes, mass, and ejection fraction in young pediatric patients with a functional single ventricle: a comparison study with cardiac magnetic resonance. Circulation. 2008;117(14):1842–8.

13. Bell A, et al. Assessment of right ventricular volumes in hypoplastic left heart syndrome by real-time three-dimensional echocardiography: comparison with cardiac magnetic resonance imaging. Eur Heart J Cardiovasc Imaging. 2013;15(3):257–66.
14. Sasikumar D, et al. Quantification of ventricular unloading by 3D echocardiography in single ventricle of left ventricular morphology following superior cavo-pulmonary anastomosis and Fontan completion—a feasibility study. Ann Pediatr Cardiol. 2017;10(3):224–9.
15. Mery CM, et al. Contemporary outcomes of the Fontan operation: a large single-institution cohort. Ann Thorac Surg. 2019;108:1439.
16. Nii M, et al. Three-dimensional tricuspid annular function provides insight into the mechanisms of tricuspid valve regurgitation in classic hypoplastic left heart syndrome. J Am Soc Echocardiogr. 2006;19(4):391–402.
17. Kutty S, et al. Tricuspid regurgitation in hypoplastic left heart syndrome: mechanistic insights from 3-dimensional echocardiography and relationship with outcomes. Circ Cardiovasc Imaging. 2014;7(5):765–72.
18. Colen T, et al. Tricuspid valve adaptation during the first Interstage period in Hypoplastic left heart syndrome. J Am Soc Echocardiogr. 2018;31(5):624–33.
19. Nguyen AV, et al. Dynamic three-dimensional geometry of the tricuspid valve annulus in hypoplastic left heart syndrome with a Fontan circulation. J Am Soc Echocardiogr. 2019;32(5):655–666.e13.
20. Mart CR. Three-dimensional echocardiographic evaluation of the Fontan conduit for Thrombus. Echocardiography. 2012;29(3):363–8.
21. Giannakoulas G, Thanopoulos V. Three-dimensional transesophageal echocardiography for guiding percutaneous Fontan fenestration closure. Echocardiography. 2014;31(7):E230–1.
22. Grattan M, Mertens L. Mechanics of the functionally univentricular heart—how little do we understand and why does it matter? Can J Cardiol. 2016;32(8):1033.e11–8.
23. Singh GK, et al. Accuracy and reproducibility of strain by speckle tracking in pediatric subjects with Normal heart and single ventricular physiology: a two-dimensional speckle-tracking echocardiography and magnetic resonance imaging correlative study. J Am Soc Echocardiogr. 2010;23(11):1143–52.
24. Moiduddin N, et al. Two-dimensional speckle strain and Dyssynchrony in single left ventricles vs. normal left ventricles. Congenit Heart Dis. 2010;5(6):579–86.
25. Moiduddin N, et al. Two-dimensional speckle strain and Dyssynchrony in single right ventricles versus Normal right ventricles. J Am Soc Echocardiogr. 2010;23(6):673–9.
26. Koopman LP, et al. Longitudinal myocardial deformation does not predict single ventricle ejection fraction assessed by cardiac magnetic resonance imaging in children with a total Cavopulmonary connection. Pediatr Cardiol. 2018;39(2):283–93.
27. Lopez C, et al. Strain and rotational mechanics in children with single left ventricles after Fontan. J Am Soc Echocardiogr. 2018;31(12):1297–306.
28. Schlangen J, et al. Two-dimensional global longitudinal strain rate is a preload independent index of systemic right ventricular contractility in hypoplastic left heart syndrome patients after fontan operation. Circ Cardiovasc Imaging. 2014;7(6):880–6.
29. Khoo NS, et al. Novel insights into RV adaptation and function in hypoplastic left heart syndrome between the first 2 stages of surgical palliation. JACC Cardiovasc Imaging. 2011;4(2):128–37.
30. Tham EB, et al. Insights into the evolution of myocardial dysfunction in the functionally single right ventricle between staged palliations using speckle-tracking echocardiography. J Am Soc Echocardiogr. 2014;27(3):314–22.
31. Suntratonpipat S, et al. Impaired single right ventricular function compared to single left ventricles during the early stages of palliation: a longitudinal study. J Am Soc Echocardiogr. 2017;30(5):468–77.
32. Michel M, et al. Decline of systolic and diastolic 2D strain rate during follow-up of HLHS patients after Fontan palliation. Pediatr Cardiol. 2016;37(7):1250–7.

33. Ghelani SJ, et al. Comparison between echocardiography and cardiac magnetic resonance imaging in predicting transplant-free survival after the Fontan operation. Am J Cardiol. 2015;116(7):1132–8.

34. Park PW, et al. Speckle-tracking echocardiography improves pre-operative risk stratification before the total Cavopulmonary connection. J Am Soc Echocardiogr. 2017;30(5):478–84.

35. Pedrizzetti G, et al. Principles of cardiovascular magnetic resonance feature tracking and echocardiographic speckle tracking for informed clinical use. J Cardiovasc Magn Reson. 2016;18(1):51.

36. Schmidt R, et al. Value of speckle-tracking echocardiography and MRI-based feature tracking analysis in adult patients after Fontan-type palliation. Congenit Heart Dis. 2014;9(5):397–406.

37. Hu L, et al. Assessment of global and regional strain left ventricular in patients with preserved ejection fraction after Fontan operation using a tissue tracking technique. Int J Cardiovasc Imaging. 2019;35(1):153–60.

38. Salehi Ravesh M, et al. Longitudinal deformation of the right ventricle in hypoplastic left heart syndrome: a comparative study of 2D-feature tracking magnetic resonance imaging and 2D-speckle tracking echocardiography. Pediatr Cardiol. 2018;39(6):1265–75.

39. Ghelani SJ, et al. Echocardiography and magnetic resonance imaging based strain analysis of functional single ventricles: a study of intra- and inter-modality reproducibility. Int J Cardiovasc Imaging. 2016;32(7):1113–20.

40. Ghelani SJ, et al. Impact of ventricular morphology on fiber stress and strain in Fontan patients. Circ Cardiovasc Imaging. 2018;11(7):e006738.

41. Ishizaki U, et al. Global strain and dyssynchrony of the single ventricle predict adverse cardiac events after the Fontan procedure: analysis using feature-tracking cine magnetic resonance imaging. J Cardiol. 2019;73(2):163–70.

42. Kato A, et al. Pediatric Fontan patients are at risk for myocardial fibrotic remodeling and dysfunction. Int J Cardiol. 2017;240:172–7.

43. Kamphuis VP, et al. Unravelling cardiovascular disease using four dimensional flow cardiovascular magnetic resonance. Int J Cardiovasc Imaging. 2017;33(7):1069–81.

44. Valverde I, et al. Systemic-to-pulmonary collateral flow in patients with palliated univentricular heart physiology: measurement using cardiovascular magnetic resonance 4D velocity acquisition. J Cardiovasc Magn Reson. 2012;14(1):25.

45. She HL, et al. Comparative evaluation of flow quantification across the atrioventricular valve in patients with functional univentricular heart after Fontan's surgery and healthy controls: measurement by 4D flow magnetic resonance imaging and streamline visualization. Congenit Heart Dis. 2017;12(1):40–8.

46. Rutkowski DR, et al. Analysis of cavopulmonary and cardiac flow characteristics in Fontan patients: comparison with healthy volunteers. J Magn Reson Imaging. 2019;49(6):1786–99.

47. Sjöberg P, et al. Decreased diastolic ventricular kinetic energy in young patients with Fontan circulation demonstrated by four-dimensional cardiac magnetic resonance imaging. Pediatr Cardiol. 2017;38(4):669–80.

48. Kamphuis VP, et al. Disproportionate intraventricular viscous energy loss in Fontan patients: analysis by 4D flow MRI. Eur Heart J Cardiovasc Imaging. 2018;20(3):323–33.

49. Kamphuis VP, et al. Stress increases intracardiac 4D flow cardiovascular magnetic resonance -derived energetics and vorticity and relates to VO2max in Fontan patients. J Cardiovasc Magn Reson. 2019;21(1):43.

50. Jarvis K, et al. Caval to pulmonary 3D flow distribution in patients with Fontan circulation and impact of potential 4D flow MRI error sources. Magn Reson Med. 2019;81(2):1205–18.

51. Dasi LP, et al. Pulmonary hepatic flow distribution in total cavopulmonary connections: extracardiac versus intracardiac. J Thorac Cardiovasc Surg. 2011;141(1):207–14.

52. Bächler P, et al. Caval blood flow distribution in patients with Fontan circulation: quantification by using particle traces from 4D flow MR imaging. Radiology. 2013;267(1):67–75.

53. Haggerty CM, et al. Fontan hemodynamics from 100 patient-specific cardiac magnetic resonance studies: a computational fluid dynamics analysis. J Thorac Cardiovasc Surg. 2014;148(4):1481–9.

54. Rijnberg Friso M, et al. Energetics of blood flow in cardiovascular disease. Circulation. 2018;137(22):2393–407.
55. Tang E, et al. Geometric characterization of patient-specific total cavopulmonary connections and its relationship to hemodynamics. J Am Coll Cardiol Img. 2014;7(3):215–24.
56. Restrepo M, et al. Energetic implications of vessel growth and flow changes over time in Fontan patients. Ann Thorac Surg. 2015;99(1):163–70.
57. Rijnberg FM, et al. Four-dimensional flow magnetic resonance imaging-derived blood flow energetics of the inferior vena cava-to-extracardiac conduit junction in Fontan patients. Eur J Cardiothorac Surg. 2019;55(6):1202–10.
58. Bossers SS, et al. Computational fluid dynamics in Fontan patients to evaluate power loss during simulated exercise. Heart. 2014;100(9):696–701.
59. Sundareswaran KS, et al. The total cavopulmonary connection resistance: a significant impact on single ventricle hemodynamics at rest and exercise. Am J Physiol Heart Circ Physiol. 2008;295(6):H2427–35.
60. Trusty PM, et al. The first cohort of prospective Fontan surgical planning patients with follow-up data: how accurate is surgical planning? J Thorac Cardiovasc Surg. 2019;157(3):1146–55.
61. Trusty PM, et al. Fontan surgical planning: previous accomplishments, current challenges, and future directions. J Cardiovasc Transl Res. 2018;11(2):133–44.
62. Frieberg P, et al. Simulation of aortopulmonary collateral flow in Fontan patients for use in prediction of interventional outcomes. Clin Physiol Funct Imaging. 2018;38(4):622–9.
63. Biglino G, et al. Computational modelling for congenital heart disease: how far are we from clinical translation? Heart. 2017;103(2):98–103.
64. Wei Z, et al. Respiratory effects on Fontan circulation during rest and exercise using real-time cardiac magnetic resonance imaging. Ann Thorac Surg. 2016;101(5):1818–25.
65. Tang E, et al. The effect of respiration-driven flow waveforms on hemodynamic metrics used in Fontan surgical planning. J Biomech. 2019;82:87–95.
66. Giannopoulos AA, et al. Applications of 3D printing in cardiovascular diseases. Nat Rev Cardiol. 2016;13:701.
67. Valverde I, et al. Three-dimensional printed models for surgical planning of complex congenital heart defects: an international multicentre study. Eur J Cardiothorac Surg. 2017;52(6):1139–48.
68. Yoo S-J, van Arsdell GS. 3D printing in surgical management of double outlet right ventricle. Front Pediatr. 2018;5:289.
69. Biglino G, et al. Piloting the use of patient-specific cardiac models as a novel tool to facilitate communication during clinical consultations. Pediatr Cardiol. 2017;38(4):813–8.
70. Biglino G, et al. Use of 3D models of congenital heart disease as an education tool for cardiac nurses. Congenit Heart Dis. 2017;12(1):113–8.
71. Carberry T, et al. Fontan revision: presurgical planning using four-dimensional (4D) flow and three-dimensional (3D) printing. World J Pediatr Congenit Heart Surg. 2019;10(2):245–9.
72. McLennan D, et al. Usefulness of 4D-flow MRI in mapping flow distribution through failing Fontan circulation prior to cardiac intervention. Pediatr Cardiol. 2019;40(5):1093–6.
73. Granegger M, et al. A long-term mechanical cavopulmonary support device for patients with Fontan circulation. Med Eng Phys. 2019;70:9–18.
74. Lui GK, et al. Diagnosis and management of noncardiac complications in adults with congenital heart disease: a scientific statement from the American Heart Association. Circulation. 2017;136(20):e348–92.
75. Rychik J, et al. End-organ consequences of the Fontan operation: liver fibrosis, protein-losing enteropathy and plastic bronchitis. Cardiol Young. 2013;23(6):831–40.
76. Krieger EV, et al. Single ventricle anatomy is associated with increased frequency of nonalcoholic cirrhosis. Int J Cardiol. 2013;167(5):1918–23.
77. Wu FM, et al. Transient elastography may identify Fontan patients with unfavorable hemodynamics and advanced hepatic fibrosis. Congenit Heart Dis. 2014;9(5):438–47.
78. Yoo S-J, et al. MR assessment of abdominal circulation in Fontan physiology. Int J Cardiovasc Imaging. 2014;30(6):1065–72.

79. Poterucha JT, et al. Magnetic resonance elastography: a novel technique for the detection of hepatic fibrosis and hepatocellular carcinoma after the Fontan operation. Mayo Clin Proc. 2015;90(7):882–94.
80. Trout AT, et al. Diagnostic performance of MR elastography for liver fibrosis in children and young adults with a spectrum of liver diseases. Radiology. 2018;287(3):824–32.
81. Silva-Sepulveda JA, et al. Evaluation of Fontan liver disease: correlation of transjugular liver biopsy with magnetic resonance and hemodynamics. Congenit Heart Dis. 2019;14(4):600–8.
82. de Lange C, et al. Increased extracellular volume in the liver of pediatric Fontan patients. J Cardiovasc Magn Reson. 2019;21(1):39.
83. Trusty PM, et al. Impact of hemodynamics and fluid energetics on liver fibrosis after Fontan operation. J Thorac Cardiovasc Surg. 2018;156(1):267–75.
84. Munsterman ID, et al. The clinical spectrum of Fontan-associated liver disease: results from a prospective multimodality screening cohort. Eur Heart J. 2019;40(13):1057–68.

Electrophysiology Interventional Planning

17

Adelina Doltra, Karina Duran, Ivo Roca-Luque,
and Susanna Prat-Gonzalez

17.1 Introduction

Cardiovascular imaging plays a determinant role in electrophysiology interventional planning. Imaging techniques can provide detailed information on anatomy, detect proarrhythmic substrate (fibrosis) and can be useful to guide interventional procedures. Although echocardiography is usually the first technique used to diagnose structural heart disease, Cardiac MR (CMR) has been established as the gold standard method for biventricular volume quantification and cardiac function assessment [1], and has also a key role in identifying fibrosis [2]. All of these characteristics make CMR an excellent technique to study adult congenital heart disease (ACHD) patients with arrhythmias. CMR is, however, limited in the presence of devices such as pacemakers or ICDs, which are common in this subset of patients. In those cases, computed tomography (CT) can provide detailed anatomical information.

In this chapter, we explain how imaging can be useful to guide complex electrophysiology procedures such as ablation of atrial fibrillation and ventricular tachycardia, and cardiac resynchronization therapy (CRT) implant in ACHD patients.

A. Doltra (✉) · K. Duran · S. Prat-Gonzalez
Cardiac Imaging Section, Cardiovascular Clinic Institute, Hospital Clinic, Barcelona, Spain
e-mail: adoltra@clinic.cat; suprat@clinic.cat

I. Roca-Luque
Arrhythmia Section, Cardiovascular Clinic Institute, Hospital Clinic, Barcelona, Spain
e-mail: iroca@clinic.cat

© Springer Nature Switzerland AG 2021
P. Gallego, I. Valverde (eds.), *Multimodality Imaging Innovations In Adult Congenital Heart Disease*, Congenital Heart Disease in Adolescents and Adults,
https://doi.org/10.1007/978-3-030-61927-5_17

17.1.1 Role of Cardiac Imaging in Congenital Heart Disease

The number of ACHD patients has increased over the past few decades due to an early diagnosis, a substantial improvement in surgical and percutaneous techniques, as well as a specialized clinical follow-up.

Atrial and ventricular arrhythmias are common in ACHD patients, and are associated with adverse events and mortality [3–5], the risk is particularly high in patients with severe defects, who have a lifetime risk of arrhythmia (particularly atrial) of 50% [5]. Arrhythmic events are also a common complication of ACHD undergoing surgery and are associated with a worse clinical outcome [6]. Regarding sudden cardiac death, its risk may reach 10% per 10 years of follow-up, with most events occurring in adult individuals with complex lesions [7]. Complex anatomic structures, the presence of conduits, patches or baffles, and fibrosis arising from either surgical repairs or chronic pressure or volume overload lead to a proarrhythmic substrate in this group of patients, and explain the high incidence of arrhythmia [3].

17.1.2 Imaging in Atrial Arrhythmia in Adult Congenital Heart Disease

Atrial arrhythmia is the leading cause of hospitalizations in adults with congenital heart disease [8]. Different subtypes of atrial arrhythmia may be present in patients with ACHD, with variable proportions according to defect complexity and age of presentation [9]. In the general ACHD population, intra-atrial reentrant tachycardia (IART) is the most common atrial arrhythmia, with increasing prevalence according to CHD complexity. Atrial fibrillation (AF) and focal atrial tachycardia are comparatively less common, although the prevalence of AF increases with age; in a multicenter cohort study, AF was the most common atrial arrhythmia in patients over 50 years [9]. Regarding AF, it has an earlier age of onset as compared to the general population [10] and is usually seen in patients with left obstructive lesions or left atrial dilatation [3]. Finally, some congenital abnormalities are associated with a higher prevalence of some particular arrhythmias (such as accessory pathways in Ebstein's anomaly) [11].

Two main mechanisms for atrial arrhythmia have been described in ACHD patients The most frequent mechanism is macro reentrant atrial arrhythmia (such as cavotricuspid isthmus dependent flutter and IART), which is usually originated around anatomic obstacles (such as vein ostia) or areas of atrial fibrosis or scarring (like suture lines or conduits); frequently, the cavotricuspid isthmus is involved [12]. Less often, increased automaticity and focal micro reentry can lead to focal atrial tachycardia, as it may be observed after Fontan or atrial switch procedures [9, 13].

Since pharmacological treatment is usually insufficient, catheter ablation is often a first-line treatment in ACHD patients with atrial arrhythmia. The efficacy of catheter ablation, however, is variable, and depends on the characteristics of the arrhythmia itself and the complexity of the CHD. In addition, because of the presence of complex anatomies and changes caused by previous surgery, the rate of complications related to the ablation is higher in ACHD as compared with other heart conditions [14]. Due to the challenging nature of many of these procedures, ablation in ACHD should be limited to high volume centers, where a dedicated multidisciplinary team (including electrophysiologists, cardiac imaging specialists, and cardiac surgeons) is available [15].

Planning catheter ablation in patients with CHD with arrhythmias needs, then, a multidisciplinary approach in order to individualize patient's strategy, guide the procedure, and limit complications.

When an ablation procedure is considered, imaging techniques can have a role by facilitating:

1. Understanding of real anatomy. This is crucial, since many patients present with anatomic variants, surgical changes or obstacles, prostheses, and baffles.
2. Vascular access knowledge.
3. Assessing the presence of arrhythmogenic substrate (fibrosis or scar).

17.1.2.1   Cardiac Imaging in Vascular Access and Underlying Anatomy

In ACHD patients, and particularly when ablation is considered, is important to understand the underlying anatomy in each particular patient, both regarding potential abnormalities and surgical corrections. In this scenario, 3D modalities, such as CMR or cardiac CT, are the techniques of choice. CMR has the advantage of offering information on cardiac volumes and function, angiography, and fibrosis/scar in the same examination. However, in cases when CMR is not possible (incompatible devices or claustrophobia, for instance), cardiac CT can be a good alternative with excellent spatial resolution. These available imaging methods (cardiac CT, angiography, and fluoroscopy) should be optimized for keeping radiation doses to patients As Low As Reasonably Achievable (ALARA) and the lowest contrast dose needed. Due to the complex nature of these studies, they should be performed in high volume centers [3].

When planning an ablation procedure, patency of vessels allowing access to the heart needs to be known. Around 6% of ACHD patients may require different vascular access than the femoral vein (due to abnormalities such as occluded femoral vessels or interrupted inferior cava vein) [16] (Fig. 17.1). Cardiac CT, CMR, or angiography should be available to complete assessment of individual anatomy and vascular access [3] (Fig. 17.2).

In addition, in certain procedures, such as AF ablation, it can be useful to identify the location, number, and size of the pulmonary veins, which typically present anatomical variants (in almost 50% of patients, according to some data [17]). In AF ablation, knowing pulmonary vein anatomy beforehand can facilitate the procedure and prevent complications [18]. For this, 3D techniques as cardiac MRI and cardiac CT are the best options (Fig. 17.3).

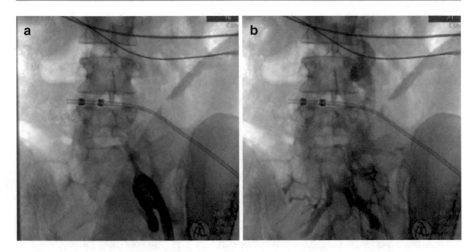

Fig. 17.1 Example of a Fontan patient who required an intra-atrial reentrant tachycardia ablation. **a** and **b** show a venogram that demonstrates an obstruction of the left iliac vein. Therefore, the right femoral vein access was impossible

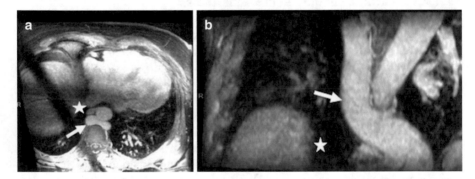

Fig. 17.2 Contrast-enhanced magnetic resonance angiography (MRA) of an atrial fibrillation patient before pulmonary vein (PV) ablation. (**a**) Gated MRA in axial plane with infrahepatic interruption of the inferior vena cava (star) with prominent hemiazygos continuation that connects to a dilated azygos vein (white arrow). (**b**) Coronal MRA view where the dilated azygos continuation drains up into the superior vena cava (arrow). Knowledge of this anatomic arrangement is important in percutaneous cardiopulmonary procedures

17.1.2.2   Identification of Arrhythmogenic Substrate

Since fibrosis or scar is associated with arrhythmia generation and recurrence, identification of those areas with gadolinium-enhanced CMR can be useful to plan ablation. Although atrial assessment of fibrosis with CMR (in contrast to ventricular fibrosis imaging) is technically challenging and not used routinely, it is feasible and can be useful in selected cases, particularly if AF ablation is considered.

In the general population, catheter ablation is an effective treatment for patients with AF, and is usually recommended in cases of symptomatic AF despite medical treatment [19]. Although the same criteria may apply for ACHD, follow-up and

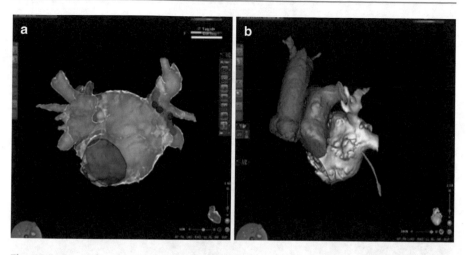

Fig. 17.3 Example of atrial fibrillation ablation in patient with TGA and situs inversus. (**a**) Integration of cardiac CT segmentation (glass shell reconstruction) with electroanatomical map is used to guide ablation and locate the PV ostia. Red dots represent the ablation points performed around the PV. (**b**) Once the integration is performed, it is possible to visualize the trajectory of the transseptal puncture (green line) and help to reintroduce the catheters into the LA in case the transseptal access is lost. *TGA* transposition of great arteries, *PV* pulmonary veins, *LA* left atria

outcomes data are limited in this population. In addition, some issues need to be taken into account in ACHD patients: on the one hand, the substrate for AF is different, with atrial wall fibrosis (instead of pulmonary veins alone) playing an important role in AF generation [10]; on the other, AF may coexist with episodes of regular atrial tachycardia [10]. However, and although evidence is limited, the treatment seems to be effective with acceptable long-term results [20].

Atrial fibrosis assessment with MR may be useful to study the arrhythmogenic substrate and predict the probability of arrhythmia recurrence. In acquired heart disease patients, larger extent of atrial fibrosis has been associated with a higher incidence of recurrence of AF after ablation [21].

The sequence used for the assessment of atrial fibrosis is a free-breathing, three-dimensional inversion recovery gradient echo, with respiratory navigator and ECG gating. The images are planned in axial orientation. This sequence is acquired 15–30 min after intravenous administration of gadolinium (0.1–0.2 mmol/kg).

Although the parameters used are variable depending on the working group, the usual thickness ranges between 1.5 and 4 mm, with an in-plane resolution between 1.2×1.2 and 1.6×1.6 mm. In our center, we use a voxel size of $1.25 \times 1.25 \times 2.5$ mm. Acquisition time is usually around 10–15 min, depending on the heart rate and respiratory pattern of the patient [22].

Once the images are acquired, post-processing is necessary to quantify the extent of atrial fibrosis. Different techniques have been described for this purpose, although most authors use semi-automatic quantification techniques with different cut-off points of signal intensity to define fibrosis [21, 23]. In order to reduce variability, a

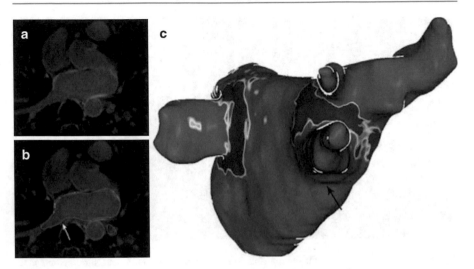

Fig. 17.4 (a) Three-dimensional (3D) late gadolinium enhancement (LGE CMR) image in axial plane (resolution 1.2 × 1.2 × 2.5 mm) of the left atria after 3 month post pulmonary vein ablation. (b) Segmentation of the LA in axial plane with post-processing software. Red color represents areas of fibrosis post-ablation. The white arrow indicates an area around the right pulmonary vein without scar (gap). (c) Reconstruction of the 3D color-coded late enhancement shell. Red areas represent scar/fibrosis post-ablation, whereas the black arrow points to a gap in the ablation line around the right pulmonary vein ostium

possible approach (used in our group) is to normalize the value of the signal strength of the atrial wall to the intensity of the blood pool [24] (Fig. 17.4).

Despite the promising results in acquired heart disease, no data is available regarding the usefulness of atrial fibrosis assessment for ablation planning in ACHD patients. However, there is emerging interest in some experienced groups to apply this methodology in a subpopulation of ACHD patients (Fig. 17.5).

17.1.2.3 Cardiac Imaging During Ablation Procedure

Although the main use of transesophageal echocardiography (TEE) is to rule out the presence of a thrombus within the left atrial appendage before the ablation is performed, it can also be useful to guide the procedure in patients with complex anatomies.

Echographic techniques, such as TEE and intracardiac echo (ICE), have a role in imaging intracardiac anatomical structures (such as the fossa ovalis), detect aneurysmal or thickened septum or previously implanted devices or surgical changes (in the interatrial septum, for instance). The use of these techniques can increase the success rate and the safety of the transseptal puncture [25]. This information is key to guide some important steps of the procedure and select an optimal puncture site (Fig. 17.6). The use of ICE to guide transseptal puncture has the potential to reduce total fluoroscopy time [26].

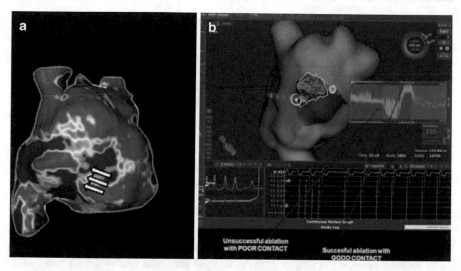

Fig. 17.5 Atrial flutter ablation in a repaired TOF patient. (**a**) Post-processed 3D LGE sequence with a right lateral view of the right atrium with fibrosis (in red) in lateral and posterolateral wall and possible voltage channel (arrows) between fibrosis regions. (**b**) Clockwise flutter in the lateral right atrium wall with slow conduction in the heterogenous tissue of the scar. Two RF applications are shown, first one with poor contact and a second one (effective) with good contact

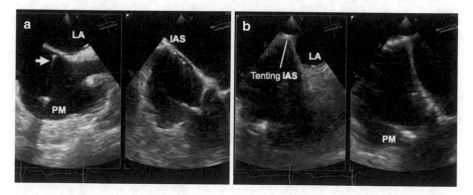

Fig. 17.6 Pulmonary vein ablation procedure in a patient with a PM and ccTGA. (**a**) TEE with X-plane in a bicaval view showing the transseptal system (white arrow). (**b**) TEE image showing tenting of the IAS with the transseptal system (needle). Once the correct position is confirmed, the electrophysiologist can perform the transseptal puncture in order to have access to the LA for the PV ablation. *PM* Pacemaker, *ccTGA* congenitally corrected transposition great arteries, *LA* left atria, *IAS* interatrial septum

Recently the real-time echocardiographic and fluoroscopic image fusion, in experienced hands, seems to be safe and can reduce the time to optimal transseptal puncture [27].

17.1.3 Imaging in Ventricular Arrhythmias in Adult Congenital Heart Disease

Ventricular arrhythmias (VA) are an important cause of late morbidity and sudden cardiac death in the growing population of ACHD patients, although their prevalence is lower than atrial tachyarrhythmias.

Sustained ventricular tachycardia (VT) (monomorphic VT, polymorphic VT) have mainly been described in patients with Tetralogy of Fallot (TOF), but also in patients with other CHD such as aortic valve disease, pulmonary valve stenosis, complex forms of d-transposition of great arteries (d-TGA), ventricular septal defect (VSD), left ventricular tract obstructive lesions and Fontan systemic right ventricle (RV) [28].

The mechanism and type of ventricular arrhythmia varies depending on the congenital defect. The arrhythmia mechanism has a direct influence in the way that VT is treated. Since available drugs to prevent recurrence of reentrant VT in structural heart disease have limited efficacy in ACHD patients, monomorphic VT can be targeted by catheter ablation. On the other hand, polymorphic VT is more associated with severe ventricular dysfunction, where ICD implantation/surgery becomes the best option [29].

If we focus on VT ablation, almost all data is related to repaired TOF patients. Recently, an international expert consensus statement on catheter ablation of ventricular tachycardia in ACHD patients recommend ablation procedure as class I of recommendation (COR) in [30]:

I. Patient with monomorphic VT or recurrent appropriate ICD therapy in repaired TOF.
I. Patient with VT and important hemodynamic lesions, treatment of hemodynamics abnormalities and consider concomitant ablation.
IIa. Surgical ablation can be considered in selected patients with VT that need surgical repair of residual hemodynamics abnormalities

It is important to remember, as we mentioned previously, that if catheter ventricular tachycardia ablation is planned in ACHD patients, real anatomy knowledge, especially in complex CHD, vascular access and arrhythmogenic substrate identification (fibrosis or scar by CMR) will be helpful for the success of the procedure.

17.1.3.1 Cardiac Imaging Pre VT Ablation Procedure: Arrhythmogenic Substrate in ACHD

Before focusing exclusively on the field of ventricular arrhythmias ablation in ACHD patients, we review shortly how CMR helps in planning and performing a ventricular tachycardia ablation on ischemic patients and non-ischemic patients. The main mechanism of ventricular tachycardia (VT) is the reentry associated with myocardial scar, both in patients with ischemic heart disease [31] and non-ischemic [32]. Several studies have demonstrated the usefulness of late gadolinium enhancement (LGE) to identify patients at risk of malignant arrhythmias [33, 34].

In patients with VT, it is especially important to identify the presence of "border zone," or presence of islets of surviving myocytes that alternate with areas of fibrotic tissue [31]. The differentiation between "border zone" and dense scar (or "core") by LGE CMR sequence is based on different signal intensity cut-off points. Thus, the dense scar (formed by fibrous tissue) will have signal intensity values higher than those of the "border zone" which, in turn, will have greater signal intensity than the healthy myocardium [35].

Regarding LGE CMR acquisition protocol, different sequences (both bidimensional and three dimensional) with different magnetic fields (1.5 T and 3 T) have been used to characterize ventricular scar. The slice thickness reported differs depending on the working group (1.4 to 8 mm). However, correct identification of the border zone channels requires high-resolution images, and 3D LGE techniques are currently preferred [36].

Using 3D acquisition and image-post-processing methods, channels involved in reentry can be identified in advance, and this information can be exported to navigation systems to guide VT ablation and plan the procedure [37] (Fig. 17.7).

If we apply the previous approach to ACHD patients, identification of the arrhythmogenic substrate could be helpful in patients with monomorphic VT who, as we mentioned before, are mostly repaired TOF patients.

Monomorphic VT secondary to a macroreentrant circuit is the most frequent cause of ventricular arrhythmia in TOF. This reentrant tachycardia in repaired TOF is known to be related to anatomical isthmuses of viable myocardium interposed between the patches (septal), the pulmonary valve and tricuspid annuli. Four isthmuses have been described [38]:

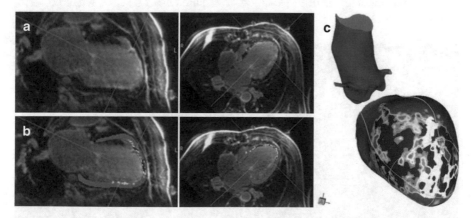

Fig. 17.7 (a) Three-dimensional (3D) late gadolinium enhancement (LGE CMR) images in two- and four-chamber views showing a subendocardial infarction of the anterior and anteroseptal wall. Image resolution is 1.4 × 1.4 × 1.4 mm. (b) Automated segmentation with a color-coded pixel signal intensity map of the left ventricle wall. Normal myocardium is depicted in blue, border zone in yellow-orange, and infarct core is red. (c) 3D reconstructed shell with the same signal intensity map obtained from LGE CMR. A heterogeneous tissue channel can be observed inside the scar (white lines inside scar)

1. Isthmus 1: bordered by tricuspid annulus and RVOT patch.
2. Isthmus 2: RV incision and pulmonary valve.
3. Isthmus 3: Pulmonary valve and ventricular septal defect (VSD) patch (most frequent type).
4. Isthmus 4: VSD patch and tricuspid annulus in cases of subaortic VSD with muscular rim.

Identification of these anatomical isthmuses by LGE CMR before VT ablation can be useful to integrate this information with the electroanatomic mapping system.

In addition, detecting the presence of arrhythmogenic substrate may offer prognostic information. Some studies have demonstrated that RV focal fibrosis after RVOT patching and resection of infundibular pulmonary stenosis is related to RV dysfunction and ventricular arrhythmias [39] (Fig. 17.8).

Moreover, the presence of a long akinetic region in the RVOT is related to episodes of sustained VT in the follow-up in TOF patients [40]. Another group have observed that RV LGE predicts sudden death and VT in a population of repaired TOF [41].

Regarding other ACHD population, although monomophic VT is uncommon, a prospective study in patients with transposition of the great arteries post atrial redirection surgery (Mustard/Senning operation), showed that non-sustained and sustained ventricular arrhythmia were associated with systemic RV LGE [42].

In the same line, in patients after Fontan procedure, LGE CMR was associated with adverse ventricular mechanics and non-sustained VT [43].

For all the above, the detection of myocardial fibrosis by LGE CMR becomes a good diagnostic and prognostic tool for ventricular arrhythmias in ACHD. Applying the same methodology as in VT ablation of acquired heart disease, when possible,

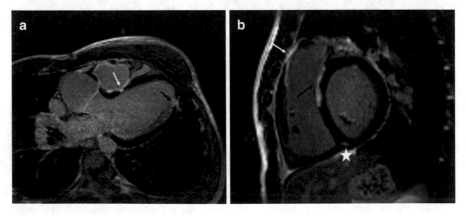

Fig. 17.8 Example of different patterns of LGE after TOF. (**a**) 3-chamber view, region of surgical patch of the ventricular septal defect (white arrow). Small myocardial infarction in the lateral apical wall, (black arrow). (**b**) Short axis view: *1* LGE in the anterior wall of the RVOT, white arrow. *2* LGE in region of surgical patch VSD, black arrow *3* LGE in the inferior septal insertion point (star). *LGE* late gadolinium enhacement, *rTOF* repaired Tetralogy of Fallot

could be beneficial if ablation is considered, although currently evidence is lacking. It has to be taken into account that these cases present some challenges: scar identification in RV is difficult, uncommon LGE patterns can be present both in RV and LV, and 3D LGE post-processing is still complex and time consuming. Therefore, further investigation and technical development are necessary.

One of the challenges that should be pointed out is that pacemakers and ICD are common in ACHD patients, and the presence of cardiac devices has been traditionally considered a contraindication for CMR imaging. Recent studies have demonstrated that LGE CMR can be safely performed in these patients [44]. However, the device generator usually creates a hyperintensity artifact that affects image quality, leading to difficulties in image interpretation and delineation of myocardium. To deal with this issue, a novel wideband LH sequence can solve part of this problem, allowing for less artifacts and a better definition of scar/fibrosis [45]. This new sequence offers new possibilities for ACHD patients who develop ventricular tachycardia and their arrhythmogenic substrate needs to be studied to guide the ablation procedure [46] (Figs. 17.9 and 17.10).

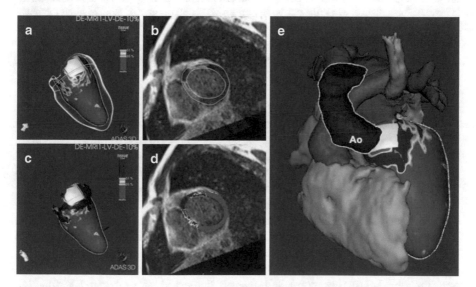

Fig. 17.9 Patient with a double-outlet right ventricle (DORV) with subpulmonary ventricular septal defect or Taussig–Bing anomaly, corrected years ago. The patient had also an aortic mechanical prosthesis, and ICD had been implanted due to a VT episode. Despite medical treatment at high doses, persistent episodes of VT were present, which recommended VT ablation. (**b**) A LGE wide band sequence was performed in stack of short axis view (5 mm thickness without gap). Interestingly, no artifact due to ICD is present in this sequence. (**a, c** and **d**) Post-processing software reconstructed a 3D image with a color-coded pixel signal intensity map, with core scar in red color, and yellow areas of viable myocardium. (**e**) Integrated contrast MRA with LGE wide band sequence shows the relationship of the scar with other structures such as the aorta (Ao) in a complex case of CHD. *VT* ventricular tachycardia, *ICD* implantable cardioverter defibrillator, *MRA* magnetic resonance angiography

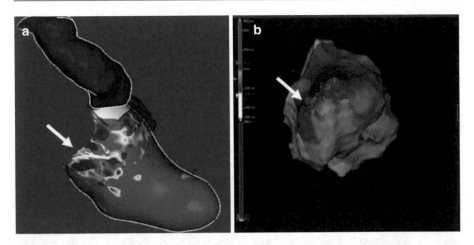

Fig. 17.10 This example shows how LGE CMR imaging was helpful to guide the VT ablation in the previous patient. (**a**) Post-processed 3D LG CMR image, where the conducting channels (white arrow and white lines) between the scar (red) and viable myocardium (yellow) can be detected. (**b**) Electroanatomical map, where the red dot (white arrow) shows the area of radiofrequency application needed to stop the macro-entry mechanism of the VT. *VT* ventricular tachycardia

17.1.4 Cardiac Resynchronization Therapy in Congenital Heart Disease

Cardiac resynchronization therapy (CRT) is one of the cornerstones of chronic heart failure treatment, with extensive evidence of arising from large randomized clinical trials and meta-analyses [47, 48]. The purpose of CRT is to restore the synchronicity in cardiac contraction. To achieve that goal, both right and left ventricle are electrically stimulated (either simultaneously or with a pre-established delay) with an added third electrode in the right atrium if the patient is in sinus rhythm.

The benefits of CRT include improvements in exercise capacity, oxygen consumption and quality of life and, even more importantly, it has been shown to reduce heart failure hospitalizations and improve long-term survival [49]. It is important to note that these benefits have been demonstrated in patients with wide QRS (especially left bundle branch block—LBBB), heart failure despite optimal medical therapy (functional class II or more), and severely depressed left ventricle (LV) function (LV ejection fraction ≤35%). Accordingly, current European Guidelines recommend implanting a CRT device in patients with LV ejection fraction (EF) ≤ 35%, NYHA functional class II-IV, and QRS width ≥ 130 ms; it constitutes a Class I indication for patients with LBBB, whereas in patients without LBBB (but otherwise wide QRS) the recommendation is Class IIa (QRS >150 ms) or IIb (<150 ms) [50].

17.1.4.1 CRT in Congenital Heart Disease

Despite the large evidence supporting the use of CRT in an adult population with left ventricular dysfunction and wide QRS, the evidence for patients with congenital heart disease (CHD) is, comparatively, much scarcer, and limited to non-randomized, small series of heterogeneous patients.

In addition to the lack of large studies, CHD patients have significant fundamental differences from patients with other kinds of cardiomyopathies; this fact makes simply applying "conventional" CRT indications to a CHD population challenging, and potentially risks avoiding implants in patients that could benefit from this therapy. On the one hand, LBBB, the conduction abnormality usually found in CRT patients and associated with good response to this therapy [51], is uncommon in a CHD population. Indeed, in CHD patients the most often found conduction abnormality is right bundle branch block [3, 52]. On the other hand, EF estimation in patients with CHD can be challenging, due to poor echocardiographic windows or complex anatomies. Finally, the indications for implanting a CRT device in CHD patients in routine clinical practice differ markedly from those in patients with other cardiomyopathies: the most common indication of CRT implant in CHD population is the upgrading of a preexisting pacemaker to avoid the detrimental effects of long-term RV pacing. In a recent report, only 12.7% of patients with CHD received CRT primarily as a heart failure treatment, whereas in 80% of the cases it was an upgrade from conventional pacing [53].

17.1.4.2 Effects of CRT on Systemic Ventricle Ejection Fraction

The studies available suggest that CHD patients obtain a benefit from CRT similar to patients with other cardiomyopathies, especially in the setting of a systemic LV. In one of the largest studies in CHD, Dubin et al. [54] studied 103 patients who underwent CRT. At a mean follow-up period of 4.8 ± 4 months, systemic ventricle ejection fraction (EF) improved 11.9 ± 12.9% units, and mean QRS width decrease was 39.1 ms. These changes in systemic EF and QRS were not statistically different from the changes observed in patients with non-CHD cardiomyopathies. No significant change in EF was observed in patients with univentricular hearts.

Similarly, CRT seems to be particularly useful in patients with conventional pacing, in which CRT is implanted to avoid pacing-induced dysfunction: in a multicentric study including 109 patients [55], improvement in EF or in fractional area change (FAC) was higher in patients upgraded from conventional pacing than in the rest of the population. Other predictors of EF or FAC improvement were the presence of systemic LV, and higher baseline degree of systemic AV valve regurgitation.

17.1.4.3 Effects of CRT on Right Ventricle Dyssynchrony and Function

Some authors have used echocardiography to assess RV dyssynchrony and its change after CRT. The most commonly used RV dyssynchrony parameter is RV septal flash, defined as a visually assessed fast movement of the interventricular septum first toward and then away from the RV during isovolumic contraction. This contraction pattern was observed in 93% of patients with repaired tetralogy of Fallot in one study [52]. Other quantitative parameters, such as RV prestretch duration and

RV basal lateral–to–midseptal delay, have been associated with RV remodeling and dysfunction [52].

Although poorly studied, the effects of CRT on RV seem to differ depending on whether the RV is subpulmonary or systemic.

In subpulmonary RV, some initial data have suggested a potential improvement of RV function and reduction of RV dyssynchrony with CRT. In a study with 6 CHD patients with RBBB, CRT improved parameters of RV performance, both acutely and at longer term follow-up. Some degree of reverse remodeling and a reduction in RV mechanical dyssynchrony was also observed [55]. Importantly, in this study CRT was delivered with single-site RV pacing in the site of latest activation, suggesting that RV CRT could lead to improvement of RV function and reverse remodeling, similiarly to what occurs with conventional CRT; these promising results need to be validated in a larger cohort of patients.

Regarding systemic RV, few studies are available with conflicting results. Although some reports have demonstrated an improvement in RV function [54], other authors failed to demonstrate a significant functional improvement despite QRS reduction [56]. In another report, patients with systemic RV showed less reduction of end-diastolic volume as compared to patients with systemic LV [57]. More studies are needed in order to define the role of CRT in systemic RV.

17.1.4.4   Single Ventricle and CRT

The evidence regarding the role of CRT in single ventricle is scarce, and the available studies have yielded conflicting results. In one study [54], patients with univentricular hearts did not present a significant change in EF at follow-up as compared to baseline despite having a significant QRS shortening. Other authors [56, 57], however, have observed a positive response to CRT in these patients, although the number of patients studied was small (less than 10 patients in all cases). Future studies should shed more light on this topic.

17.1.4.5   Current Recommendations

Despite the aforementioned limitations, and based on the data available, a recent publication from the European Society of Cardiology Working Group on CHD has sought to establish some recommendations for CRT implant in this population [3]. According to them, CRT is indicated in:

- CHD patients with LVEF ≤35%, QRS ≥150 ms with LBBB morphology, and functional class II to ambulatory IV. In patients with the same characteristics but QRS 120–149 ms, CRT can be useful (with a lesser degree of evidence).
- CHD patients with systemic EF ≤35% undergoing new device implant or replacement with anticipated requirement for significant (>40%) ventricular pacing.

In addition, CRT can be useful (although with limited evidence) in patients with functional class II to ambulatory IV, systemic ventricle EF ≤35%, and either a systemic RV with QRS ≥150 ms and RBBB morphology, or a single ventricle with

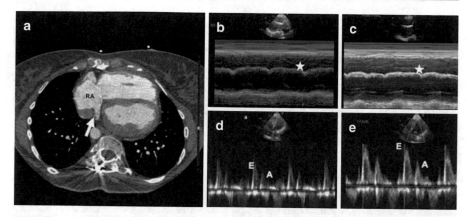

Fig. 17.11 Repaired TOF patient with right ventricle dysfunction and previous RV pacing. (**a**) Previously to resyncronization a cardiac CT was performed in order to evaluate cardiac veins anatomy; normal cardiac veins trajectory was reported. White arrow shows the coronary sinus draining in the RA. (**b**) Mode M echocardiography before CRT with abnormal contraction and relaxation of the septum, corresponding a septal flash (star)), due to RV pacing. (**c**) After optimization of the resynchronization parameters, a reduction in septal flash excursion is noted. (**d**) E and A wave pattern before optimization, indicating an impaired filling. (**e**) Improvement of filling after optimization, as observed with E/A ratio. *RV* right ventricle, *RA* right atria, *CRT* cardiac resynchronization therapy

QRS ≥150 ms and LBBB or RBBB morphology. In the same cases but QRS 120–149 ms, even less evidence exists, although CRT may be considered.

Finally, CRT is not indicated in patients with narrow (<120 ms) QRS, or those with limited life expectancy.

17.1.4.6 Cardiac Imaging to Guide CRT Implant

In complex anatomies, preprocedural imaging of the coronary sinus and cardiac veins may be necessary in order to ensure a correct CRT lead placement and avoid unnecessary interventions. Cardiac CT is the most commonly used technique in those cases [58]. This technique is able to identify cardiac veins and determine its suitability for lead placement (Figs. 17.11 and 17.12).

17.2 Conclusions

Planning electrophysiology procedures such as atrial and ventricular arrhythmias ablation in ACHD patients needs to be performed in experienced centers, where multidisciplinary team and, most commonly, a multimodality approach are available. Knowledge of the real and complex anatomy, vascular access and arrhythmogenic substrate is crucial for the success of the ablation. In this scenario CMR plays an important role. Some technical challenges, however, need to be solved regarding 3D LGE CMR sequences and post-processing tools.

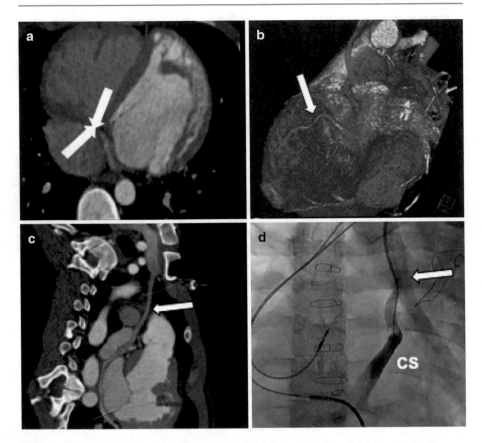

Fig. 17.12 Patient with ccTGA and dextrocardia, RBBB, and heart failure. A CRT indication was made. (**a**) Cardiac CT was performed to study cardiac veins anatomy. An atresia of the coronary sinus (CS) ostium was found (white arrows). (**b**) Also an optimal marginal vein in the CS was visualized by CT. (**c**) A prominent vein of Marshall (VM), the remnants of the left cardinal vein, draining to the CS was detected. (**d**) This vein of Marshall (white arrow) was the path that the electrophysiologist chose to implant the CRT lead in the marginal vein though the CS. *ccTGA* congenitally corrected transposition great arteries, *RBBB* right bundle branch block, *CRT* cardiac resynchronization therapy. (Images courtesy of Dr Hug Cuellar and Dra Nuria Riva. Hospital Vall Hebron. Barcelona)

Cardiac resynchronization therapy is a promising treatment in CHD patients, although its indications are not clear due to a relative lack of evidence. CRT has a role to avoid pacing-induced dysfunction, and in patients with wide QRS and systemic LV dysfunction, especially in the setting of LBBB. The role of CRT in systemic RV and univentricular hearts is less clear, and more studies are needed. In addition to determining LV and RV function, cardiac imaging can be useful to guide CRT implant in patients with complex anatomies.

References

1. Hundley WG, Bluemke DA, Finn JP, et al. ACCF/ACR/AHA/NASCI/SCMR 2010 expert consensus document on cardiovascular magnetic resonance: a report of the American College of Cardiology Foundation task force on expert consensus documents. J Am Coll Cardiol. 2010;55(23):2614–62. https://doi.org/10.1016/j.jacc.2009.11.011.
2. Kim RJ, Wu E, Rafael A, et al. The use of contrast-enhanced magnetic resonance imaging to identify reversible myocardial dysfunction. N Engl J Med. 2000;343(20):1445–53. https://doi.org/10.1056/nejm200011163432003.
3. Hernandez-Madrid A, Paul T, Abrams D, et al. Arrhythmias in congenital heart disease: a position paper of the European heart rhythm association (EHRA), Association for European Paediatric and Congenital Cardiology (AEPC), and the European Society of Cardiology (ESC) working group on grown-up congenital heart disease, endorsed by HRS, PACES, APHRS, and SOLAECE. Europace. 2018;20(11):1719–53. https://doi.org/10.1093/europace/eux380.
4. Walsh EP. Interventional electrophysiology in patients with congenital heart disease. Circulation. 2007;115(25):3224–34. https://doi.org/10.1161/circulationaha.106.655753.
5. Bouchardy J, Therrien J, Pilote L, et al. Atrial arrhythmias in adults with congenital heart disease. Circulation. 2009;120(17):1679–86. https://doi.org/10.1161/circulationaha.109.866319.
6. Koyak Z, Achterbergh RC, de Groot JR, et al. Postoperative arrhythmias in adults with congenital heart disease: incidence and risk factors. Int J Cardiol. 2013;169(2):139–44. https://doi.org/10.1016/j.ijcard.2013.08.087.
7. Walsh EP. Sudden death in adult congenital heart disease: risk stratification in 2014. Heart Rhythm. 2014;11(10):1735–42. https://doi.org/10.1016/j.hrthm.2014.07.021.
8. Verheugt CL, Uiterwaal CS, van der Velde ET, et al. The emerging burden of hospital admissions of adults with congenital heart disease. Heart. 2010;96(11):872–8. https://doi.org/10.1136/hrt.2009.185595.
9. Labombarda F, Hamilton R, Shohoudi A, et al. Increasing prevalence of atrial fibrillation and permanent atrial arrhythmias in congenital heart disease. J Am Coll Cardiol. 2017;70(7):857–65. https://doi.org/10.1016/j.jacc.2017.06.034.
10. Teuwen CP, Ramdjan TT, Gotte M, et al. Time course of atrial fibrillation in patients with congenital heart defects. Circ Arrhythm Electrophysiol. 2015;8(5):1065–72. https://doi.org/10.1161/circep.115.003272.
11. Teuwen CP, Taverne YJ, Houck C, et al. Tachyarrhythmia in patients with congenital heart disease: inevitable destiny? Neth Heart J. 2016;24(3):161–70. https://doi.org/10.1007/s12471-015-0797-z.
12. Roca-Luque I, Gándara NR, Dos Subirà L, et al. Intra-atrial re-entrant tachycardia in congenital heart disease: types and relation of isthmus to atrial voltage. Europace. 2018;20(2):353–61. https://doi.org/10.1093/europace/eux250.
13. Brouwer C, Hazekamp MG, Zeppenfeld K. Anatomical substrates and ablation of reentrant atrial and ventricular tachycardias in repaired congenital heart disease. Arrhythmia Electrophysiol Rev. 2016;5(2):150–60. https://doi.org/10.15420/aer.2016.19.2.
14. Combes N, Derval N, Hascoet S, et al. Ablation of supraventricular arrhythmias in adult congenital heart disease: a contemporary review. Arch Cardiovasc Dis. 2017;110(5):334–45. https://doi.org/10.1016/j.acvd.2017.01.007.
15. Khairy P, Van Hare GF, Balaji S, et al. PACES/HRS expert consensus statement on the recognition and Management of Arrhythmias in adult congenital heart disease: developed in partnership between the pediatric and congenital electrophysiology society (PACES) and the Heart Rhythm Society (HRS). Heart Rhythm. 2014;11(10):e102–65. https://doi.org/10.1016/j.hrthm.2014.05.009.
16. Roca-Luque I, Rivas Gandara N, Dos Subira L, et al. Intra-atrial re-entrant tachycardia in patients with congenital heart disease: factors associated with disease severity. Europace. 2018;20(8):1343–51. https://doi.org/10.1093/europace/eux180.

17. Hamdan A, Charalampos K, Roettgen R, et al. Magnetic resonance imaging versus computed tomography for characterization of pulmonary vein morphology before radiofrequency catheter ablation of atrial fibrillation. Am J Cardiol. 2009;104(11):1540–6. https://doi.org/10.1016/j.amjcard.2009.07.029.

18. Ang R, Hunter RJ, Baker V, et al. Pulmonary vein measurements on pre-procedural CT/MR imaging can predict difficult pulmonary vein isolation and phrenic nerve injury during cryoballoon ablation for paroxysmal atrial fibrillation. Int J Cardiol. 2015;195:253–8. https://doi.org/10.1016/j.ijcard.2015.05.089.

19. Kirchhof P, Benussi S, Kotecha D, et al. 2016 ESC guidelines for the management of atrial fibrillation developed in collaboration with EACTS. Eur Heart J. 2016;37(38):2893–962. https://doi.org/10.1093/eurheartj/ehw210.

20. Sohns C, Nurnberg JH, Hebe J, et al. Catheter ablation for atrial fibrillation in adults with congenital heart disease: lessons learned from more than 10 years following a sequential ablation approach. JACC Clin Electrophysiol. 2018;4(6):733–43. https://doi.org/10.1016/j.jacep.2018.01.015.

21. Marrouche NF, Wilber D, Hindricks G, et al. Association of atrial tissue fibrosis identified by delayed enhancement MRI and atrial fibrillation catheter ablation: the DECAAF study. JAMA. 2014;311(5):498–506. https://doi.org/10.1001/jama.2014.3.

22. Pontecorboli G, Figueras IVRM, Carlosena A, et al. Use of delayed-enhancement magnetic resonance imaging for fibrosis detection in the atria: a review. Europace. 2017;19(2):180–9. https://doi.org/10.1093/europace/euw053.

23. Bisbal F, Guiu E, Cabanas-Grandio P, et al. CMR-guided approach to localize and ablate gaps in repeat AF ablation procedure. JACC Cardiovasc Imaging. 2014;7(7):653–63. https://doi.org/10.1016/j.jcmg.2014.01.014.

24. Benito EM, Carlosena-Remirez A, Guasch E, et al. Left atrial fibrosis quantification by late gadolinium-enhanced magnetic resonance: a new method to standardize the thresholds for reproducibility. Europace. 2017;19(8):1272–9. https://doi.org/10.1093/europace/euw219.

25. Alkhouli M, Rihal CS, Holmes DRJ. Transseptal techniques for emerging structural heart interventions. JACC Cardiovasc Interv. 2016;9(24):2465–80. https://doi.org/10.1016/j.jcin.2016.10.035.

26. Kliger C, Cruz-Gonzalez I, Ruiz CE. The present and future of intracardiac echocardiography for guiding structural heart disease interventions. Rev Esp Cardiol (Engl Ed). 2012;65(9):791–4. https://doi.org/10.1016/j.recesp.2012.03.007.

27. Afzal S, Veulemans V, Balzer J, et al. Safety and efficacy of transseptal puncture guided by real-time fusion of echocardiography and fluoroscopy. Neth Hear J. 2017;25(2):131–6. https://doi.org/10.1007/s12471-016-0937-0.

28. Vehmeijer JT, Brouwer TF, Limpens J, et al. Implantable cardioverter-defibrillators in adults with congenital heart disease: a systematic review and meta-analysis. Eur Heart J. 2016;37(18):1439–48. https://doi.org/10.1093/eurheartj/ehv735.

29. Kapel GF, Reichlin T, Wijnmaalen AP, et al. Re-entry using anatomically determined isthmuses: a curable ventricular tachycardia in repaired congenital heart disease. Circ Arrhythm Electrophysiol. 2015;8(1):102–9. https://doi.org/10.1161/circep.114.001929.

30. Cronin EM, Bogun FM, Maury P, et al. 2019 HRS/EHRA/APHRS/LAHRS expert consensus statement on catheter ablation of ventricular arrhythmias. Europace. 2019;21(8):1143–4. https://doi.org/10.1093/europace/euz132.

31. de Bakker JM, van Capelle FJ, Janse MJ, et al. Reentry as a cause of ventricular tachycardia in patients with chronic ischemic heart disease: electrophysiologic and anatomic correlation. Circulation. 1988;77(3):589–606. https://doi.org/10.1161/01.cir.77.3.589.

32. Bogun FM, Desjardins B, Good E, et al. Delayed-enhanced magnetic resonance imaging in nonischemic cardiomyopathy: utility for identifying the ventricular arrhythmia substrate. J Am Coll Cardiol. 2009;53(13):1138–45. https://doi.org/10.1016/j.jacc.2008.11.052.

33. Klem I, Weinsaft JW, Bahnson TD, et al. Assessment of myocardial scarring improves risk stratification in patients evaluated for cardiac defibrillator implantation. J Am Coll Cardiol. 2012;60(5):408–20. https://doi.org/10.1016/j.jacc.2012.02.070.

34. Acosta J, Fernandez-Armenta J, Borras R, et al. Scar characterization to predict life-threatening arrhythmic events and sudden cardiac death in patients with cardiac resynchronization therapy: the GAUDI-CRT study. JACC Cardiovasc Imaging. 2018;11(4):561–72. https://doi.org/10.1016/j.jcmg.2017.04.021.

35. Andreu D, Berruezo A, Ortiz-Perez JT, et al. Integration of 3D electroanatomic maps and magnetic resonance scar characterization into the navigation system to guide ventricular tachycardia ablation. Circ Arrhythm Electrophysiol. 2011;4(5):674–83. https://doi.org/10.1161/circep.111.961946.

36. Perez-David E, Arenal A, Rubio-Guivernau JL, et al. Noninvasive identification of ventricular tachycardia-related conducting channels using contrast-enhanced magnetic resonance imaging in patients with chronic myocardial infarction: comparison of signal intensity scar mapping and endocardial voltage mappin. J Am Coll Cardiol. 2011;57(2):184–94. https://doi.org/10.1016/j.jacc.2010.07.043.

37. Andreu D, Ortiz-Perez JT, Boussy T, et al. Usefulness of contrast-enhanced cardiac magnetic resonance in identifying the ventricular arrhythmia substrate and the approach needed for ablation. Eur Heart J. 2014;35(20):1316–26. https://doi.org/10.1093/eurheartj/eht510.

38. Zeppenfield K, Jongbloed SM. Cardiac electrophysiology. From cell to bedside. Ventricular arrhythmias in congenital heart disease. 6th ed. Philadelphia: Elsevier Saunders; 2014. p. 1009–18.

39. Babu-Narayan SV, Kilner PJ, Li W, et al. Ventricular fibrosis suggested by cardiovascular magnetic resonance in adults with repaired tetralogy of fallot and its relationship to adverse markers of clinical outcome. Circulation. 2006;113(3):405–13. https://doi.org/10.1161/circulationaha.105.548727.

40. Bonello B, Kempny A, Uebing A, et al. Right atrial area and right ventricular outflow tract akinetic length predict sustained tachyarrhythmia in repaired tetralogy of Fallot. Int J Cardiol. 2013;168(4):3280–6. https://doi.org/10.1016/j.ijcard.2013.04.048.

41. Ghonim S, Gatzoulis MA, Smith GC, et al. 2395LGE CMR predicts sudden death and VT in adults with repaired tetralogy of Fallot - a prospective study with 3500 patient follow up years. Eur Heart J. 2019;40(Supplement_1):ehz748. https://doi.org/10.1093/eurheartj/ehz748.0148.

42. Rydman R, Gatzoulis MA, Ho SY, et al. Systemic right ventricular fibrosis detected by cardiovascular magnetic resonance is associated with clinical outcome, mainly new-onset atrial arrhythmia, in patients after atrial redirection surgery for transposition of the great arteries. Circ Cardiovasc Imaging. 2015;8(5):e002628. https://doi.org/10.1161/circimaging.114.002628.

43. Rathod RH, Prakash A, Powell AJ, Geva T. Myocardial fibrosis identified by cardiac magnetic resonance late gadolinium enhancement is associated with adverse ventricular mechanics and ventricular tachycardia late after Fontan operation. J Am Coll Cardiol. 2010;55(16):1721–8. https://doi.org/10.1016/j.jacc.2009.12.036.

44. Nordbeck P, Ertl G, Ritter O. Magnetic resonance imaging safety in pacemaker and implantable cardioverter defibrillator patients: how far have we come? Eur Heart J. 2015;36(24):1505–11. https://doi.org/10.1093/eurheartj/ehv086.

45. Rashid S, Rapacchi S, Vaseghi M, et al. Improved late gadolinium enhancement MR imaging for patients with implanted cardiac devices. Radiology. 2014;270(1):269–74. https://doi.org/10.1148/radiol.13130942.

46. Roca-Luque I, Van Breukelen A, Alarcon F, et al. Ventricular scar channel entrances identified by new wideband cardiac magnetic resonance sequence to guide ventricular tachycardia ablation in patients with cardiac defibrillators. Europace. 2020;22:598. https://doi.org/10.1093/europace/euaa021.

47. Bristow MR, Saxon LA, Boehmer J, et al. Cardiac-resynchronization therapy with or without an implantable defibrillator in advanced chronic heart failure. N Engl J Med. 2004;350(21):2140–50. https://doi.org/10.1056/NEJMoa032423.

48. Bradley DJ, Bradley EA, Baughman KL, et al. Cardiac resynchronization and death from progressive heart failure: a meta-analysis of randomized controlled trials. JAMA. 2003;289(6):730–40. https://doi.org/10.1001/jama.289.6.730.

49. Tang AS, Wells GA, Talajic M, et al. Cardiac-resynchronization therapy for mild-to-moderate heart failure. N Engl J Med. 2010;363(25):2385–95. https://doi.org/10.1056/NEJMoa1009540.
50. Ponikowski P, Voors AA, Anker SD, et al. 2016 ESC guidelines for the diagnosis and treatment of acute and chronic heart failure: the task force for the diagnosis and treatment of acute and chronic heart failure of the European Society of Cardiology (ESC)developed with the special contribution of. Eur Heart J. 2016;37(27):2129–200. https://doi.org/10.1093/eurheartj/ehw128.
51. Sipahi I, Chou JC, Hyden M, Rowland DY, Simon DI, Fang JC. Effect of QRS morphology on clinical event reduction with cardiac resynchronization therapy: meta-analysis of randomized controlled trials. Am Heart J. 2012;163(2):260–7.e3. https://doi.org/10.1016/j.ahj.2011.11.014.
52. Yim D, Hui W, Larios G, et al. Quantification of right ventricular electromechanical Dyssynchrony in relation to right ventricular function and clinical outcomes in children with repaired tetralogy of Fallot. J Am Soc Echocardiogr. 2018;31(7):822–30. https://doi.org/10.1016/j.echo.2018.03.012.
53. Flugge AK, Wasmer K, Orwat S, et al. Cardiac resynchronization therapy in congenital heart disease: results from the German National Register for congenital heart defects. Int J Cardiol. 2018;273:108–11. https://doi.org/10.1016/j.ijcard.2018.10.014.
54. Dubin AM, Janousek J, Rhee E, et al. Resynchronization therapy in pediatric and congenital heart disease patients: an international multicenter study. J Am Coll Cardiol. 2005;46(12):2277–83. https://doi.org/10.1016/j.jacc.2005.05.096.
55. Janousek J, Kovanda J, Lozek M, et al. Cardiac resynchronization therapy for treatment of chronic subpulmonary right ventricular dysfunction in congenital heart disease. Circ Arrhythm Electrophysiol. 2019;12(5):e007157. https://doi.org/10.1161/circep.119.007157.
56. Sakaguchi H, Miyazaki A, Yamada O, et al. Cardiac resynchronization therapy for various systemic ventricular morphologies in patients with congenital heart disease. Circ J. 2015;79(3):649–55. https://doi.org/10.1253/circj.CJ-14-0395.
57. Janousek J. Cardiac resynchronisation in congenital heart disease. Heart. 2009;95(11):940–7. https://doi.org/10.1136/hrt.2008.151266.
58. Ruckdeschel ES, Quaife R, Lewkowiez L, et al. Preprocedural imaging in patients with transposition of the great arteries facilitates placement of cardiac resynchronization therapy leads. Pacing Clin Electrophysiol. 2014;37(5):546–53. https://doi.org/10.1111/pace.12308.

Structural Interventional Planning

18

Pieter van der Bijl and Victoria Delgado

18.1 Introduction

Spectacular progress in the early treatment of congenital heart disease over the past decades has dramatically increased the life expectancy of these patients. Due to the prolonged life expectancy, the incidence of recurrent anatomical and/or functional defects has increased, which require structural cardiac intervention. Patients may also present de novo in adulthood with uncorrected congenital cardiac lesions, especially when not having had access to comprehensive healthcare during childhood. In many cases, these corrective procedures can now be performed with minimally invasive or percutaneous strategies, in contrast to more invasive surgery. The success of structural interventions for adult congenital heart disease (ACHD) is critically dependent on accurate multimodality imaging: both in the planning stages (including indications for intervention and procedural planning) and in-theatre procedural guidance. Multimodality imaging comprises the rational choice and combination of different cardiac imaging techniques, to take full advantage of the strengths of each particular modality. The techniques most commonly applied to the planning of structural interventions in ACHD are: (1) echocardiography, (2) cardiac computed tomography (CT) and (3) cardiac magnetic resonance (CMR) imaging. In this chapter, the role of these modalities in structural interventional planning for ACHD are reviewed, with a focus on new developments in imaging.

P. van der Bijl · V. Delgado (✉)
Department of Cardiology, Leiden University Medical Center, Leiden, The Netherlands
e-mail: V.Delgado@lumc.nl

© Springer Nature Switzerland AG 2021
P. Gallego, I. Valverde (eds.), *Multimodality Imaging Innovations In Adult Congenital Heart Disease*, Congenital Heart Disease in Adolescents and Adults,
https://doi.org/10.1007/978-3-030-61927-5_18

18.2   Echocardiography

Echocardiography is the most versatile of all cardiac imaging techniques, affording the ability to assess anatomy and function in both two and three dimensions without the use of radiation or nephrotoxic contrast agents. In addition, it is highly cost-effective and its high temporal resolution, in comparison to CT and CMR, provides an advantage for functional assessment. High frame-rate echocardiography promises to greatly improve the accuracy of deformation imaging, and has been used with speckle tracking strain [1]. Frame-by-frame tracking of "speckles" identified in the myocardium, allows deformation to be expressed as strain, i.e. the percentage change in segment length from baseline. Strain can be measured in various directions, e.g. longitudinal, circumferential and radial. It remains unknown if deformation indices derived from speckle tracking echocardiography can be interpreted in the same manner in ACHD as in acquired adult heart disease. The right ventricle, for example, normally contains only two muscle layers: circumferential subepicardial and longitudinal subendocardial fibres. In patients with tetralogy of Fallot (ToF), an additional middle layer of circular fibres has been demonstrated, which may influence strain parameters [2]. It remains to be seen how this technology will impact on ACHD and specifically the planning of structural interventions. Suboptimal echocardiographic windows and/or tissue penetration of ultrasound may limit the use of echocardiography in some patients, in which case one may have to resort to cardiac CT and/or CMR.

In planning the percutaneous closure of an atrial septal defect (ASD), contraindications to the procedure have to be identified a priori. Only septum secundum defects are suitable for percutaneous device closure, and septum primum as well as sinus venosus defects have to be recognized. The presence of anomalous pulmonary venous drainage also comprises an exclusion criterion, which requires surgical correction. Planning of the procedure itself includes description of the number and shape of the defect(s), as well as accurately measuring its size and rims. The maximum diameter amenable to device closure is 37 mm, although the final measurement is performed during sizing balloon inflation ("stretched diameter") [3]. Multiple secundum ASDs may still be closed percutaneously, but will require a dedicated device (Amplatzer Cribiform, St. Jude Medical, St. Paul, MN, USA). The following rims have to be measured: posterosuperior, atrioventricular, posteroinferior, anterior aortic, inferior and superior caval. All rims have to be at least 5 mm, except for the anterior aortic rim [3]. Three-dimensional (3D) transoesophageal echocardiography is particularly useful to assess an ASD (Fig. 18.1) [4]. The interatrial septum is a thin structure which is prone to "dropout" artefact, and therefore 3D acquisition of the interatrial septum should be performed in the mid-oesophageal four-chamber view, to maximize axial resolution. The image can then be tilted upward to provide an en-face right atrial view of the ASD, and rotated leftward to demonstrate the defect en-face from the left atrium. This image manipulation is sometimes described with the acronym TUPLE (Tilt UP and then LEft). Encompassing a structure as large as the interatrial septum in a single acquisition volume may lead to a significant decrease in volume rate—this however is not

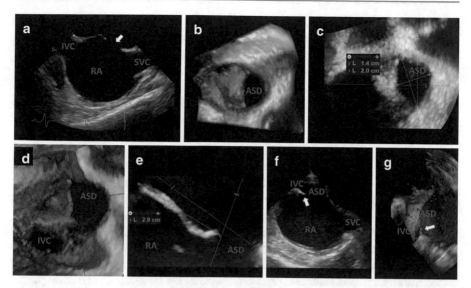

Fig. 18.1 Atrial septal defects (ASDs). A secundum ASD (white arrow) seen on a two-dimensional, bicaval transoesophageal view (**a**). The same defect as in (A) depicted on a volume-rendered, three-dimensional echocardiography image from the left atrial side of the interatrial septum (**b**). ASD dimensions measured on a multiplanar reconstruction of the three-dimensional dataset (**c**). A three-dimensional, volume-rendered image used to generate a single-plane reconstruction of the posterior ASD rim (**d**). Measurement of the posterior ASD rim on a single-plane reconstruction (**e**). An infero-posteriorly located ASD can be seen on a two-dimensional, bicaval transoesophageal view, with a deficient inferior vena cava (IVC) rim (white arrow) (**f**) that precludes percutaneous device closure. This cannot be classified as a true inferior sinus venosus defect, since the IVC does not override the defect [4]. The spatial relation between the ASD and IVC can be better appreciated on a volume-rendered, three-dimensional echocardiography image (**g**). *RA* right atrium, *SVC* superior vena cava

generally of concern, since the interatrial septum is a relatively immobile structure. Measurement of the ASD size and rims should proceed in two-dimensional (2D) images cropped from the 3D dataset with multiplanar post-processing, so as to avoid excessive blooming artefact. 3D echocardiography has been shown to correlate better with balloon sizing of ASDs than 2D echocardiography [5].

While large, residual ASDs after primary closure are very rare, stenosis at the junction of the superior vena cava and right atrium after surgical correction of a superior sinus venosus defect has been described. While this can be managed with percutaneous balloon dilatation and stenting, no specific criteria for intervention have been established.

Ventricular septal defects (VSDs) are classified according to a system proposed by the Society for Thoracic Surgery-Congenital Heart Surgery Database Committee, i.e. type I (supracristal), II (perimembranous), III (inlet) and IV (muscular). While type II VSDs have been closed percutaneously, type IV defects are best suited to device closure. Dedicated closure devices (Amplatzer Muscular/Membranous VSD Occluder, St. Jude Medical, St. Paul, MN, USA) are available for type II and IV defects. The number, type, shape and size of a VSD can be determined in a manner very similar to that described for an ASD, with transoesophageal 3D echocardiography once more being particularly suited to visualize the anatomy. Residual defects after primary surgical closure are often amenable to percutaneous device closure, and require imaging in the procedural planning.

An unrepaired patent ductus arteriosus (PDA) is not uncommon in adulthood. Before proceeding with percutaneous device (occluder/coil) closure, bidirectional flow or exclusive right-to-left flow (indicative of Eisenmenger syndrome) should be excluded with (colour) Doppler echocardiography.

Before percutaneous treatment of an unrepaired aortic coarctation, associated defects such as a bicuspid aortic valve, a parachute mitral valve and left ventricular outflow tract obstruction (often referred to as a Shone complex when multiple left-sided outflow lesions are present) requiring surgical correction, should be excluded. A high translesional gradient (>20 mmHg) in the absence of well-developed collaterals is generally accepted as an indication for treatment [3]. Although this gradient can be estimated with echocardiography, the final treatment decision is usually based on invasive measurement [3]. Percutaneous intervention involves the placement of a (covered) endovascular stent, and re-coarctation is approached similarly.

Untreated congenital valvular pulmonary stenosis (PS) may represent an acommissural, unicommissural, bicuspid or dysplastic valve. Percutaneous pulmonary balloon valvuloplasty relieves PS by commissural splitting, which can only be successfully performed in valves containing a commissure, and which are not overly dys/hypoplastic. Even though the use of 3D echocardiography has not been proven to change outcome in congenital PS, it may be valuable in the recognition of the underlying valve morphology. Treatment is only indicated in symptomatic and severe PS (peak instantaneous gradient >64 mmHg) [3] (Table 18.1)—the choice between surgery and balloon valvuloplasty depends primarily on the valve morphology.

The primary long-term complication after surgical repair of ToF is pulmonary regurgitation, especially when a transannular patch technique was used. While this is conventionally addressed with surgical placement of a homograft or valved conduit, primary percutaneous valve implantation has become feasible [6–8]. The role of percutaneous therapy for a degenerated homograft or right ventricle-to-pulmonary artery conduit, which has been placed to treat pulmonary regurgitation after ToF repair, is discussed in the section on CT. The threshold for intervention in patients with pulmonary regurgitation after ToF repair has not been resolved, and while conventionally quantified with CMR in this context, 3D echocardiography has been successfully applied to this patient population [9]. The inclusion of a dilated right

Table 18.1 Echocardiographic classification of congenital pulmonary stenosis severity

Severity	CW Doppler peak velocity (m/s)	Estimated maximum transvalvular pressure gradient (mmHg)
Mild	<3	<36
Moderate	3–4	36–64
Severe	>4	>64

CW continuous wave

Table 18.2 Classification of pulmonary regurgitation severity with echocardiography and cardiac magnetic resonance imaging (CMR) [14, 15]

Echocardiography (semiquantitative) parameters			
Severity	Colour flow PR jet width	CW signal of PR jet	Pulmonic vs. aortic flow by PW
Mild	<10 mm length with narrow origin	Faint/slow deceleration	Normal or slightly increased
Moderate	Intermediate	Dense/variable	Intermediate
Severe	Large with wide origin	Dense/steep deceleration with early termination of diastolic flow	Greatly increased

CMR (quantitative) parameters		
Severity	Regurgitant volume (mL/beat)	Regurgitant fraction (%)
Mild	<30	<25
Moderate	30–40	20–35
Severe	>40	>35

CW continuous wave, *PR* pulmonary regurgitation, *PW* pulsed wave, *CMR* cardiac magnetic resonance

ventricle in the 3D acquisition volume may be challenging, and 3D echocardiography may underestimate right ventricular volumes systematically, when compared to CMR [10–13]. Pulmonary regurgitation can be quantified with echocardiography, but CMR is generally held to be more accurate (see below) for this indication (Table 18.2) [14, 15]. Right ventricular strain is a novel functional parameter to assist in the decision to intervene on pulmonary regurgitation (Fig. 18.2). Right ventricular strain is often decreased after ToF repair, and may improve after pulmonary valve replacement, but it remains a load-dependent parameter (albeit less so than ejection fraction) [16–18]. Right ventricular strain is therefore influenced by pulmonary regurgitation (increased volume load), and CMR parametric mapping is a promising, presumably load-independent biomarker of right ventricular functional reserve (see below).

Baffle obstruction after an atrial switch procedure (Mustard or Senning) for transposition of the great arteries (TGA) can be diagnosed with transthoracic echocardiography, and entails Doppler interrogation of the connection between the venae cavae and left atrium (superior veno-caval limb and inferior veno-caval limb) and the pulmonary veins and the right atrium. High peak velocities (>1.2 m/s), mean gradients >2 mmHg and loss of a phasic flow pattern are all indicative of baffle obstruction. Agitated saline injection in the upper limb, with return of bubbles via the inferior vena cava (travelling from the superior vena cava and the azygous vein), supports obstruction of the superior veno-caval limb [3]. Similarly, return of bubbles via the superior vena cava when injected in the lower limb, suggests inferior veno-caval limb obstruction [3]. Once the diagnosis is established, baffle obstruction can often be treated percutaneously with balloon dilatation or stenting. Although no specific recommendations exist, it follows that the dimensions of the intended landing zone should be measured with imaging. Baffle leaks can also be demonstrated with transthoracic echocardiography (enhanced with an agitated saline

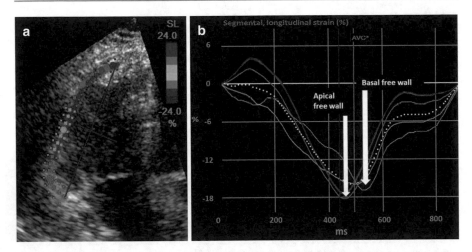

Fig. 18.2 Impaired right ventricular free wall strain in a patient with repaired tetralogy of Fallot. Longitudinal strain of the right ventricular free wall has been assessed with two-dimensional speckle tracking echocardiography in an apical, right ventricular focused view. The peak right ventricular free wall strain was decreased at −15.9%. Right ventricular free wall segmental strain is indicated by different colours, with longitudinal strain more impaired in the basal than in the apical segment of the right ventricular free wall. Arrows indicate the difference in peak longitudinal strain between the basal and apical segments of the right ventricular free wall. *AVC* aortic valve closure, *SL* longitudinal strain

infusion), and are sometimes amenable to off-label percutaneous closure with septal occluder devices or covered stents. An indirect sign of a hemodynamically significant baffle leak is a volume-overloaded left ventricle, which is expected to be a small chamber after an atrial switch procedure. Patients with TGA, pulmonary outflow tract obstruction and a VSD may be treated with a Rastelli operation, which involves insertion of a surgical conduit between the right ventricle and the pulmonary artery. Conduit failure (stenosis and/or regurgitation) is a common complication, and can be treated with percutaneous valve implantation: either a Melody (Medtronic Inc., Minneapolis, MN, USA) or an Edwards Sapien (Edwards Lifesciences, Irvine, CA, USA) valve. A peak right ventricular systolic pressure of >60 mmHg is indicative of significant conduit stenosis [3]. In the Congenital Multicenter Trial of Pulmonic Valve Regurgitation Studying the SAPIEN Transcatheter Heart Valve (COMPASSION) trial, 98.4% of patients were alive at 3 years' follow-up, while 93.7% were free from reintervention [19]. The valved conduit should be sized accurately, since a Melody valve is suitable for diameters up to 22 mm³, while an Edwards Sapien valve can be inserted into conduits of up to 25 mm. Accurate device sizing is crucial to prevent dislodgement of the stented valve, and is best performed with cardiac CT (see below). A heavily calcified conduit may prevent echocardiographic interrogation of the lumen, although Doppler data can still be obtained. Extensive calcification of the conduit is a risk for dynamic coronary artery compression, which can be best evaluated at the time of valve insertion with a balloon inflated inside the conduit.

18.3   Cardiac Computed Tomography

The high spatial resolution of CT, in addition to the acquisition of a truly 3D, isotropic dataset which can be post-processed along any imaging plane, makes this modality particularly suited to the planning of structural interventions in ACHD patients.

The sizing of ASDs and VSDs for percutaneous closure can be performed accurately with contrast-enhanced cardiac CT when echocardiography does not provide adequate windows or resolution. The drainage pattern of the pulmonary veins can also be detected with a high degree of accuracy in patients with an ASD.

Device closure of a PDA is contraindicated if the defect is very large, or in the presence of a ductal aneurysm. Assessment of the PDA size and identification of an associated ductal aneurysm is usually not feasible with echocardiography in an adult, but can be accomplished with CT.

Aortic coarctation can be depicted very well with CT, and although direct functional information cannot be derived, the presence of collaterals implies that the coarctation is hemodynamically significant. The diameter of the aorta proximal and distal to the coarctation, as well as its length, should be measured before balloon dilatation and stenting. CT allows visualization of the stent lumen, which echocardiography and CMR do not, and is therefore useful in the assessment of follow-up and re-coarctation. Stenting is also indicated for excluding an aneurysm after surgical repair or balloon dilatation, and requires accurate sizing before the intervention.

Stenosis of a right ventricular-to-pulmonary artery conduit may be underestimated by the modified Bernoulli equation when multilevel, while CT visualizes the degeneration directly (Fig. 18.3). A contraindication to percutaneous pulmonary valve replacement inside a failed right ventricular-to-pulmonary artery conduit is dynamic compression of a coronary artery by the stented pulmonary valve. Although the anatomy of the coronary arteries in relation to the planned location of stent placement and area(s) of calcification can be visualized, noninvasive cardiac imaging is unable to predict dynamic compression of a coronary artery. An invasive coronary angiogram should therefore still be performed during right ventricular outflow tract balloon inflation to recognize this potential complication. Accurate device sizing and an adequate landing zone distance to prevent pulmonary artery branch obstruction (23–26 mm required for a Melody valve; no risk with 14–16 mm frame of the Edwards Sapien valve) can be performed with cardiac CT.

Right ventricular volumes and function can be calculated with retrospectively gated cardiac CT in repaired ToF patients with implantable electronic devices (CIEDs), although it is conventionally performed with CMR (see below).

Baffle patency in recipients of an atrial switch procedure can be evaluated with contrasted cardiac CT, although it does not provide any functional information.

Major aortopulmonary collateral arteries (MAPCAs) may develop in pulmonary atresia, and require coil occlusion before surgery to prevent massive intra-operative arterial haemorrhage. MAPCAs can be sized accurately with CT before percutaneous intervention [20]. Similarly, arteriopulmonary collaterals in a patient with a Fontan circulation can be evaluated with CT before percutaneous occlusion [21].

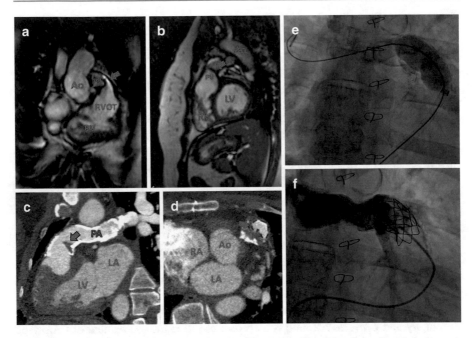

Fig. 18.3 Example of a 32-year-old female with repaired tetralogy of Fallot, who received a pulmonary artery conduit. Over the years, the conduit degenerated and the gradient through the pulmonary valve (PV) increased. Panels **a** and **b** demonstrate balanced steady-state free precession (bSSFP) cardiac magnetic resonance (CMR) images of the right ventricular outflow tract (RVOT) and PV. Note the acceleration of the flow through the stenosis (yellow arrows). On the computed tomography (CT) images, the conduit is calcified, with thickened, restrictive PV leaflets (**c**, yellow arrow). Note the close relationship of the pulmonary artery (PA) with the left main coronary artery (LM). Panel **d** shows the cross-sectional area of the stenosis (red dotted line/yellow arrow). During transcatheter implantation of a Melody (Medtronic Inc., Minneapolis, MN, USA) valve, note the calcifications of the conduit and the indentation on the balloon at the site of stenosis during dilatation (**e**, yellow arrow). The absence of regurgitation is demonstrated post-implantation by a contrast injection (**f**). *Ao* aorta, *LA* left atrium, *LV* left ventricle, *RA* right atrium, *RV* right ventricle

18.4 Cardiac Magnetic Resonance Imaging

CMR has the ability to assess both cardiac anatomy and function, without the use of ionizing radiation and along any chosen imaging plane in three dimensions. Its particular strengths for structural heart disease interventional planning lie in the accurate assessment of intracardiac flows with phase-contrast imaging and its temporal resolution, which is higher than that of CT, as well as its excellent soft tissue contrast. Routine adult cardiac CMR requires the acquisition of prespecified imaging planes, which allow for limited post-processing. Complex congenital heart disease often mandates nonstandard views, and the acquisition of 3D whole-heart images allows the offline reconstruction of planes from an isotropic dataset. Four-dimensional phase-contrast flow allows planes through which blood flow is quantified to be chosen retrospectively, greatly increasing the ability to post-process and interpret functional data. While delayed enhancement is conventionally depicted in CMR with gadolinium contrast, only focal scar can be visualized and quantified in this manner [22]. Diffuse fibrosis can be quantified with T1 parametric mapping, which represents the time constant of longitudinal myocardial spin relaxation on a pixel-by-pixel basis on a colour-coded map [22]. CMR sequences, e.g. Modified Look-Locker Inversion Recovery (MOLLI) and shortened MOLLI (ShMOLLI) are used to create pre- (native) and post-contrast T1 maps [22]. The presence of diffuse myocardial fibrosis will lead to longer native T1 values and shorter T1 values after the administration of gadolinium contrast [22]. The extracellular volume fraction (ECV) of myocardium can be estimated from the myocardial and blood pool pre- and post-contrast T1 values, and is a reflection of the size of the extracellular space [22]. Barring oedema or amyloidosis, ECV is a biomarker of fibrosis, since type I collagen is the main constituent of the extracellular space [22]. T1 mapping and ECV estimation of the thin-walled right ventricle still present technical challenges, but are feasible and are promising biomarkers for the planning of ACHD structural interventions, e.g. where the functional right ventricular reserve is sought. Although CMR has a proven safety record, caution has to be exercised in the presence of CIEDs, while metallic prostheses and implants may cause significant imaging artefacts.

While the position, number and size of ASDs are usually more readily assessed with echocardiography or cardiac CT, CMR has a role to play if doubt remains regarding the number of defects. An en-face view of the interatrial septum during phase-contrast acquisition, will clearly demarcate the number of defects. The primary uses of CMR in the planning of interventional ASD closure are the detection of anomalous pulmonary venous drainage (which will preclude percutaneous closure) and quantification of the shunt fraction. Guidelines recommend a shunt fraction of >1.5 before intervention, since this degree of shunting predisposes to the development of pulmonary hypertension [3]. Four-dimensional flow sequences have been applied to ASDs as well as anomalous pulmonary venous drainage, although the exact implications for interventional planning remain to be defined [23].

VSD imaging is performed with the same basic tenets as with ASDs, and the shunt fraction can be calculated (closure indicated if >1.5) [3]. Multiple defects, as well as type III and apical VSDs, may also be more readily visualized with CMR than with echocardiography.

While a PDA can be diagnosed on CMR when flow is visualized from the aorta into the pulmonary artery on balanced steady-state free precession (bSSFP) cine loops or phase-contrast sequences, its primary role in is quantification of shunt size by measuring flow in the aorta and pulmonary artery (distal to the defect).

Black-blood sequences are recommended for the visualization of aortic coarctation, since they do not suffer from signal loss due to high-velocity transcoarctation flow. The maximum gradient across the narrowing can be estimated with phase-contrast sequences, and the collateral flow calculated by subtracting flow distal to the coarctation from proximal flow. Since the actual gradient is dependent on volume flow, estimating the degree of collateral flow might be a valuable parameter in weighing the functional significance of a coarctation, although this has not been investigated extensively. Four-dimensional flow analysis has been applied to both uncorrected and repaired coarctation [24, 25]. The implications for structural intervention are still being explored, but include the ability to determine the maximum translesional pressure gradient more accurately (it is often located distal to the maximum stenosis, and may require multiple 2D analyses) as well as the identification of patients at higher risk of procedural complications, e.g. dissections in areas that have been exposed to high shear stress.

Congenital PS can be visualized with CMR. Transvalvular (or other) gradients may be underestimated with CMR due to: (1) the relatively low temporal resolution, (2) high velocity through a stenotic lesion exceeding the Reynolds number and causing turbulent flow, which increases phase dispersion and (3) the averaging of velocities in the voxel containing the highest velocity. Gradients estimated with CMR should therefore always be interpreted with caution, and the threshold for PS intervention has been extrapolated from echocardiographic guidelines (>3–4 m/s) but has not been validated for CMR. Planimetry is an alternative approach to the quantification of PS with CMR.

The accurate quantification of right ventricular volumes and function, as well as the severity of pulmonary regurgitation after ToF repair, is the application of CMR to ACHD per excellence (Fig. 18.4). Percutaneous pulmonary valve replacement can be performed within a stent placed to create an area of purchase, or within a dysfunctional right ventricle-to-pulmonary artery conduit or bioprosthetic valve that has already been placed for post-repair pulmonary regurgitation. Some technical aspects of the right ventricular volume determinations warrant mention. While the papillary muscles and trabeculations should be excluded from the blood pool, this is time-consuming and comes at the price of higher interobserver variability [26]. A "hood" may form where the dilated right ventricle extends beyond the atrioventricular groove, and more superior slices may have to be examined to accurately measure the right ventricular volume. Since the long axes of the right and left ventricles are not parallel, the tracing of right ventricular endocardial borders is performed on a bSSFP short axis stack which has been optimized for the left ventricle. Acquiring a separate stack which is aligned with the long axis of the right ventricle, has been shown to have superior interobserver variability. In the absence of much longitudinal and outcome data, the thresholds for intervention on a regurgitant pulmonary valve post-ToF repair remain controversial. Even though right ventricular function often does not normalize, the right ventricular dimensions usually decrease as long as the end-diastolic volume remains below 160 mL/m^2 and the end-systolic volume above 82 mL/m^2 [3, 27]. Since the high volumes/preloads at which the right ventricle operates may overestimate true systolic function, more intrinsic measures of functional reserve are being sought. T1 mapping and ECV calculation have been performed at 1.5 T and 3.0 T in patients with repaired ToF, but have not been correlated with outcomes after percutaneous pulmonary valve replacement [28, 29]. Flow abnormalities and disturbed kinetic energy in repaired ToF have been

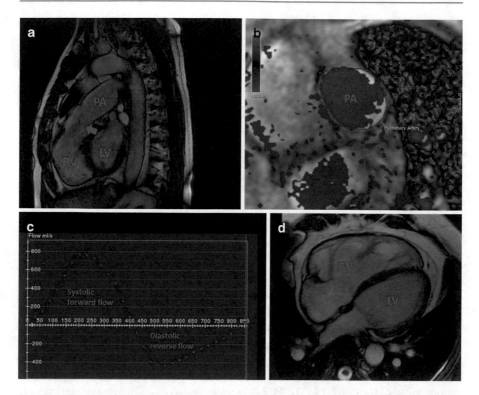

Fig. 18.4 Severe pulmonary regurgitation after tetralogy of Fallot repair. The right ventricular outflow view on balanced steady-state free precession (bSSFP) cardiac magnetic resonance (CMR) imaging demonstrates a pulmonary regurgitant jet (yellow arrow) (**a**). Pulmonary regurgitation is often underestimated visually on CMR, due to the lower flow velocities (compared to the left heart) and subsequent reduced turbulence and phase dispersion. Phase-contrast imaging demonstrates severe pulmonary regurgitation with a regurgitant volume of 107 mL and a regurgitant fraction of 58% (**b** and **c**). Colour-coded, velocity-encoded cine still frame (magnitude image) showing regurgitant flow in the pulmonary artery (PA) (**b**). The flow curve (**c**) demonstrates systolic forward and diastolic reverse flow. On a bSSFP horizontal long axis CMR view, the right ventricle (RV) is seen to be severely dilated in diastole (**d**). The RV end-diastolic volume was 407 mL, and the indexed (to body surface area) RV end-diastolic volume was 194 mL/m^2. *LV* left ventricle

characterized with four-dimensional flow CMR, both which have the potential to improve the timing of intervention [30, 31].

Baffle anatomy and obstruction after an atrial switch procedure can be visualized along any desired plane with CMR. Similar to echocardiography, elevated velocities and loss of the phasic flow profile can be used to diagnose obstruction, and baffle leaks can be identified by determining shunt fractions. It has to be kept in mind; however, that bidirectional flow can cause a near-normal shunt fraction. Technical pitfalls include the appropriate choice of velocity-encoding to characterize lower venous velocities, as well as a turbulent flow profile in the pulmonary artery which

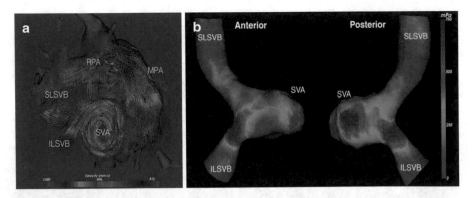

Fig. 18.5 Four-dimensional cardiovascular magnetic resonance (CMR) flow after atrial switch (Mustard) procedure. Particle tracing demonstrates increased flow velocity in the inferior limb of the systemic venous baffle (ILSVB), as well as clockwise flow in the systemic venous atrium (SVA) (**a**). Increased peak systolic wall stress can be visualized on the anterior and inferolateral aspects of the ILSVB, as well as on the posterosuperior wall of the SVA (**b**). (Adapted with permission from Van der Palen RLF et al.: *Eur Heart J Cardiovasc Imaging* 17:353, 2016). *MPA* main pulmonary artery, *RPA* right pulmonary artery, *SLSVB* superior limb of systemic venous baffle

is often angulated, and that can be circumvented by measuring and adding the caval flows and the branch pulmonary artery flows. Baffle obstruction has been demonstrated with four-dimensional flow, including areas of locally elevated peak systolic wall shear stress (Fig. 18.5) [32]. Right ventricle-to-pulmonary artery conduits may be interrogated by CMR (Fig. 18.3), but metallic valve rings and sternal wiring may generate significant artefacts.

18.5   Future Directions

3D printing allows the physical recreation of ACHD in a palpable model. While it might assist the interventionist in planning the structural heart procedure, it has not yet been proven to change outcomes. This printing technique may also have a valuable role to play in patient education and counselling.

The complex anatomic relationships between structures can be superbly appreciated by virtual/augmented reality imaging (Fig. 18.6). While outcome data are still lacking for this technology, it holds great promise.

It is expected that emerging technologies such as deformation imaging (echocardiography, CT and CMR), parametric mapping (CMR) and four-dimensional flow (CMR) will be used more frequently in ACHD as they mature, and that their value for interventional planning will become established as more evidence accrues.

Fig. 18.6 Virtual reality (VR) in interventional planning for adult congenital heart disease. VR allows interaction of the operator with a three-dimensional model via goggles. Cardiac morphology can be explored by navigation inside the model, as well as via VR dissection, where anatomical structures can be removed. VR is a promising tool for the planning of interventional procedures in adult congenital heart disease. (Image courtesy of Omar Pappalardo, Artiness S.r.l.)

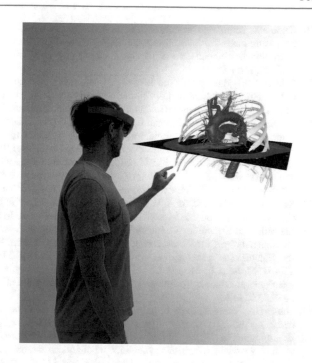

References

1. Cikes M, Tong L, Sutherland GR, et al. Ultrafast cardiac ultrasound imaging: technical principles, applications, and clinical benefits. JACC Cardiovasc Imaging. 2014;7:812–23.
2. Sanchez-Quintana D, Anderson RH, Ho SY. Ventricular myoarchitecture in tetralogy of Fallot. Heart. 1996;76:280–6.
3. Baumgartner H, Bonhoeffer P, De Groot NM, et al. ESC guidelines for the management of grown-up congenital heart disease (new version 2010). Eur Heart J. 2010;31:2915–57.
4. Plymale J, Kolinski K, Frommelt P, et al. Inferior sinus venosus defects: anatomic features and echocardiographic correlates. Pediatr Cardiol. 2013;34:322–6.
5. Hascoet S, Hadeed K, Marchal P, et al. The relation between atrial septal defect shape, diameter, and area using three-dimensional transoesophageal echocardiography and balloon sizing during percutaneous closure in children. Eur Heart J Cardiovasc Imaging. 2015;16:747–55.
6. Malekzadeh-Milani S, Ladouceur M, Cohen S, et al. Results of transcatheter pulmonary valvulation in native or patched right ventricular outflow tracts. Arch Cardiovasc Dis. 2014;107:592–8.
7. Meadows JJ, Moore PM, Berman DP, et al. Use and performance of the melody transcatheter pulmonary valve in native and postsurgical, nonconduit right ventricular outflow tracts. Circ Cardiovasc Interv. 2014;7:374–80.
8. Cools B, Brown SC, Heying R, et al. Percutaneous pulmonary valve implantation for free pulmonary regurgitation following conduit-free surgery of the right ventricular outflow tract. Int J Cardiol. 2015;186:129–35.
9. Valente AM, Cook S, Festa P, et al. Multimodality imaging guidelines for patients with repaired tetralogy of fallot: a report from the American Society of echocardiography: developed in collaboration with the Society for Cardiovascular Magnetic Resonance and the Society for Pediatric Radiology. J Am Soc Echocardiogr. 2014;27:111–41.

10. Khoo NS, Young A, Occleshaw C, et al. Assessments of right ventricular volume and function using three-dimensional echocardiography in older children and adults with congenital heart disease: comparison with cardiac magnetic resonance imaging. J Am Soc Echocardiogr. 2009;22:1279–88.

11. Grewal J, Majdalany D, Syed I, et al. Three-dimensional echocardiographic assessment of right ventricular volume and function in adult patients with congenital heart disease: comparison with magnetic resonance imaging. J Am Soc Echocardiogr. 2010;23:127–33.

12. Dragulescu A, Grosse-Wortmann L, Fackoury C, et al. Echocardiographic assessment of right ventricular volumes after surgical repair of tetralogy of Fallot: clinical validation of a new echocardiographic method. J Am Soc Echocardiogr. 2011;24:1191–8.

13. Dragulescu A, Grosse-Wortmann L, Fackoury C, et al. Echocardiographic assessment of right ventricular volumes: a comparison of different techniques in children after surgical repair of tetralogy of Fallot. Eur Heart J Cardiovasc Imaging. 2012;13:596–604.

14. Kawel-Boehm N, Maceira A, Valsangiacomo-Buechel ER, et al. Normal values for cardiovascular magnetic resonance in adults and children. J Cardiovasc Magn Reson. 2015;17:29.

15. Lancellotti P, Tribouilloy C, Hagendorff A, et al. European Association of Echocardiography recommendations for the assessment of valvular regurgitation. Part 1: aortic and pulmonary regurgitation (native valve disease). Eur J Echocardiogr. 2010;11:223–44.

16. Yim D, Mertens L, Morgan CT, et al. Impact of surgical pulmonary valve replacement on ventricular mechanics in children with repaired tetralogy of Fallot. Int J Cardiovasc Imaging. 2017;33:711–20.

17. Gursu HA, Varan B, Sade E, et al. Analysis of right ventricle function with strain imaging before and after pulmonary valve replacement. Cardiol J. 2016;23:195–201.

18. Balasubramanian S, Harrild DM, Kerur B, et al. Impact of surgical pulmonary valve replacement on ventricular strain and synchrony in patients with repaired tetralogy of Fallot: a cardiovascular magnetic resonance feature tracking study. J Cardiovasc Magn Reson. 2018;20:37.

19. Kenny D, Rhodes JF, Fleming GA, et al. 3-year outcomes of the Edwards SAPIEN transcatheter heart valve for conduit failure in the pulmonary position from the COMPASSION multicenter clinical trial. JACC Cardiovasc Interv. 2018;11:1920–9.

20. Greil GF, Schoebinger M, Kuettner A, et al. Imaging of aortopulmonary collateral arteries with high-resolution multidetector CT. Pediatr Radiol. 2006;36:502–9.

21. Grosse-Wortmann L, Al-Otay A, Yoo SJ. Aortopulmonary collaterals after bidirectional cavopulmonary connection or Fontan completion: quantification with MRI. Circ Cardiovasc Imaging. 2009;2:219–25.

22. Van der Bijl P, Podlesnikar T, Bax JJ, et al. Sudden Cardiac Death Risk Prediction: The Role of Cardiac Magnetic Resonance Imaging. Rev Esp Cardiol (Engl Ed). 2018;71:961–70.

23. Valverde I, Simpson J, Schaeffter T, et al. 4D phase-contrast flow cardiovascular magnetic resonance: comprehensive quantification and visualization of flow dynamics in atrial septal defect and partial anomalous pulmonary venous return. Pediatr Cardiol. 2010;31:1244–8.

24. Rengier F, Delles M, Eichhorn J, et al. Noninvasive pressure difference mapping derived from 4D flow MRI in patients with unrepaired and repaired aortic coarctation. Cardiovasc Diagn Ther. 2014;4:97–103.

25. Frydrychowicz A, Markl M, Hirtler D, et al. Aortic hemodynamics in patients with and without repair of aortic coarctation: in vivo analysis by 4D flow-sensitive magnetic resonance imaging. Invest Radiol. 2011;46:317–25.

26. Winter MM, Bernink FJ, Groenink M, et al. Evaluating the systemic right ventricle by CMR: the importance of consistent and reproducible delineation of the cavity. J Cardiovasc Magn Reson. 2008;10:40.

27. Oosterhof T, van Straten A, Vliegen HW, et al. Preoperative thresholds for pulmonary valve replacement in patients with corrected tetralogy of Fallot using cardiovascular magnetic resonance. Circulation. 2007;116:545–51.

28. Shiina Y, Inai K, Taniguchi K, et al. Potential value of native T1 mapping in symptomatic adults with congenital heart disease: a preliminary study of 3.0 Tesla cardiac magnetic resonance imaging. Pediatr Cardiol. 2019;41:94–100.

29. Kozak MF, Redington A, Yoo SJ, et al. Diffuse myocardial fibrosis following tetralogy of Fallot repair: a T1 mapping cardiac magnetic resonance study. Pediatr Radiol. 2014;44:403–9.
30. Geiger J, Markl M, Jung B, et al. 4D-MR flow analysis in patients after repair for tetralogy of Fallot. Eur Radiol. 2011;21:1651–7.
31. Sjoberg P, Bidhult S, Bock J, et al. Disturbed left and right ventricular kinetic energy in patients with repaired tetralogy of Fallot: pathophysiological insights using 4D-flow MRI. Eur Radiol. 2018;28:4066–76.
32. Van der Palen RL, Westenberg JJ, Hazekamp MG, et al. Four-dimensional flow cardiovascular magnetic resonance for the evaluation of the atrial baffle after mustard repair. Eur Heart J Cardiovasc Imaging. 2016;17:353.

Ebstein Anomaly

19

Lidija McGrath, Heidi M. Connolly, Dominica Zentner, and Luke Burchill

"Perhaps no other congenital heart lesion encompasses as broad a spectrum of clinical significance as does Ebstein's malformation" [1]

19.1 Introduction

Ebstein anomaly (EA) is a rare congenital heart defect that accounts for 0.37% of livebirths with congenital heart disease (CHD) [2]. EA has been described in non-syndromic single gene disorders [3] and following in-utero exposure to lithium [4] and selective serotonin reuptake inhibitors [5]. The anomaly was first described in an 1866 case report of a 19-year-old laborer who died 8 days after presenting with cachexia, severe cyanosis, a systolic murmur, and jugular veins that throbbed in synchrony with the heart's rhythm. At autopsy, Dr. Wilhelm Ebstein, a 28-year-old physician, observed a malformed tricuspid valve (TV) consisting of "at best only one cusp" with the rudimentary septal leaflet attached to the endocardium of the ventricular septum (Fig. 19.1) [6].

L. McGrath
Knight Cardiovascular Institute, Oregon Health & Science University, Portland, OR, USA
e-mail: mcgrathl@ohsu.edu

H. M. Connolly
Department of Cardiovascular Medicine, Mayo Clinic, Rochester, MN, USA
e-mail: connolly.heidi@mayo.edu

D. Zentner · L. Burchill (✉)
Department of Medicine, Royal Melbourne Hospital, Faculty of Medicine, Dentistry & Health Sciences, University of Melbourne, Melbourne, VIC, Australia
e-mail: dominica.zentner@mh.org.au; blj@unimelb.edu.au

© Springer Nature Switzerland AG 2021
P. Gallego, I. Valverde (eds.), *Multimodality Imaging Innovations In Adult Congenital Heart Disease*, Congenital Heart Disease in Adolescents and Adults, https://doi.org/10.1007/978-3-030-61927-5_19

Fig. 19.1 Ebstein anomaly as illustrated in Ebstein's original case report. The right atrium (RA) and right ventricle (RV) are opened along the right border beginning at the superior vena cava (SVC). The rudimentary septal tricuspid leaflet is seen in the middle of the diagram with its chordae tendinae inserting on the endocardium of the ventricular septum. (Reprinted from Attenhofer Jost [7]. The life story of Wilhelm Ebstein (1836–1912) and his almost overlooked description of a congenital heart disease. Mayo Clin Proc. 1979;54:197–204]. Used with permission of the Mayo Foundation for Medical Education and Research) All Rights Reserved

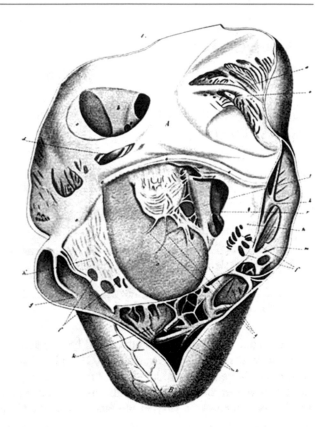

The term "Ebstein's disease" first appeared in the medical literature in 1927. It wasn't until 1951 that the first case of EA was diagnosed premortem, through a combination of cardiac catheterization and angiocardiography [8]. Subsequent advances in echocardiography revealed EA to be a remarkably heterogeneous condition encompassing a broad spectrum of disease and clinical presentations [1]. Further advances in cardiac imaging have been integral for our understanding of EA and the evolution of surgical techniques. This chapter will discuss current diagnostic and classification schema and review multimodality imaging for assessment of ventricular function, TV function, assessment around the time of cardiac surgery, and long-term surveillance.

19.2   Diagnosis and Classification

EA may be diagnosed both pre- and postnatally. Prenatal diagnosis may be coincidental during routine obstetric screening or following fetal echocardiographic assessment due to either fetal arrhythmia or maternal drug exposure. Postnatally the diagnosis may be made in the setting of investigation of cyanosis, arrhythmia, murmur or click, paradoxical embolus, reduced exercise capacity, or right heart failure.

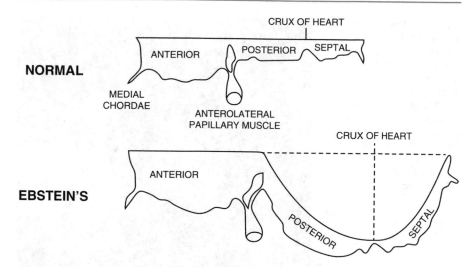

Fig. 19.2 Schematic representation of the tricuspid valve. Top, normal tricuspid valve with anterior, posterior (mural) and septal leaflets. Bottom, Ebstein tricuspid valve showing displacement of posterior and septal leaflets with maximal displacement at the crux of the posterior and septal leaflets. (Reprinted from Anderson [10]. Used with permission of the Mayo Foundation for Medical Education and Research)

19.2.1 Diagnostic Features

The normal TV has three leaflets; the posterior or mural leaflet, the septal leaflet, and the anterosuperior leaflet. The hallmark feature of EA is displacement of the septal and/or posterior leaflets from their usual annular location into the body of the right ventricle (RV) (Figs. 19.2 and 19.3). The anterior leaflet often remains normally sited, giving rise to its comparative elongated "sail-like" appearance. Displacement of the septal leaflet more than 8 mm/m^2 (indexed to body surface area) beyond the cardiac crux should lead to consideration of EA and prompt a search for other diagnostic features [9], including TV dysplasia, abnormal distal attachments, and ventricular myocardial dysfunction. Commonly, a patent foramen ovale or a secundum atrial septal defect is present and there is a strong association with accessory conduction pathways giving rise to pre-excitation [7]. Other infrequent but important congenital cardiac associations include pulmonary stenosis or atresia, ventricular septal defect, mitral stenosis, coarctation, tetralogy of Fallot, and transposition of the great arteries.

19.2.2 Classification Schema

The Congenital Heart Surgery Nomenclature and Database Project [11] classifies EA as a *spectrum diagnosis* incorporating the following features:

Fig. 19.3 Transthoracic
echocardiogram (TTE)
image from a patient with
Ebstein anomaly. Apical
4-chamber view with a
right ventricular focus
shows apically displaced
tricuspid valve leaflets with
a coaptation gap (arrow).
aRV atrialized RV, *fRV*
functional RV, *LA* left
atrium, *LV* left ventricle,
RA right atrium

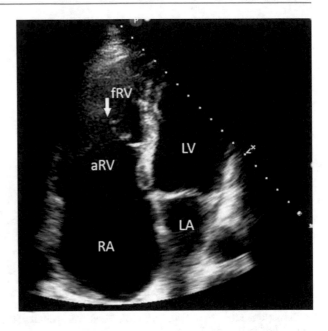

1. Failure of delamination such that the tricuspid leaflets remain adhered to the myocardium.
2. Apical displacement of the functional TV annulus.
3. Dilatation of the supra-annular atrium—which consists of both the true atrium and the "atrialized" portion of the right ventricle (aRV).
4. Abnormalities of the anterior leaflet, such as redundant tissue, fenestrations, and variable tethering and.
5. Dilatation of the true atrioventricular junction.

   The Carpentier classification describes 4 groups of findings (Type A to D) that can be used to guide the approach to surgery, particularly the suitability for surgical repair versus replacement [12]. In type A, the volume of the true RV is adequate. In type B, a large atrialized component of the RV exists, but the anterior leaflet of the TV moves freely. In type C, the anterior leaflet is severely restricted and may cause significant obstruction of the RV outflow tract. In type D, there is almost complete atrialization of the ventricle except for a small infundibular component. The Celermajer index is an echocardiographic index that calculates the ratio of the right atrium (RA) and aRV to the area of the functional RV (fRV) and left heart chambers. When applied to infants, the Celermajer index identifies increasing grades of anatomical severity and mortality risk [13]. The relevance of the Celermajer index for clinical status and outcomes in unoperated adults with EA is still under research [14].

19.3 Assessment of Tricuspid Regurgitation Severity and Ventricular Function

A comprehensive two-dimensional (2D) transthoracic echocardiogram (TTE) is the most widely used imaging tool for initial diagnosis and long-term surveillance of EA. It allows for assessment of the appearance, size and function of cardiac chambers and valves, and detection of intracardiac shunts and associated cardiac defects [15]. Additionally, comprehensive TTE provides an assessment of the left ventricular (LV) size and function, as well as the motion of the interventricular septum. In EA, progressive RV dilation can lead to paradoxical interventricular septal motion with resultant altered LV geometry and diminished LV systolic function over time [16].

19.3.1 Tricuspid Regurgitation Severity

Comprehensive TTE enables thorough assessment of the TV anatomy. This includes the extent to which the septal and/or posterior (mural) leaflets are apically displaced, the presence of TV dysplasia and tethering, leaflet coaptation, and annular dilation [9]. The anterior and septal leaflets are best visualized in the apical 4-chamber view. The posterior leaflet is best seen in the RV inflow view (Fig. 19.4), subcostal long-axis view, or RV 2-chamber view [9, 17]. Occasionally the parasternal long-axis view of the left heart provides a short-axis view of the TV due to the combination of right heart enlargement and rotation of the functional TV orifice.

Accurate assessment of tricuspid regurgitation (TR), critical for determining the severity and long-term consequences of the disease, can be challenging by standard TTE-Doppler imaging. Given the rotation of the functional TV orifice toward the RV outflow tract, regurgitation jets may be directed inferiorly/posteriorly and may

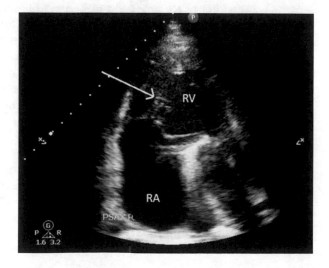

Fig. 19.4 Transthoracic echocardiogram (TTE) image from a patient with Ebstein anomaly. Off-axis parasternal short-axis right ventricular inflow view shows the posterior leaflet of the tricuspid valve (arrow), dilated right atrium (RA), apically displaced functional tricuspid valve annulus, and a dilated right ventricle (RV)

not be fully captured in the apical 4-chamber view. For this reason, subcostal sagittal or parasternal short-axis views with color and spectral Doppler are important for optimal assessment of regurgitant jet profile [9]. Leaflet fenestrations present another challenge giving rise to multiple regurgitation jets that make quantification of severity difficult [9]. In the presence of complex valve geometry, regurgitant jet density and measurement of effective regurgitant orifice area (EROA) can be unreliable [18]. With a significantly dilated and compliant aRV and RA, hepatic vein systolic flow reversal is often absent despite the presence of severe TR. A coaptation gap demonstrated in two orthogonal planes suggests the presence of severe regurgitation [9]. Additional details about the anatomy and function of the TV can be provided by three-dimensional (3D) TTE, which may be able to better characterize the posterior leaflet, delineate tethered from non-tethered segments, and more accurately assess vena contracta width and area [17, 19]. Current guidelines for management of adults with EA recommend the use of 2D and 3D transesophageal echocardiogram (TEE) for surgical planning if TTE images are inadequate to evaluate TV morphology and function [20].

Quantification of TR volume and subsequent calculation of regurgitant fraction can be achieved with cardiovascular magnetic resonance (CMR) imaging by velocity mapping perpendicular to the regurgitant jet, where a cross-section of >6 mm × 6 mm is considered severe in adults [21]. An alternative method of combining velocity mapping with cine imaging allows for quantification of regurgitant volume and regurgitant fraction by established methods [22]. A novel application for direct quantification of TR is four-dimensional (4D) flow CMR with retrospective valve tracking (Fig. 19.5), which may be helpful in follow-up of patients with EA and may have implications for the timing of intervention [23].

19.3.2 Ventricular Function

Accurate assessment of RV size and function is of utmost importance in patients with EA, as progressive RV systolic dysfunction by echocardiography or CMR imaging is an indication for surgical repair [20]. Yet, the complex geometry of the RV combined with other features of EA render 2D TTE alone unreliable, and complementary imaging modalities, particularly CMR, is now routine and standard of care for patients with EA [20]. Whereas fractional area change, tricuspid annular plane systolic excursion (TAPSE), RV tissue Doppler and measures of 2D strain have been reported to reliably assess right heart function in normal hearts under normal loading conditions, they have not been found to be reliable estimates of RV systolic function in patients with EA. As such, qualitative assessment of RV size and function in EA is most commonly used in clinical practice. Compared to CMR, qualitative assessment has a sensitivity of 77% and a specificity of 45% for identifying normal versus reduced RV ejection fraction [24]. 3D TTE can be useful but may be challenging in instances where the RV is too big for the available sector width [9]. When it can be performed, 3D TTE provides superior anatomic definition and more complete assessment of the size and volume of the fRV and aRV [17].

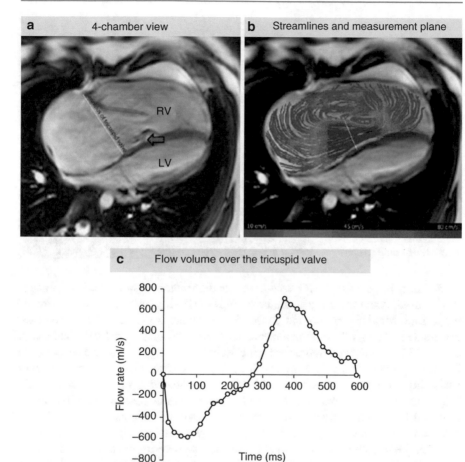

Fig. 19.5 Cardiac magnetic resonance (CMR) images and flow curves from a patient with Ebstein anomaly. Direct tricuspid regurgitation (TR) quantification by four-dimensional (4D) flow cardiac magnetic resonance (CMR) imaging with retrospective valve tracking is shown. Panel **a**: stylized representation of the tricuspid valve leaflets with the septal leaflet indicated by an arrow. Panel **b**: streamline visualization of flow patterns and the dynamic regurgitation jet. Panel **c**: The resulting flow curve allows for calculation of regurgitation fraction illustrated by the ratio between the negative versus positive area under the curve. *RV* right ventricle, *LV* left ventricle. (Reprinted from Kamphuis [23]. Used with permission from the Oxford University Press)

CMR imaging is recognized as the reference standard for assessment of RV size and function in patients with CHD including those with EA when performed by experienced cardiac imaging specialists [21]. CMR provides morphologic and functional information about the degree of TR, RV size (including aRV and fRV), RV function, as well as LV dimensions and function [9, 18, 25] (Fig. 19.6).

Due to the unique anatomic regions of aRV and fRV, assessment of RV size is more challenging in patients with EA as compared to other patients with CHD and those with normal anatomy, and considerable variability in practice exists between

Fig. 19.6 Cardiac magnetic resonance (CMR) image from a patient with Ebstein anomaly. Axial 4-chamber view shows the atrialized right ventricle (aRV) between the true atrioventricular junction (star) and the functional tricuspid valve annulus (arrow), and functional right ventricle (fRV) between the apically displaced tricuspid valve and right ventricular apex. *LA* left atrium, *LV* left ventricle, *RA* right atrium

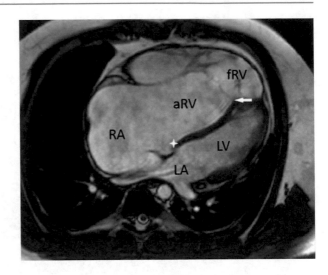

institutions. To quantify the RV volume, either axial stack or short-axis stack images can be used. Axial images provide better reproducibility and easier delineation of the atrioventricular junction and TV leaflet attachments [21, 26, 27]. In contrast, short-axis imaging allows simultaneous measurement of RV and LV volumes. A study of 32 patients with unrepaired EA concluded that right heart size and systolic function can be reliably measured with CMR, with lower inter- and intraobserver variability for data derived from axial images as compared to short-axis views [27]. This is likely because axial views allow for more accurate assessment of the atrialized and functional components of the RV by better visualization of TV leaflet insertion and coaptation points [27]. The study found no significant difference between previously established markers of disease severity by TTE and the same measurements obtained by CMR: the apical displacement of the septal TV leaflet and Celermajer severity index, calculated as (RA + aRV)/(fRV + LA + LV) [13]. The volume of aRV correlated well with both of these markers, suggesting that CMR-derived measurements could help define disease severity [27]. Additionally, the volume of aRV was found to be independently related to aerobic capacity [28], further suggesting that the volume of aRV might be a useful measure of severity of EA.

Some institutions include the aRV into the total RV volume assessment [9], whereas others measure only the fRV below the displaced TV. This can lead to considerable differences in result interpretation, emphasizing the importance of side-by-side comparison of serial examinations and the need for a standardized approach to RV volume quantification in EA. In a study of 29 adult patients with EA, CMR demonstrated RV dilation and global dysfunction with diverse regional patterns of remodeling leading to a greater contribution of short-axis fractional shortening to global RV EF, and less reliance on longitudinal shortening [29]. The latter finding explains the poor correlation between echo-derived TAPSE and CMR-derived RV ejection fraction (EF). Another study of 32 patients who underwent CMR found that the fRV is often enlarged in patients with unrepaired EA, and that the volume of fRV correlates strongly with severity of TR [30].

While RV myopathy is a cardinal feature of EA, the LV can also be affected. CMR-based studies have shown an irregularly shaped LV related to right sided dilation, globally reduced LV function, preserved LV volume, and paradoxical basal septal motion [31]. Total right to left heart volume index (RA + aRV + fRV)/(LA + LV) has been found to correlate well with clinical heart failure markers, including brain natriuretic peptide (BNP), peak oxygen consumption, ventilator response to carbon dioxide production at anaerobic threshold, as well as the severity of TR, TV apical displacement, and TAPSE [32].

LV global strain measured by CMR tissue tracking (Fig. 19.7) is reduced in patients with EA, and further reduced as LVEF declines, suggesting that strain could serve as an earlier measure of LV dysfunction [33]. Reduced LV function in EA has been attributed to a variety of causes including non-compaction cardiomyopathy, myocardial fibrosis, disruption of myofibril continuity, abnormal fiber geometry, and abnormal RV longitudinal shortening [16, 31, 34–39]. In a CMR-based study, TR was found to negatively correlate with LVEF and positively correlate with the ratio of fRV end-diastolic dimension to LV end-diastolic dimension (fRVEDD/LVEDD), suggesting that LV function, as well as LV and RV dimensional parameters could help predict the severity of EA [25].

Myocardial fibrosis can be measured focally by late gadolinium enhancement (LGE) or diffusely by calculating the extracellular volume (ECV) fraction derived from T1 mapping during CMR imaging. When assessed in EA patients, myocardial

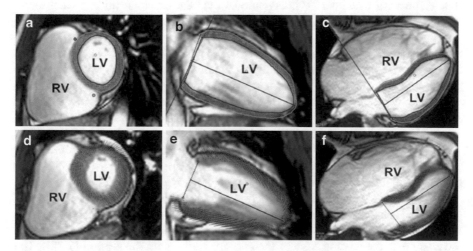

Fig. 19.7 Cardiac magnetic resonance (CMR) images from a patient with Ebstein anomaly. CMR tissue tracking using cmr42 (Circle Cardiovascular Imaging Inc., Calgary, Canada) in short-axis, two-chamber and four-chamber long-axis cine images at the end-diastole (**a–c**) and end-systole (**d–f**). The red and green curves show the endocardial and epicardial borders, respectively; the yellow dots represent the myocardial voxel points. *LV* left ventricle, *RV* right ventricle. (Reprinted from Liu [33]. Used with permission from Elsevier)

fibrosis has been associated with adverse ventricular remodeling and lower clinical status. Among 44 patients with unrepaired EA [40], ECV correlated significantly with LVEF, whereas both increased ECV and the presence of LGE were associated with larger fRV volume, larger aRV volume, increased disease severity [27], and lower NYHA functional class [40]. Other CMR-derived measures have also been found to have prognostic significance in EA patients. In a prospective study of 79 patients with unrepaired EA, RV and LV systolic dysfunction, reduced LV stroke volume, and reduced cardiac index were associated with sustained ventricular tachycardia (VT) and increased mortality [41]. Atrial tachyarrhythmias commonly preceded VT and death and were associated with right sided cardiac impairment. Moreover, first onset atrial tachyarrhythmia was strongly correlated with a composite of ventricular volumes and displacement of septal TV leaflet indexed to LV length. Taken all together, these findings highlight the importance of cardiac imaging to assess for the presence of anatomic and hemodynamic drivers of atrial arrhythmias as well as the potential for worsening right heart function following arrhythmia onset in EA patients [41].

19.4 Evaluation of Tricuspid Valve for Repair or Replacement

In general, TV repair is preferred to valve replacement in EA when feasible, primarily because of its potential longer durability and avoidance of complications related to prosthetic valves [7]. Options for surgical intervention include cone repair, alternative TV repair techniques, TV replacement, bidirectional cavopulmonary shunt (BCPS) with or without a TV intervention, or cardiac transplantation. Biventricular repair is preferred over BCPS or cardiac transplantation for all EA patients when possible.

The cone-type repair, initially described by da Silva in 2005 [42], has been employed widely by others. This surgical repair involves mobilization of all available TV leaflet tissue. The TV tissue is refashioned to create 360° of leaflet tissue (the cone) which is re-anchored at the level of the true annulus. The aRV is plicated. The cone reconstruction is the most anatomically natural of TV repairs described for EA and can be applied across a wide range of valve morphology and ages when performed by experienced surgeons. Current data suggest good durability and favorable impact on right ventricular remodeling [43].

The Danielson TV repair technique reported in 1979 consists of plication of aRV wall, posterior TV annuloplasty, reduction right atrioplasty, and creation of a monocusp valve using the anterior leaflet [44]. Subsequent modifications include approximation of the anterior leaflet papillary muscle to the ventricular septum to improve coaptation of the leading edge of the anterior leaflet with the septum [7, 45]. The most important anatomic features that allow this repair include a free leading edge of the anterior leaflet and at least a 50% delamination of the anterior leaflet [45]; this can be assessed by echocardiography or CMR.

In 1988, the Carpentier-Chauvaud monocusp method for TV repair was described, which mobilizes the tethered anterior leaflet and a portion of the posterior leaflet with reattachment of the leaflets to the true annulus, placement of annuloplasty ring, and plication of the aRV [12].

Ventricularization, characterized by reintegration of the aRV into the true RV cavity, involves orthotopic transposition of the detached septal and posterior leaflets and reimplantation such that the septal leaflet serves as an opposing structure for coaptation of the reconstructed valve [46].

BCPS is considered in selective cases of severe RV enlargement or dysfunction to provide RV volume offloading [47]. As pulmonary hypertension is rare in patients with EA, BCPS is generally feasible even in the setting of moderate LV dysfunction, though should be performed with caution in that setting. Indications for BCPS include RV end-diastolic volume index (RVEDVI) >250 mL/m², RV EF <25%, cardiothoracic ratio >65%, small and D-shaped LV, post-repair RA to LA pressure ratio >1.5:1, and post-repair low cardiac output. Additional indications include reduction of tension on complex TV repair and post-repair TV stenosis in the presence of a mean gradient >8–10 mmHg. Contraindications to BCPS include mean pulmonary artery pressure >20 mmHg, pulmonary arteriolar resistance >4 Wood units, LV end-diastolic pressure or LA pressure >12 mmHg, and significant pulmonary artery hypoplasia [47].

If the anterior TV leaflet is inadequately delaminated or if there are linear attachments of the leading edge of the anterior leaflet to the underlying myocardium, TV replacement is preferred, particularly in older patients and those with significant RV enlargement, RV dysfunction or tricuspid annular dilation [45, 48, 49]. Bioprosthetic valves are preferred to mechanical valve replacement due to good durability and the possibility to avoid lifelong anticoagulation [50]. Patients with bioprosthetic tricuspid valve replacement should be monitored for bioprosthetic valve thrombosis, an under-recognized complication of right sided bioprosthetic valves [51]. Additionally, once a bioprosthetic valve is in place, future percutaneous valve-in-valve interventions become possible, thus potentially avoiding the need for repeat surgical intervention [52]. Mechanical valve prostheses are generally avoided in EA patients, especially in the setting of significant RV dysfunction due to the risk of abnormal disc motion and thus a higher likelihood of valve thrombosis even in the presence of therapeutic anticoagulation [48].

19.5   Preoperative Assessment

The indications to proceed with surgical intervention in patients with EA include the presence of symptoms (dyspnea, progressive fatigue, and right heart failure), objective evidence of worsening exercise capacity as determined by cardiopulmonary exercise testing, and progressive RV systolic dysfunction as evidenced by echocardiography or CMR [20]. Surgery may also be beneficial in those with progressive RV enlargement, cyanosis related to the presence of right-to-left shunt, paradoxical embolism, or atrial tachyarrhythmias [20]. There are currently no standard cutoffs for RV size and function to indicate the need for surgery in patients with EA [9]. In the era predating the cone operation, the presence of moderate or greater RV dysfunction was shown to be an independent predictor of early mortality after surgical intervention [53], leading to the recommendation of proceeding with surgery prior to significant RV enlargement or dysfunction [54]. TV repair techniques are complex, and thus TV surgery is not recommended in the asymptomatic EA patient without other indications.

Prior to proceeding with surgery, a comprehensive clinical assessment and dedicated imaging focused on obtaining anatomic data to determine the best intraoperative treatment plan is required. This includes assessment of RV and LV size and function, determination of TV anatomy to assess reparability, and identification of associated lesions that might require attention during surgery [55, 56].

Comprehensive 2D TTE provides detailed assessment of the TV leaflets, degree of apical displacement and tethering, annular size, subvalvar apparatus, right sided chamber size and function, degree of TR, and associated cardiac pathology, thus remaining an essential imaging modality for preoperative evaluation [9]. The apical 4-chamber view delineates the presence and mobility of the anterior and septal leaflets and identifies areas of attachment to the myocardium. Muscularization, increased thickness and/or significant myocardial attachments of the anterior leaflet, and absence of the septal leaflet make a successful cone reconstruction more challenging [56]. A saline contrast bubble study can identify the presence, size, and directionality of an interatrial shunt, yielding important information prior to surgical intervention. Additional anatomic detail can be provided by 3D TTE, which is able to better characterize the posterior leaflet of the TV, delineate tethered from non-tethered segments, assess the fRV and aRV, and more accurately quantify the degree of TR [17, 19].

TEE is essential for intraoperative assessment and monitoring; however, it can also be used for preoperative evaluation in patients with poor acoustic windows, where TTE images are unable to fully characterize the TV morphology and function [20]. CMR has become an important adjunctive tool in preoperative assessment of patients with EA and is recommended as part of preoperative assessment. CMR often offers better visualization of the posterior TV leaflet, leaflet fenestrations, adhesions and tethering of the anterior leaflet as compared to TTE [55]. It also allows for comprehensive assessment of the complex RV geometry, the size of the RV and its atrialized and functional components, RV function, as well as quantification of TR [18]. Evaluation of the size and morphology of the aRV is important for planning technical modifications and associated procedures, such as RV plication, annular reduction, and ringed annuloplasty, which, when possible, are recommended during surgical valve repair [56].

In patients unable to undergo CMR, electrocardiogram (ECG)-gated computed tomography (CT) angiography can be used to obtain ventricular volumes and EF; however, assessment of TR severity is not possible using this technique [57]. Either coronary CT angiography or invasive coronary angiography is performed in adults for coronary artery assessment prior to proceeding with surgical intervention [9]. With advancements in percutaneous valve interventions, cardiac CT has become an essential imaging tool for detailed annular measurements and pre-procedural planning in patients undergoing percutaneous valve replacement. The presence of atrial arrhythmias and accessory pathways is high in patients with EA, and an electrophysiology consultation is recommended in all EA patients with arrhythmias to determine which patients require electrophysiology study and/or catheter ablation prior to surgical intervention [20, 48].

19.6 Intraoperative and Early Postoperative Assessment

Intraoperative and early post-bypass assessment with TEE is of critical importance during surgical valve repair or replacement in patients with EA. It helps to confirm intraoperative diagnosis, monitor hemodynamic changes and regional wall motion during surgery, evaluate the effect of TV repair immediately after the procedure, and assess postoperative RV function [58]. During intraoperative monitoring, important TEE views include the mid-esophageal 4-chamber view, which identifies the atrial and ventricular septum, mitral valve, TV with apical displacement of the functional annulus, size and function of the aRV and fRV, as well as RA size. The anterior and septal leaflets of the TV are visualized, allowing assessment of apical displacement and evaluation of leaflet attachment to the underlying myocardium. TR can be evaluated with color Doppler interrogation in this view [9, 58]. The mid-esophageal oblique view, also known as the RV inflow-outflow view, shows the anterior and posterior leaflets and the anterior rotation of the functional TV orifice into the RV outflow tract. The transgastric sagittal view is generally the best view for evaluation of the posterior TV leaflet [9]. The bicaval and transverse views can generally identify interatrial communications.

In a recent study of 164 patients undergoing intraoperative TEE during surgical intervention for EA, good agreement was found between TEE and surgical findings for apical displacement and morphologic features of the septal and posterior leaflets. However, TEE successfully identified apical displacement of the anterior leaflet only 40% of the time when compared to surgical findings, possibly due to the fact that anterior leaflet apical displacement often occurs only partially and at the junction with the posterior leaflet, making visualization more challenging [58]. Immediate post-bypass TEE is used to identify TR which allows revision of tricuspid repair with resultant improvement of the regurgitation when needed [58].

In a prospective study comparing echocardiography and CMR, 12 patients with EA underwent surgical intervention, with intraoperative TEE performed in all cases. Despite detailed preoperative evaluation with TTE and CMR, intraoperative TEE identified 3 additional cases of interatrial communications with shunting, 1 new diagnosis of cor triatriatum, 1 additional case of TV fenestrations, and one patient with hypoplastic pulmonary arteries; none of these were identified on preoperative evaluation and some led to a change in the proposed operation [55].

3D TEE is a useful complementary imaging modality for more detailed anatomic assessment during surgery, providing additional information on morphology and function of TV, pulmonary valve, and RV outflow tract [59]. One of the main advantages of 3D TEE is the ability to visualize the valve from different angles and planes, precisely delineate all valve leaflets and identify a coaptation gap, and focus on any area of interest contained within the acquired pyramidal volume of information [60] (Figs. 19.8 and 19.9). After the cone repair, the apical part of the cone-shaped valve can be difficult to visualize by 2D TEE; however, 3D TEE allows for en-face visualization from both the atrial and ventricular aspects. The repaired valve can then be evaluated for appropriate coaptation to ensure there is no significant regurgitation,

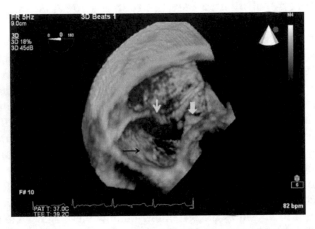

Fig. 19.8 Three-dimensional transesophageal echocardiogram (3D-TEE) image from a patient with Ebstein anomaly. 3D-TEE with en-face view of tricuspid valve (TV) through the right ventricle shows a large anterior tricuspid leaflet (thin white arrow), a small septal tricuspid leaflet (thick white arrow), a rudimentary posterior tricuspid leaflet plastered to the right ventricular wall (black arrow), with a large coaptation defect at end-systole. (Reprinted from Sujatha [60]. Used with permission from Elsevier)

Fig. 19.9 Three-dimensional transesophageal echocardiogram (3D-TEE) image from a patient with Ebstein anomaly. 3D-TEE with virtual right atriotomy performed by placing the cropping plane parallel to the anterior tricuspid leaflet (ATL) shows a fenestration in the ATL (white arrow). No portion of the posterior tricuspid leaflet (PTL) is seen in the image. *STL* septal tricuspid leaflet. (Reprinted from Sujatha [60]. Used with permission from Elsevier)

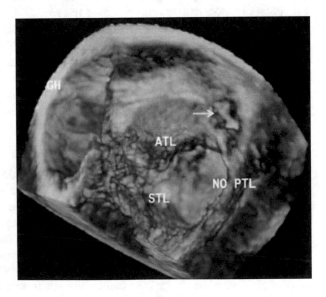

valve gradient assessed, when appropriate, valve area measured by planimetry, and the need for additional repair can be determined [60].

Recommended postoperative imaging includes a TTE prior to hospital discharge, at 3–6 months post-surgery, and annually thereafter, with detailed assessment of repaired valvular and RV function [20]. Increased TV gradient can be seen in the early postoperative period, due to anemia and tachycardia, but the gradient should improve over time [56]. CMR can also be used to assess the result of the surgical repair, allowing for determination of RV size, function, and remodeling, as well as function of the repaired or replaced TV.

19.7   Long-Term Surveillance

Neonates with EA experience high mortality that can be predicted by the presence of class IV heart failure and echocardiographic features [61], including the presence of a ventricular septal defect [62]. By contrast, EA patients presenting later in life have low operative mortality and excellent long-term survival. Among 36 EA patients (mean age 25.4 ± 15.9 years) who underwent TV repair in The Netherlands, freedom from reoperation was 80 ± 8% at 25 years. While overall survival at 25 years was excellent at 97 ± 3%, freedom from arrhythmia steadily declined from 73 ± 8% to 64 ± 9% and 53 ± 11% at 5, 10 and 25 years, respectively [63]. Evaluating 68 EA patients (mean age, 26.9 ± 7.3 years) who underwent TV repair in Germany, Hetzer et al. demonstrated significant improvement in NYHA Class, TR severity, maximal oxygen uptake, and ventricular function. Early mortality in the German series was 3% with excellent freedom from reoperation and late survival at 20 years (93% and 91%, respectively) [64].

Despite excellent long-term survival, EA patients are at increased risk of sudden death. Among 968 EA patients [mean age 25.3 years, 41.5% male; 79.8% severe EA, 18.6% accessory pathway, 0.74% implantable cardioverter-defibrillator (ICD) placement] the 10-, 50-, and 70-year cumulative incidences of sudden death from birth were 0.8%, 8.3%, and 14.6%, respectively. Prior ventricular tachycardia [hazard ratio (HR) 6.37, $P < 0.001$)], heart failure (HR 5.64, $P < 0.001$), TV surgery (HR 5.94, $P < 0.001$), syncope (HR 2.03, $P = 0.019$), pulmonic stenosis (HR 3.42, $P = 0.001$), and hemoglobin >15 g/dL (HR 2.05, $P = 0.026$) were predictors of sudden death [65]. Taken together, these findings indicate that in addition to current guidelines recommending annual TTE and CMR every 1–5 years for long-term surveillance [20], it is important to seek additional factors that place EA patients at increased risk of sudden death. Emerging data suggests this may also include CMR-derived assessment of total R/L volume index, RV/LV end-diastolic volume ratio, and apical septal leaflet displacement/total LV septal length—all of which have been shown to predict onset of atrial tachyarrhythmias leading to adverse outcomes in EA patients [41].

19.8 Conclusion

Our knowledge of EA has increased dramatically since it was first described in 1866. Fueled by advances in cardiac imaging, we understand EA to be a congenital heart defect with a seemingly infinite array of anatomic variations. Comprehensive TTE plays an essential role in recognizing the cardinal features of EA including characteristic displacement of the septal leaflet, TV dysplasia, abnormal distal attachments, ventricular myocardial dysfunction, and an atrial level shunt. While a comprehensive TTE provides important information on the mechanism and severity of TV regurgitation, CMR provides important complementary preoperative data regarding right as well as left heart size and function. EA patients with long-term survival following TV repair remain at increased risk of arrhythmias and sudden cardiac death. We anticipate that in the future cardiac imaging will assist in identifying which patients are at increased risk of adverse events and promote a highly individualized approach based on each patient's unique anatomic and hemodynamic profile.

References

1. Mair DD. Ebstein's anomaly: natural history and management. J Am Coll Cardiol. 1992;19(5):1047–8.
2. Schwedler G, Lindinger A, Lange PE, Sax U, Olchvary J, Peters B, et al. Frequency and spectrum of congenital heart defects among live births in Germany: a study of the competence network for congenital heart defects. Clin Res Cardiol. 2011;100(12):1111–7.
3. Blue GM, Kirk EP, Sholler GF, Harvey RP, Winlaw DS. Congenital heart disease: current knowledge about causes and inheritance. Med J Aust. 2012;197(3):155–9.
4. Ornoy A, Weinstein-Fudim L, Ergaz Z. Antidepressants, antipsychotics, and mood stabilizers in pregnancy: what do we know and how should we treat pregnant women with depression. Birth Defects Res. 2017;109(12):933–56.
5. Wemakor A, Casson K, Garne E, Bakker M, Addor MC, Arriola L, et al. Selective serotonin reuptake inhibitor antidepressant use in first trimester pregnancy and risk of specific congenital anomalies: a European register-based study. Eur J Epidemiol. 2015;30(11):1187–98.
6. Mazurak M, Kusa J. The two anomalies of Wilhelm Ebstein. Tex Heart Inst J. 2017;44(3):198–201.
7. Attenhofer Jost CH, Connolly HM, Dearani JA, Edwards WD, Danielson GK. Ebstein's anomaly. Circulation. 2007;115(2):277–85.
8. Soloff LA, Stauffer HM, Zatuchni J. Ebstein's disease: report of the first case diagnosed during life. Am J Med Sci. 1951;222(5):554–61.
9. Qureshi MY, O'Leary PW, Connolly HM. Cardiac imaging in Ebstein anomaly. Trends Cardiovasc Med. 2018;28(6):403–9.
10. Anderson KR, Lie JT. The right ventricular myocardium in Ebstein's anomaly: a morphometric histopathologic study. Mayo Clin Proc. 1979;54(3):181–4.
11. Dearani JA, Danielson GK. Congenital heart surgery nomenclature and database project: Ebstein's anomaly and tricuspid valve disease. Ann Thorac Surg. 2000;69(4 Suppl):S106–17.
12. Carpentier A, Chauvaud S, Mace L, Relland J, Mihaileanu S, Marino JP, et al. A new reconstructive operation for Ebstein's anomaly of the tricuspid valve. J Thorac Cardiovasc Surg. 1988;96(1):92–101.
13. Celermajer DS, Cullen S, Sullivan ID, Spiegelhalter DJ, Wyse RK, Deanfield JE. Outcome in neonates with Ebstein's anomaly. J Am Coll Cardiol. 1992;19(5):1041–6.

14. Cieplucha A, Trojnarska O, Bartczak-Rutkowska A, Kociemba A, Rajewska-Tabor J, Kramer L, et al. Severity scores for Ebstein anomaly: credibility and usefulness of echocardiographic vs magnetic resonance assessments of the Celermajer index. Can J Cardiol. 2019;35(12):1834–41.
15. Holst KA, Connolly HM, Dearani JA. Ebstein's anomaly. Methodist Debakey Cardiovasc J. 2019;15(2):138–44.
16. Oechslin E, Buchholz S, Jenni R. Ebstein's anomaly in adults: Doppler-echocardiographic evaluation. Thorac Cardiovasc Surg. 2000;48(4):209–13.
17. Booker OJ, Nanda NC. Echocardiographic assessment of Ebstein's anomaly. Echocardiography (Mount Kisco, NY). 2015;32(Suppl 2):S177–88.
18. Greutmann M, Buechel ERV, Jost CA. Editorial commentary: the caveats of cardiac imaging in Ebstein anomaly. Trends Cardiovasc Med. 2018;28(6):410–1.
19. Velayudhan DE, Brown TM, Nanda NC, Patel V, Miller AP, Mehmood F, et al. Quantification of tricuspid regurgitation by live three-dimensional transthoracic echocardiographic measurements of vena contracta area. Echocardiography (Mount Kisco, NY). 2006;23(9):793–800.
20. Stout KK, Daniels CJ, Aboulhosn JA, Bozkurt B, Broberg CS, Colman JM, et al. 2018 AHA/ACC guideline for the Management of Adults with Congenital Heart Disease. A Report of the American College of Cardiology/American Heart Association Task Force on Clinical Practice Guidelines. J Am Coll Cardiol. 2019;73(12):1494–563.
21. Kilner PJ, Geva T, Kaemmerer H, Trindade PT, Schwitter J, Webb GD. Recommendations for cardiovascular magnetic resonance in adults with congenital heart disease from the respective working groups of the European Society of Cardiology. Eur Heart J. 2010;31(7):794–805.
22. Cawley PJ, Maki JH, Otto CM. Cardiovascular magnetic resonance imaging for valvular heart disease. Technique and validation. Circulation. 2009;119(3):468–78.
23. Kamphuis VP, Westenberg JJM, van den Boogaard PJ, Clur S-AB, Roest AAW. Direct assessment of tricuspid regurgitation by 4D flow cardiovascular magnetic resonance in a patient with Ebstein's anomaly. Eur Heart J Cardiovasc Imaging. 2018;19(5):587–8.
24. Kuhn A, Meierhofer C, Rutz T, Rondak IC, Rohlig C, Schreiber C, et al. Non-volumetric echocardiographic indices and qualitative assessment of right ventricular systolic function in Ebstein's anomaly: comparison with CMR-derived ejection fraction in 49 patients. Eur Heart J Cardiovasc Imaging. 2016;17(8):930–5.
25. Liu X, Zhang Q, Yang ZG, Guo YK, Shi K, Xu HY, et al. Morphologic and functional abnormalities in patients with Ebstein's anomaly with cardiac magnetic resonance imaging: correlation with tricuspid regurgitation. Eur J Radiol. 2016;85(9):1601–6.
26. Alfakih K, Plein S, Bloomer T, Jones T, Ridgway J, Sivananthan M. Comparison of right ventricular volume measurements between axial and short axis orientation using steady-state free precession magnetic resonance imaging. J Magn Reson Imaging. 2003;18(1):25–32.
27. Yalonetsky S, Tobler D, Greutmann M, Crean AM, Wintersperger BJ, Nguyen ET, et al. Cardiac magnetic resonance imaging and the assessment of ebstein anomaly in adults. Am J Cardiol. 2011;107(5):767–73.
28. Tobler D, Yalonetsky S, Crean AM, Granton JT, Burchill L, Silversides CK, et al. Right heart characteristics and exercise parameters in adults with Ebstein anomaly: new perspectives from cardiac magnetic resonance imaging studies. Int J Cardiol. 2013;165(1):146–50.
29. Lee CM, Sheehan FH, Bouzas B, Chen SS, Gatzoulis MA, Kilner PJ. The shape and function of the right ventricle in Ebstein's anomaly. Int J Cardiol. 2013;167(3):704–10.
30. Fratz S, Janello C, Muller D, Seligmann M, Meierhofer C, Schuster T, et al. The functional right ventricle and tricuspid regurgitation in Ebstein's anomaly. Int J Cardiol. 2013;167(1):258–61.
31. Goleski PJ, Sheehan FH, Chen SS, Kilner PJ, Gatzoulis MA. The shape and function of the left ventricle in Ebstein's anomaly. Int J Cardiol. 2014;171(3):404–12.
32. Hosch O, Sohns JM, Nguyen TT, Lauerer P, Rosenberg C, Kowallick JT, et al. The total right/left-volume index: a new and simplified cardiac magnetic resonance measure to evaluate the severity of Ebstein anomaly of the tricuspid valve: a comparison with heart failure markers from various modalities. Circ Cardiovasc Imaging. 2014;7(4):601–9.

33. Liu X, Zhang Q, Yang ZG, Shi K, Xu HY, Xie LJ, et al. Assessment of left ventricular deformation in patients with Ebstein's anomaly by cardiac magnetic resonance tissue tracking. Eur J Radiol. 2017;89:20–6.
34. Benson LN, Child JS, Schwaiger M, Perloff JK, Schelbert HR. Left ventricular geometry and function in adults with Ebstein's anomaly of the tricuspid valve. Circulation. 1987;75(2):353–9.
35. Daliento L, Angelini A, Ho SY, Frescura C, Turrini P, Baratella MC, et al. Angiographic and morphologic features of the left ventricle in Ebstein's malformation. Am J Cardiol. 1997;80(8):1051–9.
36. Hurwitz RA. Left ventricular function in infants and children with symptomatic Ebstein's anomaly. Am J Cardiol. 1994;73(9):716–8.
37. Saxena A, Fong LV, Tristam M, Ackery DM, Keeton BR. Late noninvasive evaluation of cardiac performance in mildly symptomatic older patients with Ebstein's anomaly of tricuspid valve: role of radionuclide imaging. J Am Coll Cardiol. 1991;17(1):182–6.
38. Shiina A, Seward JB, Edwards WD, Hagler DJ, Tajik AJ. Two-dimensional echocardiographic spectrum of Ebstein's anomaly: detailed anatomic assessment. J Am Coll Cardiol. 1984;3(2, Part 1):356–70.
39. Yeo SY, Zhong L, Su Y, Tan RS, Ghista DN. A curvature-based approach for left ventricular shape analysis from cardiac magnetic resonance imaging. Med Biol Eng Comput. 2009;47(3):313–22.
40. Yang D, Li X, Sun J-Y, Cheng W, Greiser A, Zhang T-J, et al. Cardiovascular magnetic resonance evidence of myocardial fibrosis and its clinical significance in adolescent and adult patients with Ebstein's anomaly. J Cardiovasc Magn Reson. 2018;20(1):69.
41. Rydman R, Shiina Y, Diller GP, Niwa K, Li W, Uemura H, et al. Major adverse events and atrial tachycardia in Ebstein's anomaly predicted by cardiovascular magnetic resonance. Heart. 2018;104(1):37–44.
42. da Silva JP, Baumgratz JF, da Fonseca L, Franchi SM, Lopes LM, Tavares GM, et al. The cone reconstruction of the tricuspid valve in Ebstein's anomaly. The operation: early and midterm results. J Thorac Cardiovasc Surg. 2007;133(1):215–23.
43. Holst KA, Dearani JA, Said S, Pike RB, Connolly HM, Cannon BC, et al. Improving results of surgery for Ebstein anomaly: where are we after 235 cone repairs? Ann Thorac Surg. 2018;105(1):160–8.
44. Danielson GK, Maloney JD, Devloo RA. Surgical repair of Ebstein's anomaly. Mayo Clin Proc. 1979;54(3):185–92.
45. Dearani JA, Danielson GK. Tricuspid valve repair for Ebstein's anomaly. Oper Tech Thorac Cardiovasc Surg. 2003;8(4):188–92.
46. Ullmann MV, Born S, Sebening C, Gorenflo M, Ulmer HE, Hagl S. Ventricularization of the atrialized chamber: a concept of Ebstein's anomaly repair. Ann Thorac Surg. 2004;78(3):918–24; discussion 24-5.
47. Raju V, Dearani JA, Burkhart HM, Grogan M, Phillips SD, Ammash N, et al. Right ventricular unloading for heart failure related to Ebstein malformation. Ann Thorac Surg. 2014;98(1):167–73; discussion 73-4.
48. Dearani JA, Mora BN, Nelson TJ, Haile DT, O'Leary PW. Ebstein anomaly review: what's now, what's next? Expert Rev Cardiovasc Ther. 2015;13(10):1101–9.
49. Brown ML, Dearani JA, Danielson GK, Cetta F, Connolly HM, Warnes CA, et al. Comparison of the outcome of porcine bioprosthetic versus mechanical prosthetic replacement of the tricuspid valve in the Ebstein anomaly. Am J Cardiol. 2009;103(4):555–61.
50. Kiziltan HT, Theodoro DA, Warnes CA, O'Leary PW, Anderson BJ, Danielson GK. Late results of bioprosthetic tricuspid valve replacement in Ebstein's anomaly. Ann Thorac Surg. 1998;66(5):1539–45.
51. Egbe AC, Connolly HM, Pellikka PA, Schaff HV, Hanna R, Maleszewski JJ, et al. Outcomes of warfarin therapy for bioprosthetic valve thrombosis of surgically implanted valves: a prospective study. JACC Cardiovasc Interv. 2017;10(4):379–87.

52. Cullen MW, Cabalka AK, Alli OO, Pislaru SV, Sorajja P, Nkomo VT, et al. Transvenous, ante-grade melody valve-in-valve implantation for bioprosthetic mitral and tricuspid valve dysfunction: a case series in children and adults. JACC Cardiovasc Interv. 2013;6(6):598–605.
53. Brown ML, Dearani JA, Danielson GK, Cetta F, Connolly HM, Warnes CA, et al. The outcomes of operations for 539 patients with Ebstein anomaly. J Thorac Cardiovasc Surg. 2008;135(5):1120–36.e7.
54. Anderson HN, Dearani JA, Said SM, Norris MD, Pundi KN, Miller AR, et al. Cone reconstruction in children with Ebstein anomaly: the Mayo Clinic experience. Congenit Heart Dis. 2014;9(3):266–71.
55. Attenhofer Jost CH, Edmister WD, Julsrud PR, Dearani JA, Savas Tepe M, Warnes CA, et al. Prospective comparison of echocardiography versus cardiac magnetic resonance imaging in patients with Ebstein's anomaly. Int J Cardiovasc Imaging. 2012;28(5):1147–59.
56. Dearani JA, Said SM, O'Leary PW, Burkhart HM, Barnes RD, Cetta F. Anatomic repair of Ebstein's malformation: lessons learned with cone reconstruction. Ann Thorac Surg. 2013;95(1):220–6; discussion 6–8.
57. Chauvaud SM, Hernigou AC, Mousseaux ER, Sidi D, Hebert JL. Ventricular volumes in Ebstein's anomaly: x-ray multislice computed tomography before and after repair. Ann Thorac Surg. 2006;81(4):1443–9.
58. Tang X-J, Bao M, Zhao H, Wang L-Y, Wu Q-Y. Intraoperative transesophageal echocardiography in the operation of Ebstein's anomaly: a retrospective study. Chin Med J (Engl). 2017;130(13):1540–3.
59. van Noord PT, Scohy TV, McGhie J, Bogers AJ. Three-dimensional transesophageal echocardiography in Ebstein's anomaly. Interact Cardiovasc Thorac Surg. 2010;10(5):836–7.
60. Sujatha M, Gadhinglajkar S, Dharan BS, Sreedhar R. Role of intraoperative real-time three-dimensional transesophageal echocardiography during cone procedure for Ebstein's anomaly. J Cardiothorac Vasc Anesth. 2016;30(1):176–8.
61. Celermajer DS, Bull C, Till JA, Cullen S, Vassillikos VP, Sullivan ID, et al. Ebstein's anomaly: presentation and outcome from fetus to adult. J Am Coll Cardiol. 1994;23(1):170–6.
62. Geerdink LM, Delhaas T, Helbing WA, du Marchie Sarvaas GJ, Heide HT, Rozendaal L, et al. Paediatric Ebstein's anomaly: how clinical presentation predicts mortality. Arch Dis Child. 2018;103(9):859–63.
63. Veen KM, Mokhles MM, Roos-Hesselink JW, Rebel BR, Takkenberg JJM, Bogers A. Reconstructive surgery for Ebstein anomaly: three decades of experience. Eur J Cardiothorac Surg. 2019;56:385.
64. Hetzer R, Hacke P, Javier M, Miera O, Schmitt K, Weng Y, et al. The long-term impact of various techniques for tricuspid repair in Ebstein's anomaly. J Thorac Cardiovasc Surg. 2015;150(5):1212–9.
65. Attenhofer Jost CH, Tan NY, Hassan A, Vargas ER, Hodge DO, Dearani JA, et al. Sudden death in patients with Ebstein anomaly. Eur Heart J. 2018;39(21):1970–a.

Pulmonary Hypertension

20

Jorge Nuche and Carmen Jiménez López-Guarch

20.1 Introduction

Pulmonary hypertension (PH) is a syndrome characterized by elevated mean pulmonary artery (PA) pressure (≥ 25 mmHg). Depending on the elevation of pulmonary arterial wedge pressure it is defined as precapillary (≤ 15 mmHg) or postcapillary (>15 mmHg) PH [1, 2]. The pathological determinant of precapillary PH is the presence of pulmonary vascular remodelling leading to the proliferation of vascular wall cells and progressive obliteration of pulmonary arterioles. This determines an increase in pulmonary vascular resistance ([mean PA pressure—pulmonary arterial wedge pressure]/cardiac output, Woods Units). Thus, the complete definition of precapillary PH include:

- Mean pulmonary artery pressure ≥ 25 mmHg
- Pulmonary arterial wedge pressure ≤ 15 mmHg
- Pulmonary vascular resistance ≥ 3 Woods Units

J. Nuche
Cardiology Department, Hospital Universitario 12 de Octubre, Instituto de Investigación Sanitaria Hospital 12 de Octubre (imas12), Madrid, Spain

CIBER de enfermedades CardioVasculares (CIBERCV), Madrid, Spain

Centro Nacional de Investigaciones Cardiovasculares, Madrid, Spain
e-mail: jorge.nuche@salud.madrid.org

C. Jiménez López-Guarch (✉)
Cardiology Department, Hospital Universitario 12 de Octubre, Instituto de Investigación Sanitaria Hospital 12 de Octubre (imas12), Madrid, Spain

CIBER de enfermedades CardioVasculares (CIBERCV), Madrid, Spain

School of Medicine, Universidad Complutense de Madrid, Madrid, Spain
e-mail: cjimenez@salud.madrid.org

Table 20.1 Pulmonary
hypertension classification

1. PAH
1.1 Idiopathic PAH
1.2 Heritable PAH
1.3 Drug- and toxin-induced PAH
1.4 PAH associated with:
1.4.1 Connective tissue disease
1.4.2 HIV infection
1.4.3 Portal hypertension
1.4.4 Congenital heart disease
1.4.5 Schistosomiasis
1.5 PAH long-term responders to calcium channel blockers
1.6 PAH with overt features of venous or capillaries involvement (PVOD/PCH)
1.7 Persistent PH of the newborn syndrome
2. PH due to left heart disease
3. PH due to lung disease or hypoxia
4. PH due to pulmonary artery obstructions
5. PH with unclear or multifactorial mechanisms
5.1 Hematological disorders
5.2 Systemic and metabolic disorders
5.3 Complex congenital heart disease
5.4 Others

Adapted from [1]
PAH pulmonary arterial hypertension, *PVOD* pulmonary veno-occlusive disease, *PCH* pulmonary capillary hemangiomatosis

PH is classified into 5 groups according to its etiology [1] (Table 20.1). Group 1, or pulmonary arterial hypertension (PAH), includes several diseases with different pathophysiology but with similar histologic findings that determine the development of precapillary PH. The number of patients with congenital heart disease (CHD) who develop PH is unknown. This lack of knowledge is, at least in part, a consequence of the heterogeneous presentation of this syndrome in patients with CHD [2]:

- Eisenmenger's syndrome
- PAH associated with prevalent systemic-to-pulmonary shunts (correctable or non-correctable)
- PAH with small/coincidental defects
- PAH after defect correction

Besides these four groups, patients with complex CHD can also develop PH (group 5).

Improved survival of children born with CHD is leading to a growing prevalence of PH related to CHD. Advances in noninvasive techniques allowing an adequate evaluation of these patients is therefore mandatory. The use of most promising imaging techniques is still limited to research purposes. Further studies showing a benefit in the use of these techniques are necessary to implement its use in daily practice.

Some clinical and physiopathological concepts are important to address in order to achieve better comprehension of the different imaging techniques.

20.1.1 The Cardiopulmonary Unit

Right ventricular failure is the final determinant of PH patient's morbidity and prognosis. This ventricular failure is caused by an increased afterload secondary to pulmonary vascular remodelling. For this reason, the study of the cardiopulmonary unit, the interaction between the right ventricle (RV) and the pulmonary vasculature is of great interest. The concept of *coupling* describes the adaptation of the RV to a progressive increase in pulmonary vascular resistance (PVR) so the energy transfer is more efficient. It is determined by PA systolic elastance (Ea) and right ventricular end-systolic elastance (Ees), (coupling = Ees/Ea) and it is altered when there is a *maladaptive* right ventricular remodelling to the increased afterload [3]. Figure 20.1 summarizes the normal function of the cardiopulmonary system.

The current evaluation of the cardiopulmonary unit includes both invasive (right heart catheterization) and noninvasive (echocardiography and magnetic resonance [MR]) techniques. Measurements obtained from pressure–volume loops are not commonly used in clinical practice due to its technical complexity. A complete evaluation can be performed with a noninvasive approach [4]:

- $Ea = \dfrac{\text{Arterial end-systolic pressure}\left(ESP\right)}{\text{Stroke volume }\left(SV\right)} \approx \dfrac{mPAP}{SV}$

- $Ees = \dfrac{ESP}{\text{end-systolic volume }\left(ESV\right)} \approx \dfrac{mPAP}{ESV}$

- $RV - PA\ coupling = \dfrac{Ea}{Ees} \approx \dfrac{ESV}{SV}$

$*ESP = \text{mean PA pressure}(mPAP) - \text{PA wedge pressure} \approx mPAP$

Recently, a novel and simple echocardiographic parameter, the ratio of the tricuspid annulus plane systolic excursion (TAPSE)/systolic pulmonary artery pressure (sPAP) has shown a good correlation with invasive measurements of VA coupling (E/Ea) in patients with PAH [5]. There is a growing evidence and interest in these measurements as surrogates of RV/PA performance in patients with PH of different etiologies, and some studies have shown their ability to predict prognosis [6]. However, there is still a lack of evidence allowing specific recommendations for the use of these techniques in clinical practice [3].

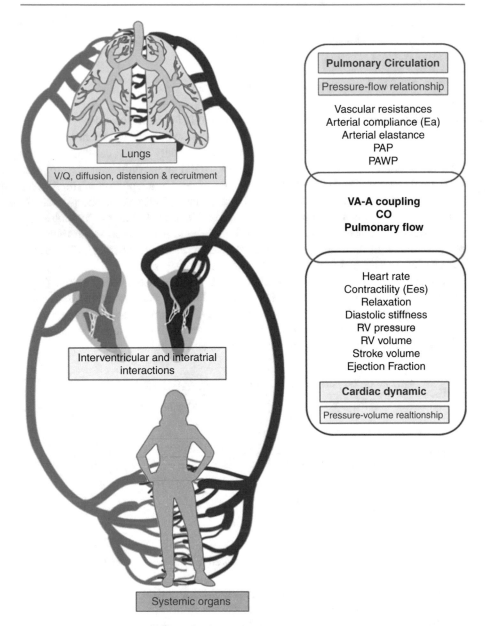

Fig. 20.1 The cardiopulmonary unit. *CO* cardiac output, *PAP* pulmonary artery pressure, *PAWP* pulmonary artery wedge pressure, *RV* right ventricle, *V-A* ventricular-arterial, *V/Q* ventilation/perfusion matching

20.1.2 PH Diagnosis

Recent registries have shown that PAH is still being diagnosed in advanced stages. The most commonly used noninvasive diagnostic tools in PH usually provide a late diagnosis, when the final consequences of the disease have already occurred (i.e., increased PA pressure and RV dysfunction) and patients are at a poor functional status. However, besides lung biopsy, there are no specific techniques allowing for an accurate diagnosis of early or even late pulmonary vascular remodelling which is the ultimate cause of the disease. In CHD patients, an imaging-based diagnosis of pulmonary vascular remodelling could help to identify those patients with uncorrected defects who are at risk of developing PH and could be candidates for surgical or percutaneous correction. Furthermore, it could help to early identify patients with corrected defects who will develop PH despite an appropriate defect closure.

20.1.3 Treatment Monitoring

Current PH guidelines recommend a prognostic assessment to guide treatment with the goal of achieving or maintaining a low-risk profile [7]. This evaluation includes clinical, analytical, functional, echocardiographic and hemodynamic variables. These scores have demonstrated to be an appropriate tool for predicting long-term survival in PH. However, the response to current or future treatments in terms of pulmonary vascular remodelling reduction or ventricular-arterial coupling improvement cannot be evaluated with currently available diagnostic techniques.

20.1.4 Prognostic Assessment

As heart failure is still the first cause of mortality among PH patients, the above-cited risk scores focus on variables able to predict clinical deterioration as a consequence of irreversible right ventricular failure. However, up to 20% of PH patients suffer sudden cardiac death during follow-up. Most commonly used prognostic scores are unable to identify patients at a higher risk of sudden cardiac death. PA dilatation has shown to be an independent risk factor for sudden cardiac death among PH patients [8]. This increased risk for sudden cardiac death could be explained by the development of potentially fatal complications in patients with a dilated PA such as left main coronary artery compression [9] or PA dissection [10]. Novel imaging techniques could help to diagnose these complications or to early identify patients at risk of developing them.

20.2   Imaging Techniques in Pulmonary Hypertension

In past years, a growing interest in the study of pulmonary vascular remodelling and the cardiopulmonary unit has led to a huge development in basic and clinical research. Advances in imaging techniques have accompanied this scientific development and appear as potential tools for diagnosis, treatment effectiveness monitoring, and prognostic assessment in PH patients. These novelties in imaging techniques have been developed for different forms of PH. Histological and clinical similarities of CHD-related PAH with other etiologic forms allow the implementation of these techniques in CHD patients.

20.2.1 Echocardiography

20.2.1.1   Three-Dimensional (3D) Echocardiography

The use of 3D echocardiography is widely extended in CHD both in children and adults due to its good spatial resolution, allowing an appropriate evaluation of the RV anatomy and function, both in uncorrected and corrected congenital defects, and live guidance during interventional procedures [11]. Its main limitation is the dependence on image quality, especially the identification of the endocardial surface of the anterior wall in patients with large RVs and previous sternotomy.

Although MRI is the gold-standard technique for the evaluation of RV volumes and function, 3D echocardiography offers some advantages in daily clinical practice: it is widely available, less expensive than MRI, portable, and its use is not hampered by the presence of prosthetic material or implantable cardiac devices [11]. Normal volumetric parameters assessed with 3D echocardiography in healthy children and teenagers have been defined in a large multicenter study and compared with MRI [12]. Normal values for RV volume and function are provided in Table 20.2. RV specific 3D echocardiography image reconstruction software has provided new insights into RV remodelling associated with progressive disease states. Furthermore, machine-learning-based quantification of volumes and ejection fraction has shown to be a promising time-saving tool to properly evaluate right ventricular function [13], and is already provided by different echocardiography vendors (Fig. 20.2).

Table 20.2 Standardized right ventricular volumetric assessment with 3D-echocardiography

	<7 years		7–18 years		Adults	
	Female	Male	Female	Male	Female	Male
RVEDV (mL/m²)	64.9 ± 11.3	64.0 ± 14.0	62.8 ± 7.9	81.7 ± 13.2	50 ± 11	59 ± 15
RVESV (mL/m²)	25.2 ± 4.8	24.8 ± 5.6	24.5 ± 3.5	30.8 ± 4.7	19 ± 7	24 ± 9
RVSV (mL/m²)	39.8 ± 6.7	39.2 ± 8.5	38.3 ± 4.8	51.0 ± 9.1	NA	NA

Adapted from [12, 67]

RVEDV right ventricular end-diastolic volume, *RVESD* right ventricular end-systolic volume, *RVSV* right ventricular stroke volume. Data are expressed as mean ± standard

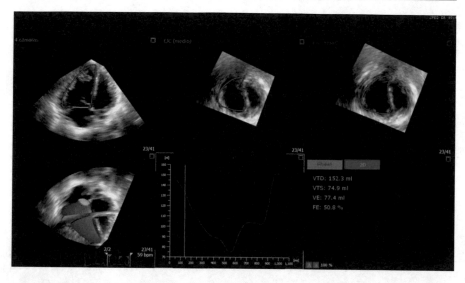

Fig. 20.2 Right ventricle automatic 3D volume measurements [Tomtec© (Philips)] in a patient with pulmonary arterial hypertension. Note the RV remodeling, with interventricular septal deviation. Volumes are obtained from multiple slices, tracking the endocardial border in both systole and diastole

Based on the good correlation in RV volumetric assessment with MRI, 3D echocardiogram also offers an accurate evaluation of right ventricle–pulmonary artery coupling despite an overestimation of elastance parameters [14].

Regarding pulmonary vasculature, 3D echocardiography also offers a good alternative to computed tomography scan and MRI for an accurate measure of PA dimensions [15].

Volumetric changes in RV and right atrium have shown to be an adequate tool to predict clinical deterioration with a higher specificity of right atrium sphericity index [16].

20.2.1.2 Deformation: Speckle Tracking Strain

Right ventricular dysfunction is the major independent prognostic predictor in PAH patients. However, RV failure is usually a late manifestation of the disease. Early diagnosis of right ventricular maladaptation to elevated afterload is therefore desirable.

Strain quantifies the change in myocardial deformation measured as a percentage from the original form, whereas strain rate measures deformation rate over time. Myocardial fiber deformation can be measured in longitudinal, radial, or circumferential planes, representing myocardial shortening, thickening and lengthening in the three dimensions in space. Two-dimensional strain measured using speckle tracking echocardiography (STE) has emerged as a sensitive and reproducible imaging technique for characterizing regional mechanical dysfunction (Fig. 20.3).

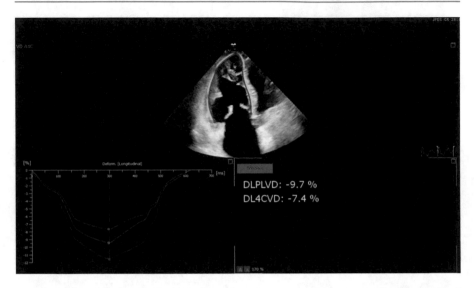

DLPLVD: -9.7 %
DL4CVD: -7.4 %

Fig. 20.3 RV automatic longitudinal strain in a patient with pulmonary hypertension. Modified apical 4 chamber view. Global longitudinal strain is automatically measured, as the mean of the three segments of the lateral RV free wall (DLPLVD). Each curve accounts for an individual segment

In patients with PAH of different etiology, including PAH-CHD, all strain and strain rate parameters are reduced when compared to healthy controls. Interestingly, global 2D longitudinal strain is also reduced in PAH patients with normal RV function assessed by volumetric parameters, such as RVEF, arising as an early marker of systolic impairment [17]. Furthermore, not only right ventricular strain magnitude provides essential information, but temporal patterns, such as the presence of post-systolic maximal strain, add prognostic information in PH patients [18]. RV deformation occurs in all three dimensions in space; therefore, a more appropriate approach should include the three axes to avoid underestimation of the true extent of deformation. Some novel 3D strain quantification techniques, such as principal strain or area strain, which include the magnitude of deformation and the direction angle, have been proposed to overcome the 2D limitations. These 3D strain parameters, have been found useful in patients with PAH [19, 20]. Whether 3D-derived strain may have an added value in the routine assessment of RV remains unclear, given the fact that only small populations have been investigated to date and normal values are yet to be established.

There is also growing interest in the assessment of RA function, and RA strain provides a physiopathological approach to the reservoir, conduit and contraction function of the RA. Two-dimensional STE has been shown to be feasible for investigating RA function.

20.2.2 Single-Photon Emission Computed Tomography (SPECT)

Novel applications of this well-known technique could help to early identify PH in CHD patients and also to evaluate the effectiveness of specific therapies.

20.2.2.1 Myocardial Perfusion

The use of myocardial perfusion imaging by SPECT has been an essential tool in the evaluation of left ventricular function and the assessment of myocardial ischemia. In PH patients, due to RV hypertrophy, SPECT might be a feasible technique to evaluate RV function and perfusion. Furthermore, in preclinical studies in a rodent model of monocrotaline-induced PH, SPECT has shown to be useful to evaluate morphological changes and variation in cardiac apoptosis reduction after resveratrol administration [21].

Recent investigations indicate that ^{99}Tc-MIBI SPECT is able to distinguish between mild and moderate to severe PH with sensitivity and specificity 86.7% and 100% respectively for a myocardial perfusion imaging target/background ratio of 1.855 [22].

20.2.2.2 Lung Perfusion

Current PH guidelines recommend ventilation/perfusion scan in the initial evaluation of patients to screen for chronic thromboembolic PH [2]. Since not all patients with abnormal ventilation/perfusion findings have thromboembolic disease, the use of SPECT offers a more accurate evaluation of lung perfusion with differentiation of thromboembolic disease, lung disorders, and veno-occlusive disease [23].

In patients with PAH, a high incidence (43.1%) of positive ventilation/perfusion SPECT scan has been documented. Furthermore, patients with global perfusion defects seem to have more severe forms of PAH with worse hemodynamic profile and higher mortality rates. On the contrary, in patients with focal and patchy perfusion defects survival and PAH severity did not differ from those with normal ventilation/perfusion SPECT scan [23]. Based on these results, the inclusion of SPECT scan in CHD patients follow-up may offer an early diagnosis of pulmonary vascular development (CHD patients with patchy and focal perfusion defects) and help to identify those patients with a higher risk (global perfusion defects). This information could be used to guide management of CHD patients allowing a prompt indication of reparative procedures or the initiation of pulmonary vasodilator therapy before right ventricular dysfunction appears.

Novel molecular SPECT imaging agent, ^{99m}Tc-Pulmobind, binds the vascular endothelium through adrenomedullin receptors which are densely expressed on the endothelial surface of alveolar capillaries. ^{99m}Tc-Pulmobind has been tested in phase 1 and phase 2 human studies [24, 25]. In PH patients, a heterogeneous distribution of the tracer was found, with zones where there was no uptake. In a murine model of PAH (mice treated with SUHx and exposed to hypoxic environment), ^{99m}Tc-Pulmobind pulmonary uptake was reduced when compared to healthy animals

Fig. 20.4 Lung vascular imaging with ⁹⁹mTc-PulmoBind. Example of whole body planar imaging of a sham rat and PAH rat 5 min after tail vein injection in a 5 min acquisition with reduced uptake in the PAH-mice. (Image obtained from [26] with the permission of the copyright holder. Published under a CC BY 4.0 license)

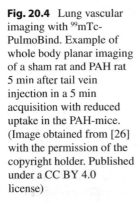
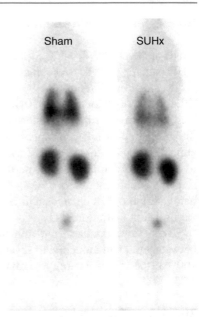

(Fig. 20.4). However, these changes in ⁹⁹ᵐTc-Pulmobind uptake were not reversed by sildenafil administration [26]. Nevertheless, the use of this novel agent could be useful in the evaluation and monitoring of future PAH therapies targeting pulmonary vascular reverse remodelling.

20.2.3 Dual Energy Computed Tomography (DECT)

DECT or spectral computed tomography involves imaging acquisition at two energy levels. Conventional computed tomography relies only on densities whereas DECT relies on the atomic number (low energy levels) and on tissue density (high energy levels) allowing a better differentiation of tissues and materials. DECT technology is based on the 90° disposition of two X-ray tubes (dual-source), in the rapid KVp switching for each X-ray single tube position or in the presence of two layers in the X-ray detectors, one for each energy level [27].

DECT-iodine maps, obtained through the calculation of the iodine concentration in each voxel, allow the evaluation of lung perfusion with a good correlation with ventilation/perfusion scan and SPECT [28, 29]. This technique is especially useful in the evaluation of patients with acute pulmonary embolism and chronic thromboembolic disease. Nevertheless, DECT-iodine maps might also be useful for the diagnosis and prognostic stratification in PAH.

In PAH patients, small, patchy and poorly defined perfusion defects have been described as in the SPECT scan [30]. These defects are different than those described in chronic thromboembolic PH where segmental and well-defined defects are seen [31]. (Fig. 20.5).

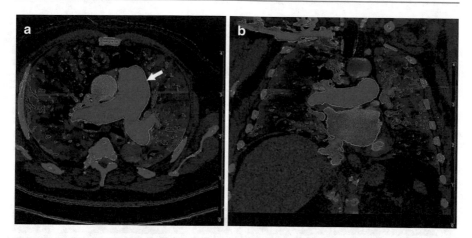

Fig. 20.5 Dual CT in pulmonary hypertension. (**a**) Axial CT perfusion image shows extensive heterogeneous and mottled perfusion (blue color) in a patient with idiopathic pulmonary arterial hypertension. Note that the main pulmonary artery (arrow) is severely dilated, measuring 4.2 cm. (**b**) Coronal CT perfusion image in the same patient shows heterogeneous perfusion with extensive areas of low perfusion (blue color). (Reprinted by permission from Springer Nature: Int J Cardiovasc Imaging; 35(8):1509–1524. State of the art: utility of multi-energy CT in the evaluation of pulmonary vasculature. Rajiah P, et al. © 2019)

In addition, DECT perfusion quantification seems to have an adequate correlation with PAH severity with a good correlation of the perfusion index with pulmonary vascular resistance, PA pressure, and right atrial pressure [32].

DECT perfusion maps can be used to evaluate left ventricular ischemia. In the same way, DECT could be used to evaluate right ventricular ischemia. However, as in the SPECT scan, the thin right ventricular wall complicates the implementation of this technique to evaluate ischemia in this scenario [33].

20.2.4 Magnetic Resonance Imaging (MRI)

MRI is a widely extended imaging technique in CHD patients and in PH patients. It offers an excellent spatial resolution of the right ventricle, evaluation of blood flow, tissue characterization, and dynamic afterload parameters.

The technical development of MRI advances constantly with the appearance of new sequences and techniques which offer new applications for the diagnosis and evaluation of PH patients. These new applications allow a better evaluation of the cardiopulmonary unit with an exhaustive assessment of cardiac function and pulmonary flow. In addition, the application of MRI maps provides useful information on the histological changes of the right ventricle (edema and extracellular volume).

20.2.4.1 Myocardial Deformation (Strain)
MRI is the gold standard for the evaluation of right ventricular global function [17], and can provide precise volumetric measurements, as well as regional and global

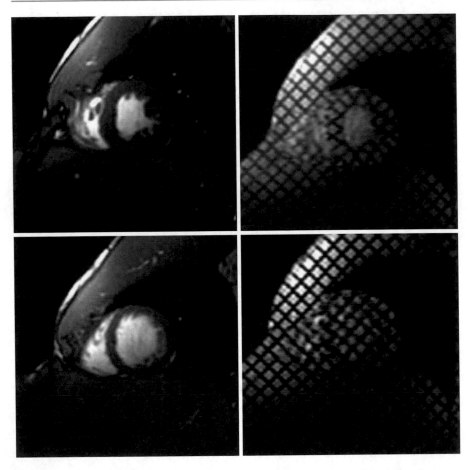

Fig. 20.6 MRI ventricular strain. Short-axis view in systole (upper images) and diastole (lower images). By modulating the magnetization gradient, the signal from the myocardium can be nulled in a grid pattern (right images) prior to the onset of image acquisition. (Images courtesy of Dr. A. Ciccone—Hospital Universitario de La Princesa, Madrid)

systolic indexes, such as myocardial deformation (strain), previously described in this chapter. Different MRI sequences, such as tagging (Fig. 20.6) or feature tracking (tissue tracking technique) (Fig. 20.7), can provide an accurate quantitative measure for deformation.

Right atrial and ventricular strain obtained by different MRI sequences have been evaluated in PAH patients, including PAH-CHD, and in patients with different non-PH CHD, such as tetralogy of Fallot or systemic right ventricles. RV strain correlates with systolic function and afterload and provides a prognostic assessment [17, 34, 35]. RV strain also presents a significant correlation with diastolic stiffness and RV-arterial uncoupling being a promising technique for noninvasive evaluation of dynamic afterload [36].

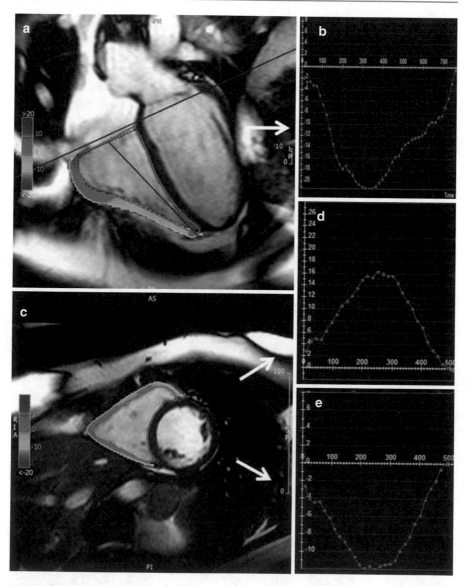

Fig. 20.7 Example of colored strain analysis with a feature-tracking software (Circle CVI42®) for the calculation of RV myocardial strain. (**a**) Four-chamber SSFP cine image, used to derive the RV longitudinal strain curve (**b**). (**c**) Short-axis SSFP cine image allows for the calculation of radial (**d**) and circumferential (**e**) RV strain curves. (Reprinted by permission from Springer Nature: Heart Fail Rev; 22:465–476. Strain imaging using cardiac magnetic resonance. Scatteia A, et al. © 2017)

Regarding PAH prognosis, abnormal RV strain has shown to be an independent predictor of poorer outcomes (death, lung transplant or worsening functional class) among PAH patients [17]. Right atrial function assessed by rapid semiautomated strain, a novel post-processing tool, is a feasible technique that may be able to identify subclinical RV failure, quantifying passive strain which corresponds to atrial conduit function [37].

20.2.4.2 Lung Perfusion

Currently, the evaluation of the pulmonary vasculature relies mostly on the use of CT and SPECT. However, the advances in MRI allow a proper evaluation of pulmonary vessels and lung perfusion [38]. Depending on the indications, contrast and non-contrast sequences may be employed. However, in this chapter, we will focus on contrast-enhanced sequences because of the limitations of non-contrast acquisition in the field of PAH [38].

Contrast-enhanced perfusion sequences are obtained using a single dose of gadolinium at a high injection rate [38] and analyze the first-pass of the contrast through the pulmonary vessels. The obtained images allow a description of the perfusion defects which, as for other perfusion techniques, are especially useful in the diagnosis of pulmonary embolism or chronic thromboembolic pulmonary hypertension [38]. Nevertheless, differences in perfusion defects assessed by MRI between CTEPH patients and PAH patients have also been described. As in SPECT and CT scan, patients with pulmonary thromboembolic disease present wedge-shaped focal defects whereas PAH patients present a diffuse reduction in perfusion [39] (Fig. 20.8).

This contrast-enhanced sequence allows the quantification of pulmonary blood flow (PBF), pulmonary blood volume (PBV), mean transit time (MTT) (calculated as PBV/PBF) and time to peak intensity. Besides its multiple applications in the

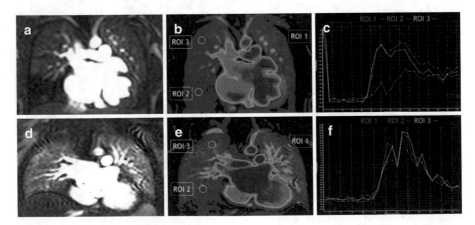

Fig. 20.8 Perfusion sequences in two patients with postcapillary pulmonary hypertension. (**a, d**): dynamic images at the maximum contrast uptake in the pulmonary tissue; (**b, e**): Parametric map representing the Area Under de Curve (AUC) resulting from the integration of the dynamic contrast curves for each pixel and it is related to the total amount of contrast that reach each image pixel. (**c, f**): Signal intensity curves representing the dynamic signal changes derived from contrast uptake at different regions in the lung parenchyma showing the lack of perfusion in the lower lung lobe of patient 2 (**d–f**). (Courtesy of J. F. Delgado (University Hospital 12 de Octubre, Spain) and J. Sánchez-González (Philips Healthcare Madrid, Spain))

field of thromboembolic disease, these parameters have demonstrated to be useful in the evaluation of PAH severity and prognosis [38]. MTT is increased in PAH patients and shows a good correlation with mean PA pressure [40]. Pulmonary transit time (PTT), calculated as the time difference between the peak signal at the pulmonary artery and the peak signal at the left atrium, has also demonstrated a significant correlation with right atrial pressure and pulmonary vascular resistance [41]. Furthermore, PTT is predictive of mortality with a good correlation with cardiac index [42].

20.2.4.3 4D-Flow

Four-dimensional phase-contrast MRI flow (4D flow MRI) consists of a volumetric time-resolved acquisition that is gated to the cardiac cycle, providing a time-varying vector field of blood flow as well as registered anatomic images. Three-directional velocity encoding enables a more accurate analysis of 3D-flow phenomena and allows the computation of secondary flow parameters like wall stress and pressure maps [43] (Fig. 20.9). In patients with PAH, a vortical flow (i.e., rotating or swirling motion occurs in the flow field with streamlines like concentric circles) in the main PA has been observed, and the duration of such vortices is positively correlated with pulmonary pressures [44]. Furthermore, when a multivariate model including vorticity, relative area change of the pulmonary artery and cardiac output was applied, an excellent correlation with pulmonary vascular resistance was obtained [45]. Moreover, different vortex patterns have been described depending on the disease severity, so that diastolic vorticity may be an indicator of mild PAH whereas systolic vorticity was found in severe PAH [44]. This technique offers special advantages in the evaluation of different CHD, allowing an excellent characterization of flows (Qp/Qs, flow direction) in simple or complex congenital heart defects, using new visualization tools such as streamlines and velocity vectors (Figs. 20.10 and 20.11).

Fig. 20.9 4D flow of the pulmonary artery in PH. Streamlines are instantaneously tangent to the velocity vector field and are useful to visualize 3D velocity fields at discrete time points

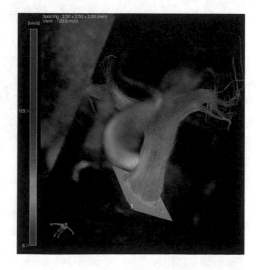

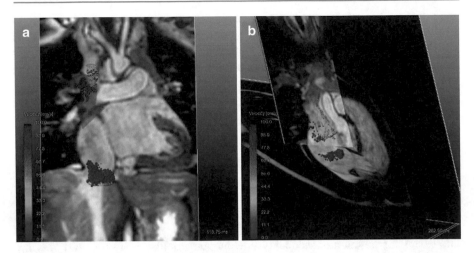

Fig. 20.10 4D flow MRI—Particle traces. Partial anomalous pulmonary venous return from the right upper pulmonary veins (red) draining into the SVC (light blue). Both flows joining together into the RA with the blood flow from the IVC (blue particles). (Images courtesy of Dr. Israel Valverde-Virgen del Rocio Hospital, Seville, Spain)

Fig. 20.11 MRI—4D flow of a sinus venous ASD. Blood flow from the left pulmonary veins (pink particles) crossing from the left atrium to the right atrium across the sinus venous ASD. (Image courtesy of Dr. Israel Valverde-Virgen del Rocio Hospital, Seville, Spain)

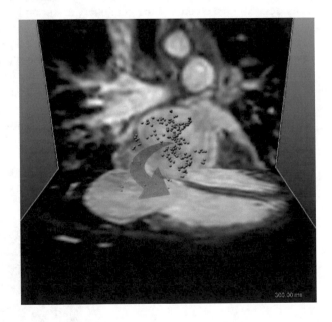

Furthermore, 4D-flow has proven to be a useful tool for the evaluation of complex CHD such as Fontan circulation or tetralogy of Fallot [46].

In PAH patients, PA stiffness is increased as a consequence of collagen accumulation or elastin loss [43]. Wall shear stress, the stress applied tangentially to the vessel wall, reflects the effect of flow changes on endothelial cells and extracellular matrix function [46], and is reduced in patients with PAH, as a consequence of the pulmonary arterial bed involvement [47]. Pulmonary artery 4D-flow characterization could help to better understand the RV-PA unit, and how such altered interaction could lead to an RV maladaptive response, and finally, systolic dysfunction [43]. It could also help to identify areas at risk of rupture in PA aneurysms [46]. Although the clinical utility of 4D flow MRI in PH is yet to be established, these techniques advance the understanding of complex pathophysiological changes occurring in the course of the disease and could help to monitor the response to therapy.

Another parameter that could be of interest in patients with PAH is pulse wave velocity (PWV), defined as the travel-time of the flow waves between two specific locations separated by a known distance. PWV was found to be higher in arteries with increased stiffness and reduced caliber [48].

Pulmonary regurgitation quantification is of paramount importance not only in CHD-PAH patients, but in other prevalent CHD such as repaired tetralogy of Fallot. 4D-flow offers a more accurate quantification of pulmonary regurgitation allowing avoidance of vertical flow [46].

20.2.4.4 T1-Mapping

Myocardial T1 relaxation time mapping is a relatively novel technique for tissue characterization offering a good evaluation of myocardial fibrosis [49] with the advantage of no needing contrast media agents use (Fig. 20.12). Several preclinical

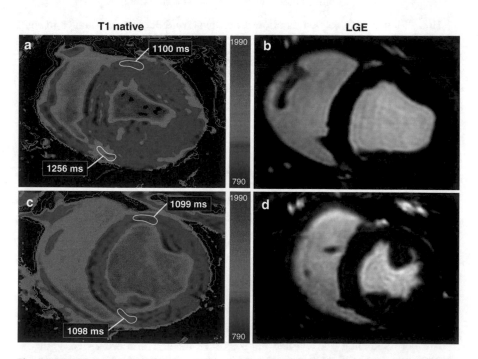

Fig. 20.12 Precontrast T1 mapping and late gadolinium enhancement in a swine with postcapillary pulmonary hypertension (**a**, **b**) and in a control swine (**c**, **d**). Figure **a** shows increased T1 recovery time in the inferior septal insertion appearing prior to extensive late gadolinium enhancement development (**b**). (Courtesy of A. García-Álvarez and I. García-Lunar (CNIC, Spain))

and clinical studies have demonstrated increased T1 times in anterior and posterior septal insertion points in both animal models of PH [50] and in PAH patients [49]. Although the results described in different studies are heterogeneous, these changes in T1 relaxation times have demonstrated a correlation with different markers of severity of the disease [49–52]. Furthermore, a recent study in patients with heart failure with preserved ejection fraction T1 relaxation times showed good correlation with PA hemodynamic parameters and increased T1 times in the anterior septal insertion were independently related to worse survival [53].

T1-mapping sequences also allow the quantification of extracellular volume which increase has shown to precede right ventricular dysfunction in a swine model of postcapillary pulmonary hypertension [50]. The calculation of extracellular volume requires the administration of gadolinium contrast media to quantify T1 relaxation times in the myocardium and blood sample before and after contrast administration [54]:

$$ECV = \left(1 - \text{hematocrit}\right) \times \frac{\left(\dfrac{1}{\text{T1 myocardial post-contrast}}\right) - \left(\dfrac{1}{\text{T1 myocardial pre-contrast}}\right)}{\left(\dfrac{1}{\text{T1 blood post-contrast}}\right) - \left(\dfrac{1}{\text{T1 blood pre-contrast}}\right)}$$

Thus, T1-mapping sequences allow a noninvasive detection of changes in right ventricular histologic composition which could help to identify those patients at higher risk of developing right ventricular failure. Extracellular volume values are increased before overt RV failure occurs and could be useful to early detect myocardial involvement in patients with increased chronic RV afterload. Whether changes in T1 relaxation times can be useful to evaluate response to therapies is still under investigation.

20.2.5 Positron-Emission Tomography

Recent investigations have demonstrated a metabolic disturbance in PAH similar to that found in cancer patients. This metabolic alteration, known as the Warburg effect or glycolytic shift, is determined by a shift in the metabolic pathway in pulmonary endothelial and smooth muscle cells toward anaerobic glycolysis instead of oxidative phosphorylation. This glycolytic shift leads to an increased concentration of lactate and a reduced concentration of radical oxygen species which confers a protective environment against apoptosis allowing a progressive proliferation of pulmonary vessel cells similar to that observed in neoplastic cells [55]. It appears as a promising new therapeutic target for PAH patients [56].

An increased lung and cardiac uptake of 18-labeled 2-fluoro-2-deoxyglucose ([18]FDG) assessed with positron-emission tomography (PET) has been observed in animal models of monocrotaline-induced PAH and patients with PAH or PH secondary to respiratory disease [57, 58]. In PH secondary to end-stage pulmonary disease a positive linear correlation of [18]FDG uptake in lung parenchyma and hemodynamic severity was found [58]. This positive correlation has also been observed with right ventricular [18]FDG uptake in PAH and CTPEH [59]. In monocrotaline-induced PAH, the administration of imatinib and dichloroacetate reduced pulmonary vascular remodelling. This effect was accompanied by a decreased [18]FDG uptake analyzed with PET [60].

Thus, evaluation of [18]FDG uptake with PET appears as an attractive tool to early diagnose the development of pulmonary vascular adverse remodelling in CHD patients, and could also be useful to monitor the response to specific PAH treatment. However, the employment of [18]FDG as a marker has several limitations due to the lack of specificity of an increased uptake, which could be secondary both to a gly-colytic shift in pulmonary wall cells and increased inflammatory activity [56]. The use of alternative markers such as 3'-deoxy-3'-[18F]-fluorothymidine ([18]FLT), which offer a better correlation with cellular proliferation, may allow an adequate differentiation between proliferation and inflammatory response [61].

20.2.6 Optical Coherence Tomography

The use of intravascular imaging techniques such as intravascular ultrasound and optical coherence tomography (OCT) is widely extended in the evaluation and treatment of coronary artery diseases. OCT offers a great spatial resolution (10 μm) which allows an accurate measure of vessel diameters and wall thickness.

In recent years, OCT has been used for the evaluation of pulmonary vasculature although available information is limited to small series [62]. Interestingly, OCT allows precise measurement of the intimal thickness and could identify pulmonary vascular remodelling [63, 64] (Fig. 20.13). Furthermore, intimal thickness has shown to have a positive correlation with hemodynamic parameters in PAH from different etiologies including CHD [63, 65]. Although a reduction of intimal thickness parallel to hemodynamic improvement after treatment optimization has been described in patients with PH, its usefulness as a marker of therapeutic response is still unknown [66].

20.3 Conclusions

Multimodality noninvasive imaging techniques play an important role in diagnosis, etiologic characterization, prognostic evaluation, and follow-up of patients with PH, and particularly in those patients with PAH-CHD. Novel new techniques and applications such as 3D echocardiography, deformation, tissue and metabolic characterization, flow pattern or lung and myocardial perfusion are already available and constantly developing so they may help to provide new insights into pathophysiological processes of the right heart-pulmonary circulation unit. Although imaging techniques have great potential, further investigation is still necessary to improve clinical practice and prognosis, allowing early disease detection, assessing the severity, and guiding response to therapy.

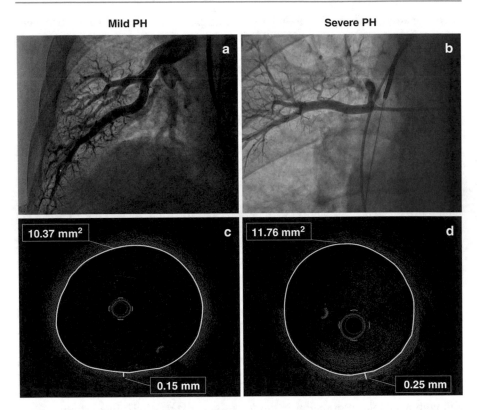

Fig. 20.13 Pulmonary angiography and simultaneous optic coherence tomography in patients with mild (**a**, **c**) and severe (**b**, **d**) pulmonary hypertension showing a wider intimal thickness in the patient with severe PH. (Courtesy of L. García-Cosío and F. Sarnago (University Hospital 12 de Octubre, Spain))

References

1. Simonneau G, Montani D, Celermajer DS, Denton CP, Gatzoulis MA, Krowka M, et al. Haemodynamic definitions and updated clinical classification of pulmonary hypertension. Eur Respir J. 2019;53(1):1801913.
2. Galiè N, Humbert M, Vachiery JL, Gibbs S, Lang I, Torbicki A, et al. 2015 ESC/ERS guidelines for the diagnosis and treatment of pulmonary hypertension: the joint task force for the diagnosis and treatment of pulmonary hypertension of the European Society of Cardiology (ESC) and the European Respiratory Society (ERS): endorsed by: Association for European Paediatric and Congenital Cardiology (AEPC), International Society for Heart and Lung Transplantation (ISHLT). Eur Heart J. 2016;37(1):67–119.
3. Vonk Noordegraaf A, Chin KM, Haddad F, Hassoun PM, Hemnes AR, Hopkins SR, et al. Pathophysiology of the right ventricle and of the pulmonary circulation in pulmonary hypertension: an update. Eur Respir J. 2019;53(1):1801900.
4. Sanz J, García-Alvarez A, Fernández-Friera L, Nair A, Mirelis JG, Sawit ST, et al. Right ventriculo-arterial coupling in pulmonary hypertension: a magnetic resonance study. Heart. 2012;98(3):238–43.

5. Richter MJ, Peters D, Ghofrani HA, Naeije R, Roller F, Sommer N, et al. Evaluation and prognostic relevance of right ventricular-arterial coupling in pulmonary hypertension. Am J Respir Crit Care Med. 2019;201(1):116–9.

6. Jone PN, Schäfer M, Pan Z, Ivy DD. Right ventricular-arterial coupling ratio derived from 3-dimensional echocardiography predicts outcomes in pediatric pulmonary hypertension. Circ Cardiovasc Imaging. 2019;12(1):e008176.

7. Benza RL, Gomberg-Maitland M, Elliott CG, Farber HW, Foreman AJ, Frost AE, et al. Predicting survival in patients with pulmonary arterial hypertension: the REVEAL Risk Score Calculator 2.0 and comparison with ESC/ERS-based risk assessment strategies. Chest. 2019;156(2):323–37.

8. Żyłkowska J, Kurzyna M, Florczyk M, Burakowska B, Grzegorczyk F, Burakowski J, et al. Pulmonary artery dilatation correlates with the risk of unexpected death in chronic arterial or thromboembolic pulmonary hypertension. Chest. 2012;142(6):1406–16.

9. Galiè N, Saia F, Palazzini M, Manes A, Russo V, Bacchi Reggiani ML, et al. Left main coronary artery compression in patients with pulmonary arterial hypertension and angina. J Am Coll Cardiol. 2017;69(23):2808–17.

10. Nuche J, Montero Cabezas JM, Alonso Charterina S, Escribano SP. Management of incidentally diagnosed pulmonary artery dissection in patients with pulmonary arterial hypertension. Eur J Cardiothorac Surg. 2019;56(1):210–2.

11. Simpson JM, van den Bosch A. Educational series in congenital heart disease: three-dimensional echocardiography in congenital heart disease. Echo Res Pract. 2019;6(2):R75–86.

12. Laser KT, Karabiyik A, Körperich H, Horst JP, Barth P, Kececioglu D, et al. Validation and reference values for three-dimensional echocardiographic right ventricular volumetry in children: a multicenter study. J Am Soc Echocardiogr. 2018;31(9):1050–63.

13. Genovese D, Rashedi N, Weinert L, Narang A, Addetia K, Patel AR, et al. Machine learning-based three-dimensional echocardiographic quantification of right ventricular size and function: validation against cardiac magnetic resonance. J Am Soc Echocardiogr. 2019;32(8):969–77.

14. Aubert R, Venner C, Huttin O, Haine D, Filippetti L, Guillaumot A, et al. Three-dimensional echocardiography for the assessment of right Ventriculo-arterial coupling. J Am Soc Echocardiogr. 2018;31(8):905–15.

15. Anwar AM, Soliman O, van den Bosch AE, McGhie JS, Geleijnse ML, ten Cate FJ, et al. Assessment of pulmonary valve and right ventricular outflow tract with real-time three-dimensional echocardiography. Int J Cardiovasc Imaging. 2007;23(2):167–75.

16. Grapsa J, Gibbs JS, Cabrita IZ, Watson GF, Pavlopoulos H, Dawson D, et al. The association of clinical outcome with right atrial and ventricular remodelling in patients with pulmonary arterial hypertension: study with real-time three-dimensional echocardiography. Eur Heart J Cardiovasc Imaging. 2012;13(8):666–72.

17. de Siqueira ME, Pozo E, Fernandes VR, Sengupta PP, Modesto K, Gupta SS, et al. Characterization and clinical significance of right ventricular mechanics in pulmonary hypertension evaluated with cardiovascular magnetic resonance feature tracking. J Cardiovasc Magn Reson. 2016;18(1):39.

18. Moceri P, Duchateau N, Baudouy D, Schouver ED, Leroy S, Squara F, et al. Three-dimensional right-ventricular regional deformation and survival in pulmonary hypertension. Eur Heart J Cardiovasc Imaging. 2018;19(4):450–8.

19. Satriano A, Pournazari P, Hirani N, Helmersen D, Thakrar M, Weatherald J, et al. Characterization of right ventricular deformation in pulmonary arterial hypertension using three-dimensional principal strain analysis. J Am Soc Echocardiogr. 2019;32(3):385–93.

20. Smith BC, Dobson G, Dawson D, Charalampopoulos A, Grapsa J, Nihoyannopoulos P. Three-dimensional speckle tracking of the right ventricle: toward optimal quantification of right ventricular dysfunction in pulmonary hypertension. J Am Coll Cardiol. 2014;64(1):41–51.

21. Paffett ML, Hesterman J, Candelaria G, Lucas S, Anderson T, Irwin D, et al. Longitudinal in vivo SPECT/CT imaging reveals morphological changes and cardiopulmonary apoptosis in a rodent model of pulmonary arterial hypertension. PLoS One. 2012;7(7):e40910.

22. Liu M, Qin C, Xia X, Li M, Wang Y, Wang L, et al. Semi-quantitative assessment of pulmonary arterial hypertension associated with congenital heart disease through myocardial perfusion imaging. Hell J Nucl Med. 2017;20(3):204–10.

23. Chan K, Ioannidis S, Coghlan JG, Hall M, Schreiber BE. Pulmonary arterial hypertension with abnormal V/Q single-photon emission computed tomography. JACC Cardiovasc Imaging. 2018;11(10):1487–93.

24. Harel F, Langleben D, Provencher S, Fournier A, Finnerty V, Nguyen QT, et al. Molecular imaging of the human pulmonary vascular endothelium in pulmonary hypertension: a phase II safety and proof of principle trial. Eur J Nucl Med Mol Imaging. 2017;44(7):1136–44.

25. Harel F, Levac X, Nguyen QT, Létourneau M, Marcil S, Finnerty V, et al. Molecular imaging of the human pulmonary vascular endothelium using an adrenomedullin receptor ligand. Mol Imaging. 2015;14.

26. Merabet N, Nsaibia MJ, Nguyen QT, Shi YF, Letourneau M, Fournier A, et al. PulmoBind imaging measures reduction of vascular Adrenomedullin receptor activity with lack of effect of sildenafil in pulmonary hypertension. Sci Rep. 2019;9(1):6609.

27. Rajiah P, Tanabe Y, Partovi S, Moore A. State of the art: utility of multi-energy CT in the evaluation of pulmonary vasculature. Int J Cardiovasc Imaging. 2019;35(8):1509–24.

28. Thieme SF, Graute V, Nikolaou K, Maxien D, Reiser MF, Hacker M, et al. Dual energy CT lung perfusion imaging—correlation with SPECT/CT. Eur J Radiol. 2012;81(2):360–5.

29. Nakazawa T, Watanabe Y, Hori Y, Kiso K, Higashi M, Itoh T, et al. Lung perfused blood volume images with dual-energy computed tomography for chronic thromboembolic pulmonary hypertension: correlation to scintigraphy with single-photon emission computed tomography. J Comput Assist Tomogr. 2011;35(5):590–5.

30. Giordano J, Khung S, Duhamel A, Hossein-Foucher C, Bellèvre D, Lamblin N, et al. Lung perfusion characteristics in pulmonary arterial hypertension (PAH) and peripheral forms of chronic thromboembolic pulmonary hypertension (pCTEPH): dual-energy CT experience in 31 patients. Eur Radiol. 2017;27(4):1631–9.

31. Hachulla AL, Lador F, Soccal PM, Montet X, Beghetti M. Dual-energy computed tomographic imaging of pulmonary hypertension. Swiss Med Wkly. 2016;146:w14328.

32. Talwar A, Sarkar P, Patel N, Shah R, Babchyck B, Palestro CJ. Correlation of a scintigraphic pulmonary perfusion index with hemodynamic parameters in patients with pulmonary arterial hypertension. J Thorac Imaging. 2010;25(4):320–5.

33. Ameli-Renani S, Rahman F, Nair A, Ramsay L, Bacon JL, Weller A, et al. Dual-energy CT for imaging of pulmonary hypertension: challenges and opportunities. Radiographics. 2014;34(7):1769–90.

34. Diller GP, Radojevic J, Kempny A, Alonso-Gonzalez R, Emmanouil L, Orwat S, et al. Systemic right ventricular longitudinal strain is reduced in adults with transposition of the great arteries, relates to subpulmonary ventricular function, and predicts adverse clinical outcome. Am Heart J. 2012;163(5):859–66.

35. Orwat S, Diller GP, Kempny A, Radke R, Peters B, Kühne T, et al. Myocardial deformation parameters predict outcome in patients with repaired tetralogy of Fallot. Heart. 2016;102(3):209–15.

36. Tello K, Dalmer A, Vanderpool R, Ghofrani HA, Naeije R, Roller F, et al. Cardiac magnetic resonance imaging-based right ventricular strain analysis for assessment of coupling and diastolic function in pulmonary hypertension. JACC Cardiovasc Imaging. 2019;12(11 Pt 1):2155–64.

37. Leng S, Dong Y, Wu Y, Zhao X, Ruan W, Zhang G, et al. Impaired cardiovascular magnetic resonance-derived rapid semiautomated right atrial longitudinal strain is associated with decompensated hemodynamics in pulmonary arterial hypertension. Circ Cardiovasc Imaging. 2019;12(5):e008582.

38. Johns CS, Swift AJ, Hughes PJC, Ohno Y, Schiebler M, Wild JM. Pulmonary MR angiography and perfusion imaging-a review of methods and applications. Eur J Radiol. 2017;86:361–70.

39. Ley S, Fink C, Zaporozhan J, Borst MM, Meyer FJ, Puderbach M, et al. Value of high spatial and high temporal resolution magnetic resonance angiography for differentiation

between idiopathic and thromboembolic pulmonary hypertension: initial results. Eur Radiol. 2005;15(11):2256–63.

40. Ley S, Mereles D, Risse F, Grünig E, Ley-Zaporozhan J, Tecer Z, et al. Quantitative 3D pulmonary MR-perfusion in patients with pulmonary arterial hypertension: correlation with invasive pressure measurements. Eur J Radiol. 2007;61(2):251–5.

41. Skrok J, Shehata ML, Mathai S, Girgis RE, Zaiman A, Mudd JO, et al. Pulmonary arterial hypertension: MR imaging-derived first-pass bolus kinetic parameters are biomarkers for pulmonary hemodynamics, cardiac function, and ventricular remodelling. Radiology. 2012;263(3):678–87.

42. Swift AJ, Telfer A, Rajaram S, Condliffe R, Marshall H, Capener D, et al. Dynamic contrast-enhanced magnetic resonance imaging in patients with pulmonary arterial hypertension. Pulm Circ. 2014;4(1):61–70.

43. Barker AJ, Roldán-Alzate A, Entezari P, Shah SJ, Chesler NC, Wieben O, et al. Four-dimensional flow assessment of pulmonary artery flow and wall shear stress in adult pulmonary arterial hypertension: results from two institutions. Magn Reson Med. 2015;73(5):1904–13.

44. Reiter G, Reiter U, Kovacs G, Olschewski H, Fuchsjäger M. Blood flow vortices along the main pulmonary artery measured with MR imaging for diagnosis of pulmonary hypertension. Radiology. 2015;275(1):71–9.

45. Kheyfets VO, Schafer M, Podgorski CA, Schroeder JD, Browning J, Hertzberg J, et al. 4D magnetic resonance flow imaging for estimating pulmonary vascular resistance in pulmonary hypertension. J Magn Reson Imaging. 2016;44(4):914–22.

46. Azarine A, Garçon P, Stansal A, Canepa N, Angelopoulos G, Silvera S, et al. Four-dimensional flow MRI: principles and cardiovascular applications. Radiographics. 2019;39(3):632–48.

47. Odagiri K, Inui N, Hakamata A, Inoue Y, Suda T, Takehara Y, et al. Non-invasive evaluation of pulmonary arterial blood flow and wall shear stress in pulmonary arterial hypertension with 3D phase contrast magnetic resonance imaging. SpringerPlus. 2016;5(1):1071.

48. Forouzan O, Dinges E, Runo JR, Keevil JG, Eickhoff JC, Francois C, et al. Exercise-induced changes in pulmonary artery stiffness in pulmonary hypertension. Front Physiol. 2019;10:269.

49. Reiter U, Reiter G, Kovacs G, Adelsmayr G, Greiser A, Olschewski H, et al. Native myocardial T1 mapping in pulmonary hypertension: correlations with cardiac function and hemodynamics. Eur Radiol. 2017;27(1):157–66.

50. García-Álvarez A, García-Lunar I, Pereda D, Fernández-Jimenez R, Sánchez-González J, Mirelis JG, et al. Association of myocardial T1-mapping CMR with hemodynamics and RV performance in pulmonary hypertension. JACC Cardiovasc Imaging. 2015;8(1):76–82.

51. Nasrallah A, Goussous Y, El-Said G, Garcia E, Hall RJ. Pulmonary artery compression due to acute dissecting aortic aneurysm: clinical and angiographic diagnosis. Chest. 1975;67(2):228–30.

52. Chen YY, Yun H, Jin H, Kong H, Long YL, Fu CX, et al. Association of native T1 times with biventricular function and hemodynamics in precapillary pulmonary hypertension. Int J Cardiovasc Imaging. 2017;33(8):1179–89.

53. Nitsche C, Kammerlander AA, Binder C, Duca F, Aschauer S, Koschutnik M, et al. Native T1 time of right ventricular insertion points by cardiac magnetic resonance: relation with invasive haemodynamics and outcome in heart failure with preserved ejection fraction. Eur Heart J Cardiovasc Imaging. 2019;21(6):683–91.

54. Flett AS, Hayward MP, Ashworth MT, Hansen MS, Taylor AM, Elliott PM, et al. Equilibrium contrast cardiovascular magnetic resonance for the measurement of diffuse myocardial fibrosis: preliminary validation in humans. Circulation. 2010;122(2):138–44.

55. Peng H, Xiao Y, Deng X, Luo J, Hong C, Qin X. The Warburg effect: a new story in pulmonary arterial hypertension. Clin Chim Acta. 2016;461:53–8.

56. Guignabert C, Tu L, Girerd B, Ricard N, Huertas A, Montani D, et al. New molecular targets of pulmonary vascular remodelling in pulmonary arterial hypertension: importance of endothelial communication. Chest. 2015;147(2):529–37.

57. Zhao L, Ashek A, Wang L, Fang W, Dabral S, Dubois O, et al. Heterogeneity in lung (18)FDG uptake in pulmonary arterial hypertension: potential of dynamic (18)FDG positron emission

tomography with kinetic analysis as a bridging biomarker for pulmonary vascular remodelling targeted treatments. Circulation. 2013;128(11):1214–24.

58. Frille A, Steinhoff KG, Hesse S, Grachtrup S, Wald A, Wirtz H, et al. Thoracic [18F]fluoro-deoxyglucose uptake measured by positron emission tomography/computed tomography in pulmonary hypertension. Medicine (Baltimore). 2016;95(25):e3976.

59. Oikawa M, Kagaya Y, Otani H, Sakuma M, Demachi J, Suzuki J, et al. Increased [18F]fluoro-deoxyglucose accumulation in right ventricular free wall in patients with pulmonary hyperten-sion and the effect of epoprostenol. J Am Coll Cardiol. 2005;45(11):1849–55.

60. Zhao Y, Li ZA, Henein MY. PDA with Eisenmenger complicated by pulmonary artery dissec-tion. Eur J Echocardiogr. 2010;11(8):E32.

61. Ashek A, Spruijt OA, Harms HJ, Lammertsma AA, Cupitt J, Dubois O, et al. 3′-Deoxy-3′-[18F]Fluorothymidine positron emission tomography depicts heterogeneous prolifera-tion pathology in idiopathic pulmonary arterial hypertension patient lung. Circ Cardiovasc Imaging. 2018;11(8):e007402.

62. Jorge E, Baptista R, Calisto J, Faria H, Monteiro P, Pan M, et al. Optical coherence tomogra-phy of the pulmonary arteries: a systematic review. J Cardiol. 2016;67(1):6–14.

63. Jiang X, Peng FH, Liu QQ, Zhao QH, He J, Jiang R, et al. Optical coherence tomography for hypertensive pulmonary vasculature. Int J Cardiol. 2016;222:494–8.

64. Brunner NW, Zamanian RT, Ikeno F, Mitsutake Y, Connolly AJ, Shuffle E, et al. Optical coher-ence tomography of pulmonary arterial walls in humans and pigs (Sus scrofa domesticus). Comp Med. 2015;65(3):217–24.

65. Homma Y, Hayabuchi Y, Ono A, Kagami S. Pulmonary artery wall thickness assessed by opti-cal coherence tomography correlates with pulmonary hemodynamics in children with con-genital heart disease. Circ J. 2018;82(9):2350–7.

66. Dai Z, Sugimura K, Fukumoto Y, Tatebe S, Miura Y, Nochioka K, et al. Visualization of com-plete regression of pulmonary arterial remodelling on optical coherence tomography in a patient with pulmonary arterial hypertension. Circ J. 2014;78(11):2771–3.

67. Maffessanti F, Muraru D, Esposito R, Gripari P, Ermacora D, Santoro C, et al. Age-, body size-, and sex-specific reference values for right ventricular volumes and ejection fraction by three-dimensional echocardiography: a multicenter echocardiographic study in 507 healthy volunteers. Circ Cardiovasc Imaging. 2013;6(5):700–10.

Printed in the United States
by Baker & Taylor Publisher Services